AF838583

MISCELLANEA ON ENCEPHALOPATHIES

Edited by **Radu Tanasescu**

Miscellanea on Encephalopathies
Edited by Radu Tanasescu

Published by InTech
Janeza Trdine 9, 51000 Rijeka, Croatia

Copyright © 2012 InTech
All chapters are distributed under the Creative Commons Attribution 3.0 license, which allows users to download, copy and build upon published articles even for commercial purposes, as long as the author and publisher are properly credited, which ensures maximum dissemination and a wider impact of our publications. After this work has been published by InTech, authors have the right to republish it, in whole or part, in any publication of which they are the author, and to make other personal use of the work. Any republication, referencing or personal use of the work must explicitly identify the original source.

As for readers, this license allows users to download, copy and build upon published chapters even for commercial purposes, as long as the author and publisher are properly credited, which ensures maximum dissemination and a wider impact of our publications.

Notice
Statements and opinions expressed in the chapters are these of the individual contributors and not necessarily those of the editors or publisher. No responsibility is accepted for the accuracy of information contained in the published chapters. The publisher assumes no responsibility for any damage or injury to persons or property arising out of the use of any materials, instructions, methods or ideas contained in the book.

Publishing Process Manager Molly Kaliman

Technical Editor Teodora Smiljanic

Cover Designer InTech Design Team

Additional hard copies can be obtained from orders@intechopen.com

Miscellanea on Encephalopathies, Edited by Radu Tanasescu
p. cm.
ISBN 978-953-51-0499-5

We are IntechOpen, the world's leading publisher of Open Access books

Built by scientists, for scientists

4,100+
Open access books available

116,000+
International authors and editors

120M+
Downloads

151
Countries delivered to

Our authors are among the
Top 1%
most cited scientists

12.2%
Contributors from top 500 universities

CLARIVATE ANALYTICS BOOK CITATION INDEX INDEXED

WEB OF SCIENCE™

Selection of our books indexed in the Book Citation Index
in Web of Science™ Core Collection (BKCI)

Interested in publishing with us?
Contact book.department@intechopen.com

Numbers displayed above are based on latest data collected.
For more information visit www.intechopen.com

For EU product safety concerns:
IN TECH d.o.o., Prolaz Marije Krucifikse Kozulić 3, 51000 Rijeka, Croatia,
info@intechopen.com or visit our website at intechopen.com.

Meet the editor

Dr Radu Tanasescu is Senior Lecturer in the Department of Neurology, "Carol Davila "University of Medicine and Pharmacy, Colentina Hospital - Bucharest, Romania. Dr Tanasescu fulfilled his clinical training in France (2001-2003, Central Hospital Nancy). He pursued training in neurophysiology (University of Bristol, UK) and immunology of multiple sclerosis (Division of Clinical Neurology University Hospital, Nottingham, UK). In 2010 and 2011, he was awarded by the European Neurological Society and the European Federation of Neurological Societies with two scientific Fellowship research grants for projects studying advanced imaging techniques and stem cell therapy in multiple sclerosis (University of Nottingham, UK). He conducted the firsts studies in Romania on neurological manifestations associated with antiphospholipid antibodies, being awarded with a PhD degree in 2007. He is author of more than 100 published scientific contributions and was contributor to 6 medical books. As a member of EFNS scientific Panels of Neuroimmunology and Neurotoxicology he co-authored two Guideline Papers of the EFNS.

Contents

"There is only one good, knowledge, and one evil, ignorance"
Socrates

Preface

Along the years the concept of encephalopathy evolved from a clinical syndrome translating a more or less diffuse and more or less reversible or even progressive structural or only functional impairment of the brain, to a multitude of syndromes corresponding to one or several overlapping etiologies, ranging from toxic (endogenous or exogenous), to metabolic (genetic or acquired), hypoxic and/or ischemic, dysimmune, infectious and neurodegenerative, and having more or less understood pathogenic mechanisms, therefore describing distinct diseases. One may argue that a book on this subject is futile: the term encephalopathies encompasses such a broad, heterogeneous and constantly expanding spectrum; the focus of the current medical practice is changing from holistic to increasingly specialized; and the current literature revolves around diseases and not syndromes.

A challenge for a nowadays neurologist is to cover all the complex field of brain disturbances by mastering the clinical features, knowing the right treatment and understanding the underlying mechanisms of those conditions. It is no doubt that this somewhat exhaustive attempt is difficult, if not impossible. The quantity of information laying at our disposal makes things more difficult than simplifying them, since the Socratic quote "Information is not Knowledge" implies integration of information as a crucial step on the path of understanding. Notwithstanding, while synthesizing and sedimenting information is an individual process, gathering the 'right kind' of information – the one which is not only accurate or complete but most of all relevant for the topic tackled- implies having access to 'appropriate' information sources.

Nevertheless, brain disease implies multidisciplinary approach. For incumbent mechanisms understanding integration of basic science notions is required, while for circumscribing a broader context which facilitate brain disease (such as a metabolic one), a look gathering multi-specialty angles is needed.

With this particular clinical approach in mind I propose to the reader the present book as the first part of a book project on various aspects of encephalopathies. This book groups mainly but not solely encephalopathies associated to infectious conditions, while a future one will be mainly dedicated to some various aspects regarding metabolic and hypoxic encephalopathies. As the title 'Miscellanea on

Encephalopathies' states, the book does not aspire to be exhaustive, nor didactic, but rather a unique collection of chapters, written by different authors, discussing several particular aspects of certain encephalopathies as understood through the own experience of each author. By contributing to a book designed to have an atypical and less rigid structure, each author was allowed to write on a chosen subject that best reflects his/hers own expertise in the field. This approach is pertinent in the contemporaneous world when the access to information is facile, and of greater value than a uniform approach of all encephalopathies. Moreover, I consider it to be in agreement with the above-mentioned increasingly specialization tendency. Though not unitary in structure and in the quantity and quality of the offered information, the present book covers many of the important aspects regarding common and also rare encephalopathies, mostly in respect to their classic and novel diagnostic techniques and up to date therapies, and thus the book tries to respond in detail to some of the questions encountered in the clinical practice. Therefore the book is less than a sum of the current information and less than a review of the literature, but at the same time is more than that, transmitting valuable information filtered through the real life clinical and research experience of the authors, to which I thank for their willingness and effort in sharing their knowledge. Since many encephalopathies appear in the setting of systemic disease (e.g. organ failure, infectious diseases) and/or sometimes of their therapy (e.g. chemotherapy), the book addresses not only neurologists, but also fellow colleagues of other specialties, and into a lesser degree, medical researchers in the fields of neuroscience, genetics, immunology and infectious diseases and medical students. With this being said, the authors and I hope that the book will become a valuable source of information allowing to a more comprehensive view on such a vast subject as encephalopathies.

Radu Tanasescu
University of Medicine and Pharmacy "Carol Davila" Bucharest,
Department of Neurology, Colentina Hospital,
Romania

1

Posttransplantation Encephalopaties

Daniela Anghel[1,2], Laura Dumitrescu[3], Catalina Coclitu[4], Amalia Ene[4], Ovidiu Bajenaru[1,4] and Radu Tanasescu[1,3]
[1]*University of Medicine and Pharmacy "Carol Davila" Bucharest,*
[2]*Department of Neurology, Fundeni Clinical Institute,*
[3]*Department of Neurology, Colentina Hospital,*
[4]*Department of Neurology, University Emergency Hospital,*
Romania

1. Introduction

Neurological complications may occur in 30 to 60% of the patients undergoing organ transplantation, especially liver and bone marrow (Padovan et al. 2000). Because of the constantly changing protocols regarding the transplantation procedure and the subsequent immunosuppression required for the prevention of graft rejection and graft versus host disease, the nature of the neurologic complications has changed over time.

Recipients of solid organ or bone marrow cell transplants are at risk of life-threatening neurological complications including encephalopathies, seizures, brain infections and malignancies, stroke, central pontine myelinolysis and neuromuscular disorders. Many of these disorders are linked directly or indirectly to the immunosuppressive therapy. However, they may also result from graft versus host disease, from pretransplantation radiation or chemotherapy, and from injuries induced during surgery and intensive care unit(ICU) stay. In rare cases neuroinfectious pathogens may be transmitted with the transplanted tissue. Though most of the neurological complications occur disrespectful of the transplanted organ, transplant-specific complications also exist. Heart and pulmonary transplants are frequently associated to cerebral hypoxia, ischemia and bleeding. Bone marrow transplant is commonly associated with prolonged thrombocytopenia that may lead to catastrophic cerebral haemorrhage (Bashir 2001).

In spite of the advances that have been made in the management of transplanted patients, the so-called posttransplantation encephalopathy (PTE), a complex syndrome with various etiologies characterized especially by disturbance of consciousness, is still frequently observed. The spectrum of PTE is vast and changes along in relationship with the time that has passed since transplantation (see Table1). Metabolic disturbances (secondary to the underlying or associated systemic disease or iatrogenic), drug neurotoxicity (caused by immunosuppressant, but also by antibiotics or other drugs), disimmunity and opportunistic central nervous system infections are frequent PTE etiologies. Though commonly the encephalopathies with these etiologies are well circumscribed clinical entities, highlighting the diagnostic and therapeutic particularities arising from their occurrence in the posttransplantation setting is of great utility for the current clinical practice. Moreover, encephalopathies of different etiologies may overlap in the same transplanted patient (Mathew and Rosenfeld 2007).

The etiological diagnosis of PTE is challenging because the clinical presentation and the neuroimagistic findings lack specificity and the unique circumstances related to the underlying disease, the transplant procedure and the subsequent management may give rise to less typical presentations. Most clinical signs of PTE are nonspecific and do not reliably identify a particular etiology. Humoral or tissue samples are often required for definite diagnosis.

The major clinical feature is impaired attention, but the clinical findings can range from subtle cognitive difficulties to delirium or coma. A characteristic abnormality is marked fluctuation in the level of consciousness. The motor signs are variable and include tremor, asterixis and multifocal myoclonus, the latter particularly involving the face and the proximal muscles. In the severely affected subjects decorticate and decerebrate posturing may occur. Computed tomography (CT) or magnetic resonance imaging (MRI) of the brain is mandatory when signs suggestive for diffuse or focal brain injury are present. If clinical examination shows no focal signs and brain MRI is normal, the most probable causes of the encephalopathy are systemic metabolic abnormalities or drug toxicity (commonly related to cyclosporine, tacrolimus or amphotericin-B). In postransplatation encephalopathic patients with normal MRI cytomegalovirus (CMV) infection should also be considered. In the setting of CNS signs and symptoms the electroencephalogram (EEG) is a useful investigation since it can identify diffuse non-specific slowing of the normal activity translating diffuse brain injury, and it can confirm the presence of non-convulsive seizures which may be difficult to differentiate from confusion or other mental status changes on clinical grounds only. The required laboratory investigations include complete blood count, coagulation studies, electrolyte panel, glucose, renal and liver function parameters and arterial blood gases. Assessment of the blood immunosuppressive drug levels should be performed when overdose may have occurred and blood and CSF cultures should be obtained when infection is suspected.

Early posttransplantation period (first 30 days)	Subacute posttransplantation period (1-6 months)	Chronic posttransplantation period (>6 months)
METABOLIC DISTURBANCES	OPPORTUNISTIC INFECTION (SOLID ORGAN ALLOGRAFTS)	OPPORTUNISTIC INFECTION (SOLID ORGAN ALLOGRAFTS)
HYPOXIC-ISCHEMIC ENCEPHALOPATHY	METABOLIC DISTURBANCES	METABOLIC DISTURBANCES
IMMUNOSUPPRESSIVE DRUG TOXICITY	IMMUNOSUPPRESSIVE DRUG TOXICITY	IMMUNOSUPPRESSIVE DRUG TOXICITY
OPPORTUNISTIC INFECTION (BONE MARROW TRANSPLANTATION)		

Table 1. The time relationship with the transplant procedure of the common causes of PTE

The patient's management should be centered on preventing further neurological injury, administering etiology-targeted therapy, and balancing the benefits and toxicities of the specific immunosuppressive agents used. Knowledge regarding the etiologies of PTE and their incidence in relationship with the posttransplantation period in which they occur is essential for the adequate medical approach (Mathew and Rosenfeld 2007). Without the objective of being exhaustive, the present chapter offers an updated overview on the subject.

2. Encephalopathy related to the underlying disease

In a significant number of cases the disease that imposed transplantation also predisposes to brain injury, some patients having a certain degree of encephalopathy when the transplant procedure takes place. Moreover, hyperacute, acute or cronic graft rejection may also lead to encephalopathy secondary to organ failure (but also, see 'Rejection Encephalopathy' below).

Patients with end-stage cardiomyopathy may develop encephalopathy secondary to global cerebral hypoperfusion.

Patients with chronic renal failure may develop pretransplant uremic encephalopathy and acute renal rejection encephalopathy (Brouns et De Deyn 2004).

The patients undergoing liver transplant may continue to experience hepatic encephalopathy if the graft fails acutely and/or may suffer hypoxic ischemic brain injury. In the majority of cases the clinical picture is the expression of the intracranial hypertension caused by brain edema, i.e. the net increase in brain water that may occur in the cellular (cytotoxic edema) or interstitial (vasogenic edema) compartments of the brain. Toxic, metabolic, inflammatory and infectious humoral factors may play a pathogenic role in the development of brain edema. Therefore, measurement of arterial ammonia levels is important for estimating the risk for the development of intracranial hypertension. It has been reported that worsening of hepatic encephalopathy may precede the detection of bacterial infection by an average of 24 hours, so, is recommended that patients experiencing worsening of hepatic encephalopathy should be treated with empiric wide-spectrum antibiotics. In those with hepatic insufficiency the translocation of bacteria from the intestine to regional lymph nodes may be an important pathogenic pathway, but endovenous catheters are also important routes of infection. Acute hyponatremia can induce brain edema by itself, therefore electrolytes levels should be routinely checked (Londono et al. 2006).

Brain edema leads to impaired consciousness ranging from sleepiness to stupor and coma and correlates with severe encephalopathy. The presence of long tract signs, decerebrate posturing, alterations in pupillary reactivity, or abnormalities in oculovestibular reflexes are specific though not sensitive indicators of the presence of an increased intracranial pressure. Radiological detection of brain edema can provide useful information, but the sensitivity is low. For identifying the presence of intracranial hypertension, intracranial pressure monitoring is the most accurate tool.

The therapeutic measures include treatment of the underlying disease and correction of the metabolic disturbances. Ammonia can be removed by dialytic methods. N-acetylcysteine administered over 3-days infusion may lead to a significant improvement in the survival of those with mild hepatic encephalopathy. The management of elevated intracranial pressure includes correcting the patient's position, temperature, ventilation and hemodynamics and when present removal of the excessive fluid. Osmotic therapy (e.g. mannitol 0.25 to 2 g/kg as 20% solution IV over at least 30 minutes, administered not more frequently than every 6 to 8 hours) is commonly administered. In selected cases forced hyperventilation (aiming a $paCO_2$ lower than 25 mmHg), barbiturate coma, high dose indomethacin administration and bilateral decompressive craniectomy should be taken into consideration (Jantzen 2007).

3. Cranial irradiation encephalopathy

Cranial irradiation is commonly used before bone marrow transplantation. Encephalopathy related to cranial irradiation has been reported. The clinical picture is that of an acute encephalopathy characterized by fever, headache, nausea, somnolence and seizures. The cause is diffuse cerebral edema. The treatment comprises of corticosteroids administration. In those with hematologic malignancies, pretransplant cranial irradiation and intrathecal chemotherapy may also cause a delayed leukoencephalopathy, which may occur even several years after these procedures.

4. PTE due to transplantation procedures

Hypoxic-ischemic encephalopathy is a potential posttransplantation complication common to most of the transplant procedures.

Hypoxia describes a reduction in oxygen supply or tissue utilisation, which leads to an increase in cerebral blood flow that aims at providing glucose to the brain and clearing toxic metabolites.

Ischemia refers to a reduction in blood supply, which leads to decreased oxygen delivery, impaired clearance of the accumulating toxic cellular metabolites (lactate, H^+, glutamate) and subsequent exacerbation of the pre-existent brain injury. Global cerebral ischemia is usually due to: cardiac arrest, profound hypotension associated with surgery, shock, sepsis, metabolic encephalopathy, prolonged hypoxia or hypoglycemia and severe anemia (Liang 2000). Precaution should be taken to avoid the occurrence of these precipitating factors. Elevated cerebral metabolic rate may also play a role in the etiology of hypoxic-ischemic encephalopathy. Global cerebral ischemia quickly leads to impaired synaptic transmission and axonal conduction. The degree of neuronal susceptibility to the hypoxic/ischemic injury is not uniform within the brain, particularly vulnerable regions being the hippocampus, the neocortex, the reticular nucleus of the thalamus, the amygdala, the cerebellar vermis and some neurons in the caudate nucleus and pars reticulata of the substantia nigra. This different topographic susceptibility to ischemic injury seems to be caused by the specific properties of the neurons in those brain regions, and not by uneven circulation. An impaired cerebral oxygen supply may lead to transient or irreversible neurologic changes, depending on the severity of the initial insult and on the post-resuscitation management.

The clinical picture of hypoxic ischemic encephalopathy consists of impaired consciousness ranging from coma to vegetative state or minimally conscious state and epileptic seizures. Generalised tonic-clonic seizures may be masked in the first days, due to sedation. Focal seizures may be restricted to blinking, eye deviations or small repetitive facial or limb movements, which can be easily overlooked. Multifocal generalised myoclonus (posthypoxic myoclonic status) may start immediately after injury, responds unsatisfactory to medication and translates a poor prognosis. Focal myoclonus, action or startle sensitive (Lance-Adams syndrome), may appear in the first 24-48 hours after the injury, responds well to antiepileptic drugs (valproate, levetiracetam, clonazepam) and carries a favourable prognosis(Chabolla et al. 2003).

The investigations required when facing hypoxic-ischemic encephalopathy include:

Neurophysiological tests (EEG, somatosensory evoked potentials), which are valuable in assessing the diagnosis and prognosis.

Imaging studies, which in the first days commonly show brain edema (hypodensity on CT or hyperintensity on MRI - DWI, FLAIR- localised in the cortical grey matter, basal ganglia and subcortical white matter). In the subacute phase there is progressive resolution of brain edema, normalisation of DWI, but persistence of cortical, basal ganglia and white matter hyperintensity on T2 and FLAIR images. Cortical laminar necrosis and boundary zone infarctions may also appear.

The treatment should be adapted for each particular situation, but several approaches are commonly required. As mentioned above, if raised intracranial pressure is clinically suspected, several measures should be taken: adequate positioning of the head, osmotherapy (mannitol, hypertonic saline), controlled hyperventilation and metabolic control (fever, seizures, hypoglycaemia, hypokalemia). Systemic coagulopathy can occur, due to an increase in cytokines, so antithrombotic therapy should be given. For the patients in coma, hypothermia should be tried, as it increases the chances for a good outcome, if the possible complications are avoided (i.e. cardiac arrhytmias, sepsis, hypotension during rewarming, renal failure, hypokalemia).

The outcomes of hypoxic-ischemic brain injury include death, coma, vegetative state (VS), minimally conscious state (MCS), severe neurological or cognitive deficits, with chronic dependence on nursing care or, in some cases, recovery. The factors that correlate with worse prognosis are: duration of coma over 6 hours, absence of spontaneous limb movements or localisation to painful stimuli in the first hours, prolonged loss of pupillary responses, ocular abnormalities (e.g. sustained conjugate eye deviation, up- or downbeat nystagmus, ping-pong gaze, periodic alternating nystagmus), myoclonic seizures, absent reflexes of lower cranial nerves (cough and gag reflexes). Biomarkers that may predict outcome have been searched. So far, the only one that appears to be related to a poor prognosis seems to be neuron specific enolase (NSE), if it rises over 80ng/ml in the first days.

Among the types of transplant, lung transplantation is associated with increased risk of hypoxic-ischemic encephalopathy. A particular situation is that of heart transplantation which has similar neurological complications as other open-heart procedures, including encephalopathy. The manifestations of the perioperative cerebral injury include ischemic (or, less commonly, hemorrhagic) stroke, encephalopathy and neurocognitive dysfunction occurring in the first month after surgery. Brain injury secondary to cardiac surgery is primarily ischemic. The etiology of ischemic brain injury secondary to cardiac transplant includes:

1. Cerebral embolism: cerebral macroembolism arising from the ascending aorta causes stroke, while cerebral microembolism causes encephalopathy and neurocognitive dysfunction; microemboli are either gaseous or particulate.

2. Cerebral hypoperfusion: induces injury caused by the combination of systemic hypotension and cerebral venous hypertension (traction on the superior vena cava), occuring during off-pump surgery.
3. Atherosclerosis of the aorta: atherosclerotic lesions injury during surgery can result in emboli and may expose lipidic prothrombotic material, which promotes thrombus formation postoperatively. On the other hand, atherosclerosis of the ascending aorta is a marker for severe atherosclerosis of the cerebral arteries, which prones to cerebral injury during hypoperfusion.
4. Perioperative anemia reduces cerebral oxygen delivery and/or causes increased cerebral blood flow, increasing the number of potential emboli.

5. PTE related to the immunosuppressive medication

Immunosupresive therapy is required in all transplanted patients for the prevention of graft rejection and graft versus host disease. Commonly used drugs include calcineurin inhibitors, corticosteroids and biological agents. It is widely recognized that the immunosuppressive therapy is associated with an increased incidence of sepsis (and thus of sepsis encephalopathy) and of central nervous system opportunistic infections, both of which are briefly discussed in separate sub-chapters. The literature is abundant in case reports of encephalopathy occurring in the absence of sepsis or neuroinfections. As detailed further on, these encephalopathies appear to be specifically related to several drugs. Their evolution is typically favourable, providing the offending drug is stopped. It is important to note that even if metabolic disturbances or other causes that may explain the encephalopathy are identified, the blood levels of the potential neurotoxic drugs that the patient is receiving should be assessed.

Certain particularities in respect with the organ being transplanted have been reported.

The patients undergoing liver transplantation commonly have an advanced stage of the disease resulting in immunodepression and coagulopathy (Watt et al. 2010). Disrespectful of the technique used, the surgical procedure required by liver transplantation is very complex and has high risk of blood loss or massive fluid shifts. In the days following the transplant, the engrafted liver releases immunologically active cells (T-cells, macrophages, stem cells), which can react with the host immune system, already affected by the preexistent liver failure and by the immunosuppressive medication. Liver transplanted patients commonly develop PRES related to calcineurin inhibitors administration early after transplantation and usually have associated favouring factors such as serious bacterial infection, organ rejection or CMV infection (reactivation or new infection). The arterial blood pressure is normal in most cases.

Because the possibility of adequately substituting the impaired renal function via periodic dialysis, the patients requiring kidney transplantation are usually "healthier" than those with liver failure. At the same time, the transplant procedure is less laborious than in the case of liver transplantation. These patients may develop late PRES related to calcineurin inhibitors administration and usually have high blood pressure, episodes of severe systemic infection or rejection. Probably the chronic exposure to the graft endothelium promotes a minimal inflammatory response (increased leukocyte trafficking and activation of endothelial adhesion molecules). These changes can receive a boost when the immune system is stimulated by an infection or an episode of rejection.

Patients with allogenic bone marrow transplantation have the highest risk for infection and neurotoxicity, because of the aggressive chemotheraphy and total body irradiation (both can cause endothelial injury) and because of the potential developement of graft versus host disease, requiring high doses of neurotoxic immunosupressants.

5.1 Calcineurin inhibitors

Calcineurin inhibitors (i.e. cyclosporine and tacrolimus) are drugs with immunosuppresive effects, frequently administered in transplant receivers. They act as blockers of calcineurin, which is a T lymphocyte calmodulin-dependent protein. The principal role of calcineurin consists of increasing the quantity of interleukin 2 (IL-2) released by the activated T lymphocyte. The blockage of this signal stops the clonal expansion of the T lymphocytes, thus decreasing the amplitude of the immune response (Gerald 2001). Cyclosporine and tacrolimus are frequently administered in transplant recipients, especially in those with allogeneic hematopoietic stem cell transplant for the prophylaxis of graft versus host disease. Cyclosporine and tacrolimus are absorbed in jejunum, metabolised by P450 cytocrome and excreted mostly through bile. Their plasma levels are increased by certain drugs which are metabolised by the same pathways (e.g. calcium channel blockers, macrolides, conasoles, amiodarone, metoclopramide, colchicine, allopurinolum). The drugs that are enzyme inducers (e.g. phenytoin, phenobarbital, rifampicin, carbamazepine, sulfonylureas) lower the plasma level of cyclosporine and tacrolimus. The optimum blood level of cyclosporine is between 250-350 ng/ml in the first 3 months after transplantation, with progressive reduction to 100-150 ng/ml after one year, required for minimizing the adverse effects. Its potential adverse effects include arterial hypertension, nephrotoxicity and neurotoxicity. For tacrolimus, the optimum blood level is 10ng/ml in the first 3 months after transplantation, with progressive reduction to 5ng/ml at one year for the same rationale as above. Its potential adverse effects are arterial hypertension, nephrotoxicity, neurotoxicity and diabetes mellitus. Both drugs cause similar neurotoxicity, which particularly occurs in the first months after transplant when the administered doses are higher.

Cyclosporine and tacrolimus are lipophilic molecules which pass the blood-brain barrier, sometimes reaching higher concentrations in the corticospinal fluid (CSF) than those present in the blood. That is why neurotoxicity can appear early and may not correlate with the presence of high blood concentrations. It is commonly accepted that early calcineurin inhibitor-induced neurotoxicity occurs within the first 4 weeks since treatment initiation (and since transplantation). Their neurotoxicity occurs through various mechanisms, one of which is the release of endothelin, which causes intense cerebral vasospasm, sympathetic activation and local coagulation disturbances, finally determining vasogenic edema affecting predominantly (but not exclusively) the subcortical white matter of the posterior regions of the brain. Both cyclosporine and tacrolimus decrease endothelial cell viability (Illsinger et al. 2010) and increase endothelial permeability (i.e. endotheliotoxic dysfunction), with secondary failure of the cerebral vascular autoregulation and impaired function of the blood-brain barrier. Both drugs inhibit P-glycoprotein, which could result in the enhancement of the brain distribution of these drugs and thus increased neurotoxicity. Factors favouring these alterations induced by cyclosporine and tacrolimus include arterial hypertension, concomitant treatment with corticosteroids, hypocholesterolemia, hypomagnesemia, concomitant graft versus host disease (as it needs high doses of immunosuppressant therapy) and high aluminium blood levels- occuring especially in the patients from developing countries where contaminated dialysis water is still used or in those taking over-the-counter aluminium-containing phosphate binders(Bechstein 2000).

The neurotoxicity induced by calcineurin inhibitors occurs more frequently in liver transplanted patients. The neurotoxic effects of cyclosporine and tacrolimus may be divided in minor symptoms (mild postural and action tremor of the extremities, distal burning paresthesia, somnolence or insomnia, headache, dysarthria, agitation, depression) and major symptoms (auditive or visual hallucinations, cortical blindness, akinetic mutism, speech apraxia, psychosis, seizures, coma, polineuropathy, myopathy). The exclusion of other potential causes (stroke, central nervous system infection, central pontine myelinolisis) is mandatory. Following dose modification or swiching to another calcineurin inhibitor there is an obvious clinical improvement. Tremor and paresthesias are the most common side effects of calcineurin inhibitors, occurring in up to 30% and respectively 11% of the patients. These commonly subside when the dose is decreased. Isolated seizures are reported in up to 5% of patients and may sometimes be associated with hypomagnesemia (nota bene: imipenem, cefepime and levofloxacine administration is also associated with seizures). Although more severe neurological complications are rare, two CNS syndromes have been reported: posterior reversible encephalopathy syndrome (PRES) and a syndrome predominantly characterized by motor features of parkinsonism or ataxia. A similar syndrome consisting of confusion, tremor and parkinsonism may be caused by amphotericin-B.

PRES is caused by potentially reversible, predominantly vasogenic edema of the white matter, with a predilection to the brain regions supplied by the posterior arteries(Wijdicks 2001).

PRES can manifest with seizures, disturbed vision, headache and altered mental status. Severe hypertension is sometimes present, but usually the mean arterial pressure is normal. Because acutely raised blood pressure is found in many PRES patients, it is sometimes considered to be an important causal factor. On the other hand, patients with normal blood pressure may also develop PRES. Perhaps, therefore, the raised blood pressure is required to sustain cerebral blood flow and is reactive rather than a cause. The symptoms usually develop quite quickly over a few hours, reaching their worst in 12 to 48 hours since onset. Confusion and altered mental status are very frequent findings and may hide other symptoms such as disturbed vision and nausea. Patients can be confused, lethargic with slowed motor responses or deeply stuporous. As mentioned, seizures, including non-convulsive status epilepticus, may occur in those with PRES.Differentiating altered mental status from non-convulsive status epilepticus on clinical grounds only may be difficult. Using EEG monitoring in all patients with altered mental status can help detecting non-convulsive electroencephalographic seizures. PRES patients with status epilepticus show rhythmic delta and sharp waves, mostly in the parieto-occipital and temporal regions. The EEG abnormalities resolve along with clinical improvement(Cruz-Martinez et Gilmore 2002). Visual disturbances occur frequently due to the involvement of the occipital lobe. PRES patients may experience not only cortical blindness or homonymous hemianopsia, but also blurred vision, visual neglect and visual hallucinations. Headache, usually bilateral and dull in nature, commonly occurs in PRES. Tremor of the extremities is a minor but very important sign, because most of the patients with altered consciousness due to calcineurin inhibitor neurotoxicity have this sign, which is not so often present when other causes are involved. Other clinical features of PRES include nausea and vomiting. These occur less frequently. The tendon reflexes are often brisk but symmetrical. Hemiparesis, Babinski's sign and brainstem features may occur occasionally.

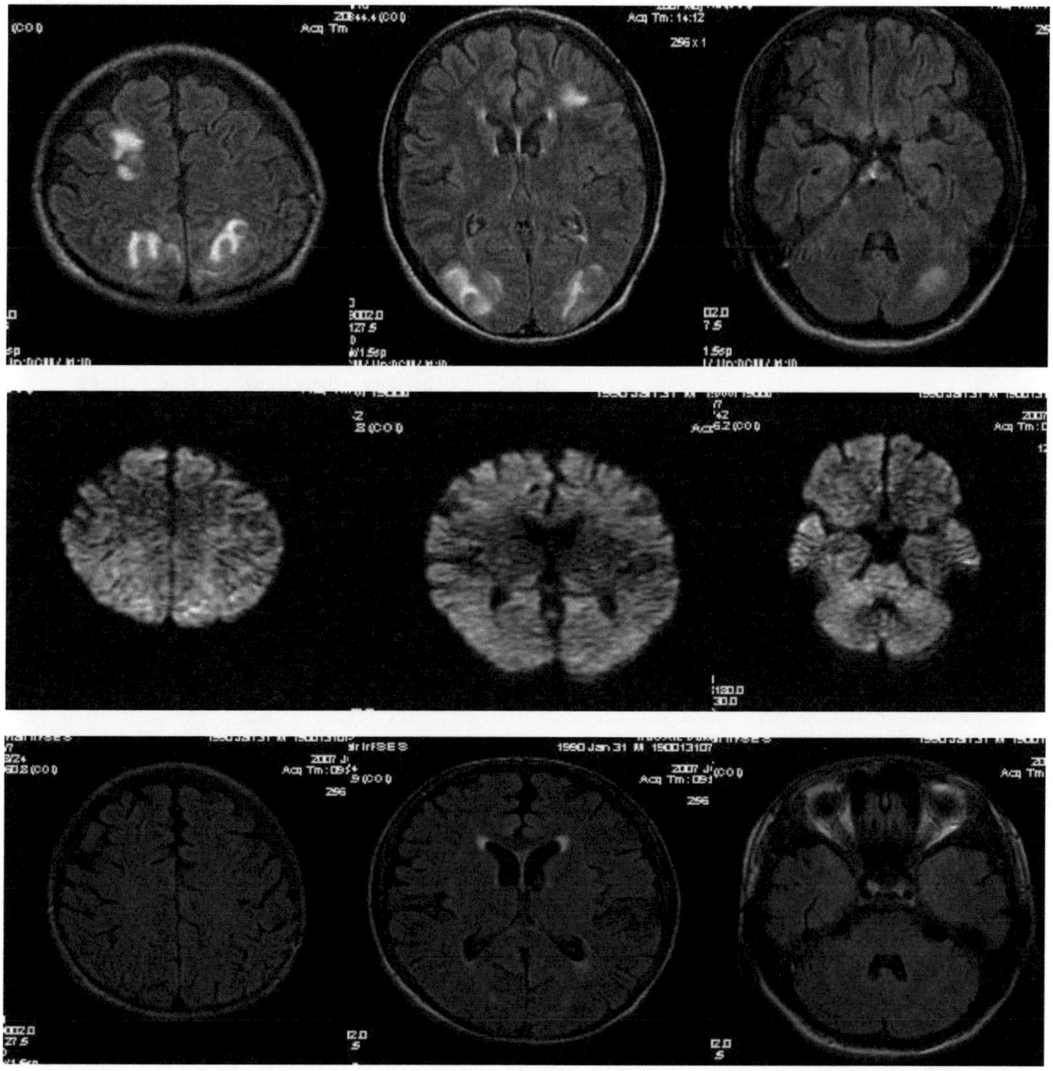

Fig. 1. PRES in a 17-year-old male who developed headache, seizures, visual disturbances and altered mental status 14 days after cadaveric renal transplant for glomerulonephritis-related chronic renal failure. He was treated for pneumonia just before toxicity occurred. The MR imaging was obtained 4 days after the onset of PRES. (A) FLAIR sequences showing bilateral frontal and occipital hyperintensity, translating vasogenic edema. (B) Diffusion weighted imaging showing isointensity of the affected areas (i.e. no cytotoxic edema). (C) Follow-up FLAIR sequences obtained one month later show resolution of the vasogenic edema.

The CSF may be normal or show slightly raised protein level.

Brain imagistic studies (CT or preferably MRI) are required. The common neuroradiological abnormalities comprise of the subcortical white matter hyperintensities typically bilaterally, nonenhanced and involving mainly the posterior lobes-parietal and/or occipital(Bartynsky et al. 2008). Involvement of the anterior brain (frontal lobes, along the superior frontal sulcus), cerebellum, and brain stem may also be observed. A typical PRES pattern mostly spares the paramedian occipital structures below the sulcus calcarinus. Although PRES is often thought to be a leukoencephalopathy, the cortex and deep gray mater can often be involved.

SYNDROME	PARTICULAR CHARACTERISTICS
Posterior circulation stroke - "top of the basilar syndrome"	MRI: hyperintensity on DWI images and low signal on ADC map; involvement of calcarine and paramedian areas
Primary CNS vasculitis	Insidious onset Abnormal CSF, with inflammatory changes MRI: multiple infarcts, of different ages
Reversible cerebral vasoconstriction syndrome	Severe headache (thunderclap headache) Progression of symptoms in days, not hours Angiography: multiple segmental stenoses, reversible after few weeks
Viral Encephalitis- (herpetic)	Systemic inflammation signs: fever, blood tests, inflammatory CSF changes

Table 2. The differential diagnosis of PRES

Although the blood levels of cyclosporine and tacrolimus tend not to correlate with PRES and normal serum levels do not rule out drug-related neurotoicity, both clinical and radiologic findings can resolve as the blood levels of the offending drug are reduced(Singh et al. 2000). Therefore the specific therapeutic approach comprises of lowering of the dose or discontinuation of the offending drug, which interestingly can be switched with the other calcineurin inhibitor without PRES reoccurring. The encephalopathy is almost always reversible but it may not resolve until several weeks after the drug has been stopped. There are reports of a potential protective effect of soya bean oil administration (Kentaro et al. 2007). The lipids contained by this oil may impair the passage of the calcineurin inhibitors through the blood-brain barrier, and therefore diminish their accumulation in the central nervous system. Symptomatic treatment is also required and should be adapted to each case. The minor symptoms related to calcineurin inhibitors neurotoxicity are usually self-limited and responsive to symptomatic drugs. However, refractory headache leading to change of the immunosuppressive drug has been reported. When facing major symptoms the usual therapeutic approach is changing the immunosuppressive treatment: either substituting calcineurin inhibitor with a non-calcineurin inhibitor (e.g. sirolimus, mycophenolate mofetil) or changing the calcineurin inhibitors between each other - cyclosporine with tacrolimus or tacrolimus with cyclosporine (Guarino et al. 2006). Syndrome-specific treatments are mandatory. These include administration of cerebral depletive drugs and administration of antiepileptic drugs adapted to the type of seizures according to the local guidelines but also adapted to the patient (i.e. lacking either hepatotoxicity or nephrotoxicity and not interfering with the patient's immunosuppressant drugs). Since it does not induce hepatic metabolism of cyclosporine or tacrolimus and can be given either orally or intravenously in the absence of liver dysfunction valproic acid may be optimal for treatment of seizures. The antiepileptic treatment may be stopped after about 6 months, unless the seizures reappear. Administration of anxiolytics (for agitation) or neuroleptics (for psychotic episodes) may sometimes be required.

5.2 Corticosteroids

Corticosteroids prevent interleukin IL–1 and IL-6 production by macrophages and inhibit all stages of T-cell activation. In transplanted patients, they are commonly used for the induction and maintenance of immunosuppression and for the treatment of acute rejection. Corticosteroid administration may cause insomnia, irritability, impaired concentration, and mood changes, and sometimes they may even cause psychotic episodes. The treatment of corticosteroid-related neurological side effects consists of lowering the dose and administering antipsychotic agents.

5.3 Biologic agents

The biologic agents include polyclonal and monoclonal antibodies with immunomodulatory/immunosuppressive effects. They are used for the induction of immunosupresion and for the treatment of graft rejection.

The polyclonal antibodies (e.g. antithymocyte globulins) are produced by injecting animals with human lymphoid cells, then harvesting and purifying the resultant antibody. Polyclonal antibodies induce lysis of lymphocytes and mask the lymphoid cell-surface receptors. The available pharmaceutical preparations include horse antithymocyte globulin (ATGAM) and rabbit antithymocyte globulin (Thymoglobulin). These agents are used for immunosupresion induction and treatment of acute graft rejection. Adverse effects include fever, chills, thrombocytopenia, leukopenia, hemolysis, respiratory distress, serum sickness, and anaphylaxis. Some adverse effects are ameliorated with steroids, acetaminophen, and diphenhydramine.

The monoclonal antibodies used in transplanted patients include monoclonal anti-CD3 antibody (i.e. muromonab-CD3), monoclonoal anti-CD25 antibody (i.e.basiliximab and daclizumab), monoclonal anti-CD20 antibody (i.e. rituximab). Except for muromonab their administration in transplanted patients is associated with a very low prevalence of neurologic adverse effects.

Muromonab-CD3 (Orthoklone OKT3) is a murine monoclonal antibody directed to the CD3 portion of the T-cell receptor. It blocks T-cell function and has limited reactions with other tissues or cells. This agent is used for induction and acute rejection (primary treatment or steroid-resistant). Its adverse effects include cytokine release syndrome (fever, dyspnea, wheezing, headache, hypotension, diarrhea, vomiting, nausea, tremor, generalized weakness) and pulmonary edema, usually following the first few doses. Sometimes patients experience "shock-like" reactions, which may include cardiovascular and central nervous system manifestations. All patients must be carefully evaluated for excessive fluid retention and hypertension before the initiation of Muromonab therapy. Close monitoring for neuro-psychiatric symptoms must be observed during the first 24 hours following the first injection. Patients who may be at greater risk for CNS adverse events include those with history of seizures, with cerebrovascular disease, head trauma, uraemia, or who are receiving a medication concomitantly that may affect the central nervous system. Premedication with steroids (first 2 doses only), acetaminophen, and diphenhydramine avoids cytokine release syndrome. The possible neuro-psychiatric events include headache, seizures, aseptic meningitis, encephalopathy and cerebral edema/herniation. Seizures, which have been occasionally accompanied by cardiorespiratory arrest, have occurred independently or in conjunction with any of the neurologic syndromes described below. Patients predisposed to seizures are those with the following conditions: uraemia, fever, infection, fluid overload, hypertension, hypoglycaemia, history of seizures, and electrolyte imbalances. Symptoms of aseptic meningitis include fever, headache, stiff neck and photophobia. The cerebrospinal fluid shows leucocytosis, elevated protein and normal or decreased glucose, with negative viral, bacterial and fungal cultures. Most patients with aseptic meningitis have a benign course, but infectious meningitis must be taken into account in the differential diagnosis of an immunosuppressed transplant patient with any signs or symptoms of meningitis. Manifestations of encephalopathy may include impaired cognition, confusion, altered mental status, auditory/visual hallucinations, psychosis (delirium, paranoia), mood changes (mania, agitation), hyperreflexia, myoclonus, tremor, asterixis, involuntary movements, major motor seizures, lethargy/stupor/coma and diffuse weakness. All these side effects are usually reversible.

6. Rejection encephalopathy

Rejection Encephalopathy is a pathogenic entity seen in patients with systemic features of acute graft rejection. Commonly the symptoms appear in the first 3 months post transplantation. The presumed pathology is cytokine production secondary to the rejection process. The clinical picture includes headache, confusion, seizures, and papilledema. The lumbar puncture reveals increased CSF opening pressure and the cerebral CT/MRI reveals diffuse cerebral edema. The EEG shows diffuse or focal rhythm slowing. The overall prognosis is good, with rapid and complete recovery after the immunosuppressive treatment of the rejection episode.

7. Graft versus host disease

Graft versus host disease is a complex complication of allogenic hematopoieic stem cell transplantation. It occurs in 40 to 75% of the patients undergoing this procedure. The underlying mechanism comprises of donor T cells reaction against host antigens. Neurological complications associated with graft versus host disease occur several months after the transplantation, in chronic phase of the disease, and typically involve the peripheral nervous system, causing polymiositis, myasthenia gravis and peripheral neuropathies compatible with acute Guillain-Barre syndrome or chronic idiopathic demyelinating polyneuropathy(Echaniz-Laguna et al. 2004). Brain MRI abnormalities comprising mainly of atrophy and white matter lesions are not uncommon in patients with chronic graft versus host disease, but their etiopathogeny is difficult to establish since these patients associate several factors that may result in brain injury. According to the current knowledge, the brain does not express major histocompatibility complex antigens, and therefore is expected to be protected from the potential damage induced by autoreactive T cells. However, a few cases of possible central nervous system involvement related to graft versus host disease have been reported. These patients presented with subacute encephalopathy developing in the setting of systemic involvement. The neuropathological examination revealed widespread T-cell infiltrates in the absence of conclusive evidence for viral infection. Imagistic features compatible with CNS vasculitis (one case with pathological confirmation) were reported to occur in several patients with chronic graft versus host disease. The authors that reported the latter series of cases proposed that an angeitis-like syndrome involving the CNS may occur as a complication of chronic graft versus host disease and may be responsible for the clinical and brain MRI findings encountered in some of these patients (Padovan et al. 1999).

8. Septic encephalopathy

Sepsis is defined as a known or suspected infection leading to the systemic inflammatory response syndrome. Due to the associated immunodepresion sepsis has higher incidence in transplanted patients. It frequently presents with delirium and represents perhaps the most common causal factor for intensive care unit delirium. Encephalopathy occuring in the setting of sepsis may have several causes, being either a direct consequence of sepsis, or secondary to various of its associated complications, such as liver or renal failure (resulting in metabolic disturbances), or induced by the pharmacologic agents required for its treatment. The evolution is usually acute. Though commonly diffuse brain involvement is observed, focal brain lesions may also occur.

The physiopathology of sepsis-associated encephalopathy is complex and involves inflammatory and non-inflammatory processes that affect endothelial cells, glial cells and neurons and that induce blood-brain barrier breakdown, dysfunction of intracellular metabolism, and cell death. The ongoing inflammatory cascade may impair capillary blood flow and therefore decrease the brain's supply of oxygen and essential nutrients and the clearance of toxic by-products. Elevated levels of tumour necrosis factor-alpha, interleukin-1, and other cytokines and chemokines that are released in response to the presence of bacterial lipopolysaccharides promote leukocyte–vascular endothelium adhesion and induce endothelial damage, sometimes resulting in disseminated intravascular coagulation. The endothelial dysfunction may lead to blood-brain barrier disruption with its subsequent consequences on brain parenchyma. Peri-microvessel edema impairs the transfer of oxygen, nutrients, and metabolites, while increased blood-brain barrier permeability facilitates the passage of various neurotoxic factors. The sepsis-related damage of the blood-brain barrier is attenuated by glial cells, dexamethasone or nitric oxid syntethase inhibition. Mitochondrial dysfunction, oxidative stress, and apoptosis also occur. The formation of reactive oxygen species compromises cell function and survival. A major consequence of oxidative stress is apoptosis. Neuronal apoptosis can also be secondary to glial cell dysfunction. Neurons are also vulnerable to other disturbances that frequently accompany sepsis, such as hypoxemia, hyperglycemia, hypoglycemia and consequences of organ dysfunction. Liver dysfunction increases plasma levels of ammonium, which interferes with neurotransmission. Exposure to lipopolysaccharide causes accumulation of calcium in brain cells, impairs synaptic transmission and depresses neuronal excitability.

Patients with sepsis-associated encephalopathy have altered state of consciousness; they can be disoriented, agitated, confused, or delirious but also somnolent, stuporous or comatose.

Agitation and somnolence occur alternatively. Confusion and agitation are associated with hypoxia; despite hypoxia correction the state of consciousness remains altered, usually correlated with septic hypotension. Neurological examination should assess neck stiffness, motor responses, muscular strength, plantar and deep tendon reflexes and cranial nerves to disclose a focal neurologic sign. Seizures should be considered in the presence of abnormal movements or eyelid twitching. In heavily sedated patients, detection of brain dysfunction is challenging. Interruption of sedation is necessary for the evaluation of mental status, but it is very difficult to discriminate between a sepsis associated encephalopathy and an effect of sedative accumulation or withdrawal. In patients who cannot tolerate sedative interruption, the diagnosis of brain dysfunction relies on electrophysiology (somatosensory evoked potentials, electroencephalogram), serum brain biomarkers (neuron-speciffic enolase, S-100b protein) or brain imaging. Routine biochemical tests are mandatory to rule out a metabolic disturbance. An EEG may be helpful to detect non-convulsive status epilepticus. In sepsis-associated encephalopathy, the electroencephalogram may be normal or show excessive theta, predominantly delta, triphasic waves, or burst suppression (the two latter patterns are associated with increased mortality). Lumbar puncture should be performed if meningitis or encephalitis is suspected. In septic encephalopathy, cerebrospinal fluid is usually normal. Brain imaging is indicated in the presence of a focal neurologic sign or seizure. In comparison with the CT scan, the MRI allows an accurate exploration of the brain, especially of the white matter and blood-brain barrier. MRI can reveal ischemic or hemorrhagic lesions, white matter lesions including PRES or leukoencephalopathy related to blood-brain barrier breakdown affecting predominately the areas around the Virchow-Robin spaces, as well as grey matter lesions involving the basal ganglia and thalami.

Treatment consists of controlling the underlying infection and general supportive measures, management of organ failure and metabolic disturbances and avoidance of neurotoxic drugs.

9. Wernicke's encephalopathy

Wernicke's Encephalopathy is caused by the impairment of thiamine-dependent enzymatic activity in the susceptible brain cells. The classical clinical picture comprises of mental status changes, ocular motility signs and axial and/or gait ataxia developing acutely or subacutely in individuals prone to thiamine (vitamin B1) deficiency (e.g. alcoholics). Atypical clinical presentations ranging from unexplained hypothermia to coma may occur, especially in non-alcoholics. In the majority of cases the clinical picture is completely reversible providing adequate parenteral thiamine is promptly supplied (Galvin et al. 2010; Tanasescu 2009; Thorarinsson et al. 2011; Thomson et al. 2002). Due to factors related to the underlying disease (including increased metabolic requirements, impaired intestinal absorption and persistent vomiting) and sometimes to the inadequate diet, transplanted patients have increased risk of developing thiamine deficiency and therefore Wernicke's Encephalopathy (Bleggi-Torres et al. 2000; Thomson and Marshall 2006). Moreover, several drugs that may be required for the transplanted patients (e.g. 5-fluorouracil, cisplatin, erbulozole, ifosfamide metronidazole, antacids, phenytoin, cephalosporins, diuretics and tetracycline) may impair thiamine's absorption or utilization or may increase its elimination, thus increasing the risk of developing Wernicke's Encephalopaty (Kondo et al. 1996; Imtiaz and Muzaffar 2010; Hamadani and Awan 2006; Van Belle et al. 1993; Cho et al. 2009). Special attention should be paid that those on total parenteral nutrition receive adequate amounts of thiamine. In marginally thiamine deficient patients, the administration of high doses of intravenous glucose solution may precipitate the developement of Wernicke's Encephalopathy. Iatrogenic hyperalimentation without adequate thiamine supplementation may also precipitate it (Serra et al. 2007; Watson et al. 1981; Sechi and Serra 2007). The diagnosis is supported by the presence of characteristic imagistic findings (i.e. symmetrical periaqueductal and periventricular gray matter signal changes on brain MRI translating cytotoxic and subsequently vasogenic edema and blood brain barrier disruption) and by the identification of low thiamine blood levels. However, since parenteral thiamine administration is cheap, has virtually no contraindications (except for prior allergic reactions) and might be a life saving intervention, its administration should be started on clinical grounds only. The presence of concomitant hypomagnesaemia should be searched for and corrected. The 2010 EFNS guideline recommends that 200 miligrams of thiamine hydrochloride diluted in 100 millilitres of normal saline or glucose solution should be administered intravenously, thrice a day, until there is no further clinical improvement and advocates the maintenance of a low threshold for thiamine administration and a high index of suspicion for Wernicke's Encephalopathy (Galvin et al. 2010; Tanasescu 2009; Thorarinsson et al. 2011; Thomson et al. 2002).

10. Posttransplantation opportunistic infection involving the CNS

The incidence of bacterial, fungal, viral and parasitic opportunistic infections is high in transplant recipients, especially in those with persistent neutropenia. The prophylactic use of broad spectrum antibiotics increases the risk of fungal infections (e.g. various Candida or Aspergillus species). Considering the poor prognosis of these infections prophylactic approaches are justified. The identification of the pathogen may sometimes be difficult and the treatment should be empirically started prior to the identification of the causative organism. Though the detailed discussion of the opportunistic infections involving the CNS is above the objective of the present chapter, several important aspects are detailed bellow.

Encephalitis caused by Listeria, Toxoplasma, Varicella Zoster virus, Cytomegalovirus and Cryptococcus may present with clinical and paraclinical findings similar to that of posttransplantation encephalopathies of other causes. In the cronic posttransplant period JC virus activation resulting in progressive multifocal leucoencephalopathy (PML) may also occur. Viral CNS oportunistic infections are most likely caused by herpes group viruses. Adenoviruses are also frequently involved. Routine prophylaxis with acyclovir has been reported to significantly reduce the incidence of herpes simplex type I, Varicella Zoster virus and Cytomegaovirus infections in transplanted patients(Shanahan et al. 2009). Human herpesvirus-6 has been reported to cause limbic encephalitis, commonly responsive to gancyclovir or foscarnet, in several transplant recipients. Septic Aspergillus brain embolism may be encountered, being reported to account for 15% of the neurological complications observed at necropsy in hematopoietic stem cells transplanted patients.

The brain MRI reveals multiple lesions preferentially involving the cerebral hemispheres, basal ganglia and corpus callosum. The microbiological isolation of the organism is especially difficult, the prognosis is poor and treatment (e.g. voriconazole and surgical management) should be started as soon as possible (Schwartz et al. 2005). CNS toxoplasmosis (i.e. infection with Toxoplasma gondii) is the most frequent parasitic CNS infection occurring in transplanted patients. The clinical picture comprises of various degrees of mental status changes associated or not with the presence of focal signs. The brain MRI reveals multiple mass lesions, with different characteristics than those seen in AIDS-related toxoplasmosis, because in transplant patients contrast enhancement and haemorrhage are only rarely encountered(Portegies et al. 2004). Toxoplasma gondii DNA may be identified in the CSF of these patients by various tehniques of polymerase chain reaction. Though it does not completely eliminate the risk of developing CNS toxoplasmosis, the prophylactic administration of trimethoprim/sulfamethoxazole should be considered in transplanted patients. Rarely Listeria monocytogenes, Mycobacterium tuberculosis and Cryptococcus neoformans may cause meningitis in transplanted patients. Brain abscesses caused by Nocardia asteroides, Mucorales or Candida species have been reported to occur in transplanted patients (Singh and Husain 2000).

11. Conclusions

Transplantation medicine is a constantly changing field. PTE is a common neurologic complication with a broad spectrum of causes and presentations. Knowledge of all the potential etiologies and of the particularities of transplanted patients are a sine qua non condition for the optimal management of these patients.

12. References

Bartynski WS, Tan HP, Boardman JF, Shapiro R, Marsh JW(2008) Posterior reversible encephalopathy syndrome after solid organ transplantation. American Journal of Neuroradiology;29:924–930

Bashir RM (2001) Neurologic Complications of Organ Transplantation. Current treatment options in neurology 3 (6):543-554

Bechstein WO(2000) Neurotoxicity of calcineurin inhibitors: impact and clinical management. Transplant International; 5:313-326.

Bleggi-Torres LF, de Medeiros BC, Werner B, Neto JZ, Loddo G, Pasquini R, de Medeiros CR (2000) Neuropathological findings after bone marrow transplantation: an autopsy study of 180 cases. Bone marrow transplantation 25 (3):301-307.

Brouns R, De Deyn PP(2004) Neurological complications in renal failure: a review. Clinical Neurology and Neurosurgery ; 107: 1–16

Chabolla DR, Harnois DM, Meschia JF(2003) Levetiracetam monotherapy for liver transplant patients with seizures.Transplant Proc; 35: 1480–1481

Cho IJ, Chang HJ, Lee KE, Won HS, Choi MY, Nam EM, Mun YC, Lee SN, Seong CM (2009) A case of Wernicke's encephalopathy following fluorouracil-based chemotherapy. Journal of Korean medical science 24 (4):747-750.

Cruz-Martinez E, Gilmore RL(2002). Transplantation and seizures. In: Ettinger AB and Devinsky O, eds. Managing epilepsy and co-existing disorders. Boston: Butterworth-Heinemann;75-82.

Echaniz-Laguna A, Battaglia F, Ellero B, Mohr M, Jaeck D(2004) Chronic inflammatory demyelinating polyradiculoneuropathy in patients with liver transplantation. Muscle and Nerve; 30: 501–504.

Galvin R, Brathen G, Ivashynka A, Hillbom M, Tanasescu R, Leone MA (2010) EFNS guidelines for diagnosis, therapy and prevention of Wernicke encephalopathy. European journal of neurology : the official journal of the European Federation of Neurological Societies 17 (12):1408-1418.

Gerald R. Crabtree (2001). Calcium, Calcineurin and the Control of Transcription. Journal of Biological Chemistry; 276(4): 2313-2316.

Guarino M, J. Benito-Leon, J. Decruyenaere, E. Schmutzhard, K. Weissenborn, A. Stracciari(2006) EFNS guidelines on management of neurological problems in liver transplantation. European Journal of Neurology; 13: 2–9

Hamadani M, Awan F (2006) Role of thiamine in managing ifosfamide-induced encephalopathy. Journal of oncology pharmacy practice : official publication of the International Society of Oncology Pharmacy Practitioners 12 (4):237-239.

Illsinger S, Janzen N, LÃ¼cke T, Bednarczyk J, Schmidt K-H, Hoy L, Sander J, Das nAM(2010). Cyclosporine A:impact on mitochondrial function in endothelial cells. Clinical Transplantation; 25(4)

Imtiaz S, Muzaffar N (2010) Ifosfamide neurotoxicty in a young female with a remarkable response to thiamine. JPMA The Journal of the Pakistan Medical Association 60 (10):867-869

Jantzen JP (2007) Prevention and treatment of intracranial hypertension. Best Pract Res Clin Anaesthesiol 21 (4):517-538

Kentaro I, Hideki O, Hiroyuki T, Kohei I, Masayuki S, Toshimitsu I, Masahiro O, HirotakaT(2007) Possible therapeutic effect of lipid supplementation on neurological complications in liver transplant recipients.Transplant International; 20 (7): 632–635.

Kondo K, Fujiwara M, Murase M, Kodera Y, Akiyama S, Ito K, Takagi H (1996) Severe acute metabolic acidosis and Wernicke's encephalopathy following chemotherapy with 5-fluorouracil and cisplatin: case report and review of the literature. Japanese journal of clinical oncology 26 (4):234-236

Liang BC(2000) Neurologic complications of orthotopic liver transplantation. Hospital Physician: 43-46

Londono MC, Guevara M, Rimola A, Navasa M, Taura P, Mas A, Garcia–Valdecasas JC, Arroyo V, Gines P(2006) Hyponatremia Impairs Early Posttransplantation Outcome in Patients With Cirrhosis Undergoing Liver Transplantation. Gastroenterology;130 :1135–1143

Mathew RM, Rosenfeld MR (2007) Neurologic Complications of Bone Marrow and Stem-cell Transplantation in Patients with Cancer. Current treatment options in neurology 9 (4):308-314

Padovan CS, Bise K, Hahn J, Sostak P, Holler E, Kolb HJ, Straube A (1999) Angiitis of the central nervous system after allogeneic bone marrow transplantation? Stroke; a journal of cerebral circulation 30 (8):1651-1656

Padovan CS, Sostak P, Straube A (2000) [Neurological complications after organ transplantation]. Der Nervenarzt 71 (4):249-258

Portegies P, Solod L, Cinque P, et al(2004) Guidelines for the diagnosis and management of neurological complications of HIV infection. European Journal of Neurology 11:297–304

Sechi G, Serra A (2007) Wernicke's encephalopathy: new clinical settings and recent advances in diagnosis and management. Lancet neurology 6 (5):442-455. Serra A, Sechi G, Singh S, Kumar A (2007) Wernicke encephalopathy after obesity surgery: a systematic review. Neurology 69 (6):615; author reply 615-616.

Singh N, Bonham A, Fukui M(2000) Immunosuppressive-associated leukoencephalopathy in organ transplant recipients. Transplantation;69:467

Singh N, Husain S (2000) Infections of the central nervous system in transplant recipients. Transpl Infect Dis 2 (3):101-111.

Shanahan A, Malani PN, Kaul DR(2009) Relapsing cytomegalovirus infection in solid organ transplant recipients. Transplant Infectious Disease;11(6)

Tanasescu R (2009) Wernicke's Encephalopathy In General Neurological Practice: Short Considerations On The Need For Revision (I). Romanian Journal of Neurology VIII (3):3

Thomson AD, Cook CC, Touquet R, Henry JA (2002) The Royal College of Physicians report on alcohol: guidelines for managing Wernicke's encephalopathy in the accident and Emergency Department. Alcohol Alcohol 37 (6):513-521

Thomson AD, Marshall EJ (2006) The treatment of patients at risk of developing Wernicke's encephalopathy in the community. Alcohol Alcohol 41 (2):159-167.

Thorarinsson BL, Olafsson E, Kjartansson O, Blondal H (2011) [Wernicke's encephalopathy in chronic alcoholics]. Laeknabladid 97 (1):21-29

Van Belle SJ, Distelmans W, Vandebroek J, Bruynseels J, Van Ginckel R, Storme GA (1993) Phase I trial of erbulozole (R55104). Anticancer research 13 (6B):2389-2391

Watson AJ, Walker JF, Tomkin GH, Finn MM, Keogh JA (1981) Acute Wernicke's encephalopathy precipitated by glucose loading. Irish journal of medical science 150 (10):301-303

Watt KD, Pedersen RA, Kremers WK, Heimbach JK, Charlton MR(2010). Evolution of Causes and Risk Factors for Mortality Post-Liver Transplant: Results of the NIDDK Long-Term Follow-Up Study. American Journal of Transplantation; 10(6):1420-1427 Wijdicks EF (2001)Neurotoxicity of imunosuppressive drugs. Liver Transplantation; 7: 937-942

2

HIV Encephalopathy – Now and Then

Cristina Loredana Benea, Ana-Maria Petrescu
and Ruxandra Moroti-Constantinescu
*National Institute of Infectious Diseases "Prof Dr. Matei Bals",
Bucharest,
Romania*

1. Introduction

HIV can cause a wide range of neurocognitive complications recently grouped under the name of HAND (HIV associated neurocognitive disorders). Depending on the degree of the impairment, there are three categories, progressing in disabilities from asymptomatic neurocognitive impairment (ANI) to HIV associated mild neurocognitive impairment (MND) and to HIV associated dementia (HAD)[1].

The introduction of HAART (highly active antiretroviral therapy) has led to a marked decrease in the incidence of HAND. But also the spectrum of HAND has changed in the HAART era; it seemed that minor cognitive impairment slightly increased. HAND consists of a triad of cognitive, behavioral and motor dysfunctions. With the exception of dementia, the symptoms are generally mild but can impact the quality of life and treatment adherence.

Diagnosis of HAND is based on a combination of careful history and neurological examination, neuropsychological testing, neuroimaging (especially magnetic resonance: MRI) and cerebrospinal fluid (CSF) analyses. The last two have a crucial role in differentiating from other etiologies. The differential diagnosis is quite broad in HIV patient with neurological impairment including HIV- related causes and also metabolic disturbances, substance abuse and psychiatric disorders.

Initiation of HAART with a good CNS penetration is the most effective mean of treating cognitive impairment.[2]

2. Epidemiology

HIV-encephalitis (HIVE) is the most frequent neurologic disorder of the brain in HIV-1 infection and is the principal cause of HAND. Neurocognitive impairments in overall HIV population appear to be nearly 50% [1], varying considerably by the region, due to the tests used for detection, HIV infection stage and comorbidities, virus subtype and treatment schedules.

The large majority of HIV-associated neurocognitive disorders (HAND) are asymptomatic (ANI) or mild (MND), but around 5% are severe, representing an AIDS-related illness: HIV-associated dementia (HAD). [3,4]

Paradoxically, HAART introduction didn't decrease the occurrence of HAND, but there was a shift from severe to moderate and mild forms [5]. Causes of continuing high rates of HAND despite HAART, have multiple possible explanations:

- the presence of irreversible brain injury prior to initiating ART;
- the possible neurotoxicity of some antiretroviral drugs;
- the persistence of minimal HIV replication in CNS and
- the effect of chronic immune activation, condition that lead to metabolic disorders and vascular degeneration, inclusive of CNS tissue.[6]

Risk factors for developing HAND included

- host factors: low educational status, older age, genetic predisposition, metabolic disorders, coinfection with hepatitis C virus and iv drug abuse.
- viral factors: virus subtype (subtypes B, C and D more related to HAND than subtype A; subtype F also associated with high prevalence of HAND) [1,7]
- relation host-virus: AIDS stage and presence of chronic immune activation - measured by different serum markers such as TNF-alpha and monocyte chemo-attractant protein 1 (MCP-1), hsCRP, IL6 and soluble CD14 - which leads to metabolic disorders and accelerated senescence; low nadir of CD4 T cell counts [8, 9]; HIV-DNA load in circulant macrophages and higher CSF viral load compared to serum viral load.[10,11]

Although HIV penetrates CNS early (during the acute HIV infection), the onset of HAND is delayed for years, superposing with moderate and advanced immune-suppression stages [12, 5]. It emerges gradually, in weeks or months.

There are no conclusive data regarding the HAND outcome: there is a variable degree of reversibility for ANI and MND, unlike typical neurodegenerative syndromes and MND doesn't progress necessarily to HAD.[1]. Although it is considered to be a treatable condition, HAND is associated with a shortened survival [13].

3. Pathogenesis of HIV encephalitis

HIV-encephalitis (HIVE) represents the mainly HAND substrate.

HIV enters the central nervous system early during the infection [12,5], transported by CD4 T lymphocytes and monocytes, that cross the blood-brain barrier (BBB). The infected monocytes become perivascular macrophages in nervous tissue. Then, HIV infects local macrophages (microglia). Perivascular macrophages and microglia fused together, forming multinucleated giant cells (MGCs). MGCs replicate the virus (serving as HIV-reservoir) and express neurotoxic molecules: viral (gp-120 and tat protein) and cellular [14]. These neurotoxins have at least two properties:

- they activate astrocytes, which in turn release cytokines and increase BBB permeability, promoting migration of more HIV-infected cells from blood to brain.
- they damage the neurons, with demyelination and neuronal loss.

Therefore, the picture of local histopathology in HIVE shows inflammatory changes and neuronal destructions: perivascular macrophages accumulation, reactive gliosis with microglial nodules and MGCs formation and focal neuronal necrosis with demyelination and neuroatrophy [15,1].

Macroscopically, in HIVE, there is global white matter pallor, a reduction in nervous substance thickness, especially in deep grey matter structures and in subcortical frontal white matter. Mostly affected are basal ganglia (especially caudate nucleus), corpus callosum and hippocampus, which correlate well with clinical cognitive and behavioral syndromes - but in a lesser extent with motor manifestations [1]

HIV proved to damage the neurons directly, via viral neurotoxins and indirectly, via immunologic pathways. The lasts consist in local changes (already mentioned cellular neurotoxins and BBB deterioration) and systemic changes, which means chronic immune activation.

The chronic immune activation can be done by any persistent infectious or noninfectious inflammation. The repercussion is an accelerated immune-mediated global vascular senescence (endothelial dysfunction with subsequent atherosclerosis) which has as consequences many metabolic disorders[16], including neuro-degeneration (subclinical atherosclerotic disease of the brain vessels)

In HIV infection, chronic immune activation takes place even in HIV-treated patients, with a good control of the plasma viral load, but with a poor control of viral sanctuary (reservoirs). It is demonstrated that despite plasma level suppression, HIV could continue to replicate in brain tissues with a rate of 3-10% [1]. This replication (as low as 2 copies/ml) is capable to maintain a persistent immune activation [8] with its consequences. The HIV presence/ persistence in the brain in the HAART era has a series of explanations:

- incomplete suppression: the virus can not be totally suppressed in the brain tissues because of the poor penetration of antiretrovirals through BBB, thus too low drug's concentrations achieve there allowing the development of different HIV (resistant) cvasispecies in CNS. [8].
- viral afflux from peripheral reservoirs: there could exists a permanent traffic of the mononuclear infected cells (with pro-viral DNA: HIV-DNA) from peripheral reservoirs (bone marrow) to the brain. Even in patients with undetectable plasma viral load, we can find HIV-DNA in circulating monocytes, with the same viral signature as in the bone marrow and in the deep brain structures.

Other factors that may contribute to neurocognitive disorders in HIV patients with HIVE in HAART era are:

- the medication per se (antiretrovirals or miscellanea), which can have neurotoxic effects
- aging - there is an accelerated neuro-degeneration in older HIV subjects, which has similarities with neurodegenerative syndromes, with abnormal accumulation of beta-amyloid apolipoproteinE4, tau protein and synuclein[1,5]
- hepatitis C virus coinfection: both viruses invade SNC and cause synergic neurotoxic effects.
- iv drug abuse contribute to neuro-degeneration

A particular situation in HIV treated patients is IRIS (immune reconstitution syndrome). A severe HIVE development can be observed in patients receiving HAART, with a low basal CD4 T lymphocytes count and high initial HIV-RNA level, despite the good suppression obtained under treatment. Histo-pathologically numerous CD8-positive lymphocytes were found close to the neurons, in the perivascular areas and in the parenchyma. This condition may be interpreted as an immune reconstitution phenomenon directed against HIV itself [17], leading to an extensive white matter destruction, with vacuolar leucoencephalopathy [12]

The neuro-injury in HIVE can be paraclinically appreciated by:

- biochemical and molecular analysis of plasma and CSF: uncontrolled viral replication increases the HAND risk; discordances in viral loads, with higher CSF load represent a particular risk; the presence of high levels of neopterin and beta-microglobulin in CSF (neuro-degeneration and macrophage/microglial activation markers) even in the absence of a CSF viral replication correspond to neuronal impairment; the low number of CD4 T lymphocytes in peripheral blood increases the risk of HAND (especially at CD4 below 200/mmc)[3]; presence of the chronic immune activation markers in peripheral blood is also a predictive factor for HAND, measured by hsCRP, soluble CD14, D-dimers, IL6, TNF-alpha and MCP-1; high level of HIV DNA in peripheral monocytes correlates well with HAND.
- histological, biochemical and molecular analysis of the nervous parenchima: there is reported HIV presence in brain tissue more frequently than in CSF [18,1-16], suggesting that CSF levels may underestimate HIV replication in brain tissue.
- imaging-based methods which can appreciate the nervous tissue injuries in HIVE

At present, the main goal of treatment is the effective suppression of the HIV from reservoirs, that can disrupt the vicious circle of chronic immune activation and reverse (partially) HIVE.

4. HIV-associated neurocognitive disorders – Nomenclature and staging

In 1991 the American Academy of Neurology AIDS Task Force developed a consensus nomenclature and case definition for HIV associated dementia (HAD) complex. Several terms are still used interchangeably, including AIDS dementia complex, HIV encephalopathy, HIV subacute encephalitis, and HAD. The severity of dementia in the consensus nomenclature (mild, moderate, and severe) reflects functional deficits that affect the activities of daily living.(19)

A milder form of cognitive impairment, HIV-1-associated minor cognitive/motor disorder (MCMD), was also introduced in 1996; however, it was not determined whether this represented an intermediate step in the progression to dementia. Subsequent research has shown that MCMD is a risk factor for HAD [20].

Since the introduction of HAART in 1996, the incidence of moderate or severe dementia fell from about 7% in 1989 to only 1% in 2000, and the severity of neurological disease appears to have been attenuated (21). Despite this remarkable effect on incidence rates, the prevalence of HIV Associated Neurocognitive Disorders (HAND) continues at very high rates. In response to the changes, in 2007 the National Institutes of Health created a working group to critically review the adequacy and utility of current definitions and diagnostic criteria (22). The report provides a new nosology (Table 1) witch distinguishes among patients with subclinical dysfunctions categorized as suffering asymptomatic neurocognitive impairments (ANI) , patients with greater cognitive decline that have mild adverse effects on daily living activities categorized as HIV-associated mild neurocognitive disorder (MND) and patients with significant functional impairment who can be categorized as having HIV – associated dementia (HAD). An algorithm is proposed to assist in standardized diagnostic classification of HAND. The clinical algorithms give guidelines for decision making regarding: (1) cognitive impairment, (2) functional decline, (3) factoring in comorbidities, and alternative approaches when full neurodiagnostic assessment capabilities are not available (22).

HIV-associated asymptomatic neurocognitive impairment (ANI)
Acquired impairment in two or more cognitive domains, with evidence of performance >1.0 SD below the mean for age- and education-appropriate norms on standardized neuropsychological tests
Cognitive impairment does not interfere with everyday functioning
Cognitive impairment does not meet the criteria for delirium or dementia
No evidence of another preexisting cause for the ANI
If prior ANI existed, but no longer does, a diagnosis of ANI in remission is made
Diagnosis deferred for patients with major depression or substance abuse on examination
HIV-associated mild neurocognitive disorder (MND)
Acquired impairment in two or more cognitive domains, with evidence of performance >1.0 SD below the mean for age- and education-appropriate norms on standardized neuropsychological tests
Typically, impairment staging corresponds to an MSK scale stage of 0.5 to 1
The cognitive impairment produces at least mild interference in daily functioning (at least one of the following): (a) self-report of reduced mental acuity, inefficiency in work, homemaking, or social functioning; (b) observation by knowledgeable others that the individual had undergone at least mild decline in mental acuity with resultant inefficiency in work, homemaking, or social functioning
The cognitive impairment does not meet the criteria for delirium or dementia
No evidence of another preexisting cause for the MND
Remission and comorbid psychiatric disturbance criteria similar to that for ANI
HIV-associated dementia (HAD)
Marked acquired impairment in at least two cognitive domains. Typically impairments involve multiple domains, especially in learning of new information, slowed information processing, and defective attention/concentration
The impairments must be >2 SD below average on neuropsychological testing
Correspond to an MSK scale stage of 2.0 or greater
The cognitive impairment markedly interferes with daily functioning
The impairments do not meet the criteria for delirium
No evidence of another preexisting cause for dementia, such as CNS infection, neoplasm, etc.,or severe substance abuse compatible with CNS disorder
Remission and comorbid psychiatric disturbance criteria similar to that for ANI and MND.
However, if dementia persists after one month on remission of major depression, a reassessment should be conducted to reassess for dementia

Table 1. Nosology of HIV-associated neurocognitive impairment (22).

5. Clinical manifestations

Neurocognitive impairment in people with HIV is characterized by a triad of cognitive, psychological, and motor dysfunctions. Symptoms may include any combination of the following: distractibility, poor concentration or attention, memory problems on short-term or long-term, impaired problem-solving or calculation ability, reduced ability to plan ahead, difficulty learning new things, problems with speech and language comprehension, abnormal visual perception, psychomotor slowness, poor balance, clumsiness, changes in mood (e.g., apathy, depression), social withdrawal, altered behaviour.

Specific neurological manifestations depend on which parts of the brain are affected. Impairment can range from so mild that it is not apparent without specialized testing, to so severe that it prevents independent living.

HIV-associated dementia **(HAD)** is diagnosed when there is evidence of marked declines in function in at least two separate cognitive domains, along with evidence of functional deterioration affecting activities of daily living (ADL) and self care. By definition, there must be evidence of significant declines from premorbid abilities.

The early described cases of HAD presented clinical features different from "classic" dementias such as Alzheimer's disease and other cortical degenerative diseases (23). HAD is considered a "subcortical" type of dementia", the neuropsychological profile involving : executive functions (ability of planning, decision-making, mental flexibility), concentration and complex attention (sustained attention, divided attention, selective attention, processing speed), verbal memory, learning and memory recall (24,25). Cortical dementia is more likely to involve memory loss, language comprehension, visual- spatial dysfunction and deficient conceptual abilities. Most patients with HAD do not present primary amnestic disturbances. Impairments of memory and learning are different from those seen in Alzheimer's disease: usually is retained the ability to store new memory but the efficiency for learning is diminished and the recognition memory is better preserved than recall memory, suggesting that the hippocampus is less affected.

Some patients with HAD may experience severe memory impairments or cortical symptoms that are virtually impossible to distinguish from Alzheimer's disease and related dementia. The cognitive domains most commonly affected are those of attention and executive functions (23, 26, 27). Impaired reaction time and reduced processing speed determining cognitive slowing reflects the effects of HIV on subcortical white and the basal ganglia, most notably the caudate nucleus (the caudate has been shown to be particularly vulnerable to HIV) (28, 29,30). Primary language functions are not very affected in HAD, severe aphasia being rare present but verbal fluency is frequently impaired as an expression of executive dysfunction (31).

Patients with HAD frequently show impaired motor abilities even when other cognitive functions are relatively intact (26). They can present: psychomotor slowing, poor coordination, tremors, impaired fine motor skills (egg, handwriting, buttoning etc). The presence of motor problems along with other cognitive problems is one of the key factors that distinguished AIDS–dementia from Alzheimer's disease and related dementias (32).

Behavioral changes include irritability, apathy, reduced social contact, decreased libido, and altered sleeping patterns. Mild to moderate depressive symptoms may precede the onset of

HAD (33); however, significant depression may confound the diagnosis of HAD and needs to be considered along with HAD since depressive symptoms can be ameliorated with both pharmacological and nonpharmacological intervention.

Patients with mild to moderate cognitive impairment often have a normal neurological exam. Early neurological findings include abnormal pursuit and saccadic eye movements and reduced rapid alternating and sequential hand movements. Later, patients develop gait abnormalities, hyperreflexia (ankle reflexes may be normal or reduced if HIV-associated neuropathy coexists) and postural instability. As HAD progresses, ataxia, tremor, hypertonia, and frontal release signs appear.

5.1 Milder neurocognitive disorders (ANI or MCD)

For milder forms of HAND, difficulties in concentration, attention, and memory may be present while the neurologic examination is unremarkable (34). Affected individuals are easily distracted, make errors in tasks regularly conducted, lose their train of thought, complain of increased fatigue due to effort to organize, plan and making decision, require repeated prompting. Activities of daily living may take longer and become more laborious. Overall the clinical manifestations are similar to those of HAD but of lesser severity.

6. Diagnostic workup

6.1 Biomarkers of HIV- Related Central Nervous System Disease

CSF analysis is critical in ruling out alternative etiologies. Tests useful for differential diagnosis include: opening pressure, culture (particularly fungal and mycobacterium), cell count, protein, cryptococcal antigen, VDRL for neurosyphilis and polymerase chain reaction testing for toxoplasma, cytomegalovirus, Epstein Barr virus, John Cunningham virus, and herpes virus.

The CSF profile of patients with HAND is often indistinguishable from HIV-infected individuals without cognitive impairment. The nonspecific abnormalities may include mild elevated total protein and mild mononuclear pleocytosis. Almost all patients with HAD have elevated protein levels. A CSF leucocytosis greater than 50 cell/μL is unlikely to be due to HIV alone, especially when the CD4 is below 200 cell/ μL (35). A polymorphonuclear pleocytosis is unlikely with HAD and raised the possibility of bacterial meningitis or cytomegalovirus ventriculitis (36).

Many biomarkers have been described but the discovery of reliable diagnostic markers has been elusive (37). These biomarkers can be divided into those related to pathogenesis and those reflecting the state of relevant cells. Recent studies have shown that both markers of immune activation (neopterin and beta-2 microglobulin) and neuronal destruction (neurofilament light chain) are elevated in HAD (38).

β-2-microglobulin (light chain of the HLA I expressed on the surface of all nucleated cells with the exception of neurons) presents elevated concentrations in CSF in both inflammatory and lymphoproliferative conditions (39). CSF β-2-microglobulin correlates well with the severity of HAD and the levels decrease with successful treatment of HIV (39).

Neopterin (a product of guanosine triphosphate metabolism, mainly produced by activated monocytes, macrophages, and microglia) presents high CSF concentrations in patients with opportunistic CNS infections as well as HAD. The CSF concentrations correlate with HAD severity and decrease with antiretroviral therapy (40). In one study after 2 years of virologic suppression, only 55% had normal CSF neopterin levels (41).

Neurofilament-Light (a major structural element of large myelinated neurons) presents CSF levels significantly but nonspecifically raised in HAD and rise with HAART interruption (42, 43). It seems that levels fall to normal in the majority of patients initiated on HAART (44).

HIV RNA

Plasma HIV RNA levels are not specific or sensitive to HAND. In HAART-treated patients, an undetectable plasma RNA level seems to occur more often in HAD for reasons that are unclear (45).

CSF HIV RNA is also nonspecific, with elevated levels in HAD, asymptomatic patients and those with opportunistic infections (45,46,47). Prior to HAART, higher CSF HIV RNA correlated with lower neuropsychological scores in subjects with more advanced disease (48). HAD can occur in the absence of an elevated HIV RNA in CSF (49, 50,51). Possible explanations for this situation are: residual deficits despite HAART (49); the presence of confounding conditions like hepatitis C or substance abuse or autonomous immune activation in response to the initial HIV infection (50) .

6.2 Neuroimaging

HAD is a diagnostic of exclusion. Computed tomography (CT) and magnetic resonance imaging (MRI) studies of the brain can support a diagnosis of HIV encephalopathy (HIVE) and rule out HIV-associated opportunistic infections or neoplasm.

CT scan reveals diffuse cortical atrophy, ventricular enlargement, and hypodensities in white matter in later stages. Basal ganglia calcifications are seen in adults but are more common in children. Usually computer tomography investigations offer normal results in ANI and MND.

MRI: When the infection becomes clinically symptomatic, the most common MRI findings are general atrophy in both cortical and subcortical regions of the brain (52). More specifically, these regions include frontal white matter and basal ganglia (53,54), with modifications in this area becoming more prominent in most advanced HAND stages. Caudate nucleus atrophy is a common finding (54,55,56). Another common imaging finding, although not a defining MRI feature of HIVE, is the presence of T2-weighted hyperintenses images in white matter of the CNS (white matter signal abnormalities WMSA) (52,57,58). These lesions without mass effect can be solitary, diffuse unilateral or large bilateral, and are located predominantly in the periventricular white matter and centrum semiovale These usually do not enhance after iv contrast administration and are better reveled on FLAIR MR sequences. WMSA corresponding loci of demyelization and vacuolation was shown to be related to HIV infection (dendrite pruning) (59) but also to vascular risk factors among older HIV infected patients (60). MRI findings are often but not always associated with performance on cognitive tests and are not always correlated with immunological function (CD4) or disease activity (viral load). Structural changes are sensitive to later stage of HAND but do not characterize very well the asymptomatic or the milder stages of the HIVE.

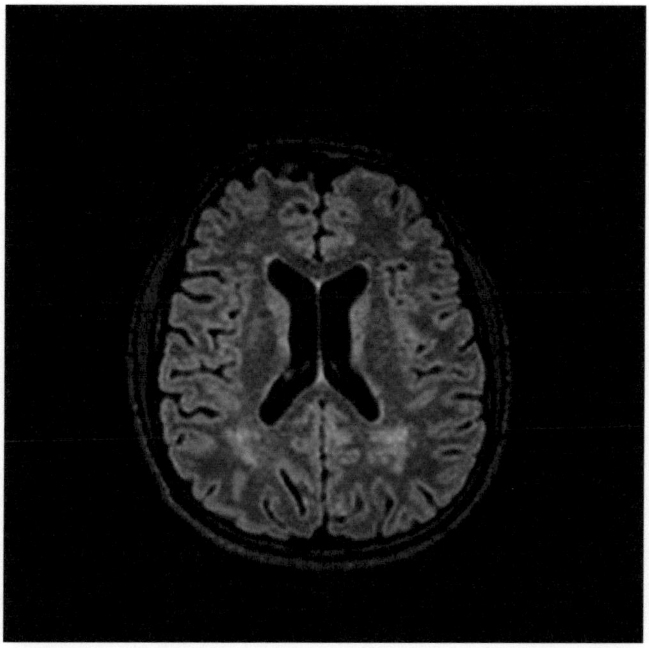

Fig. 1. HIVE. MRI (T2-w FLAIR) transversal section: symmetric high signals in subcortical profound white matter and in periventricular areas (INBI Matei Bals collection, courtesy of Dr. M. Mardarescu)

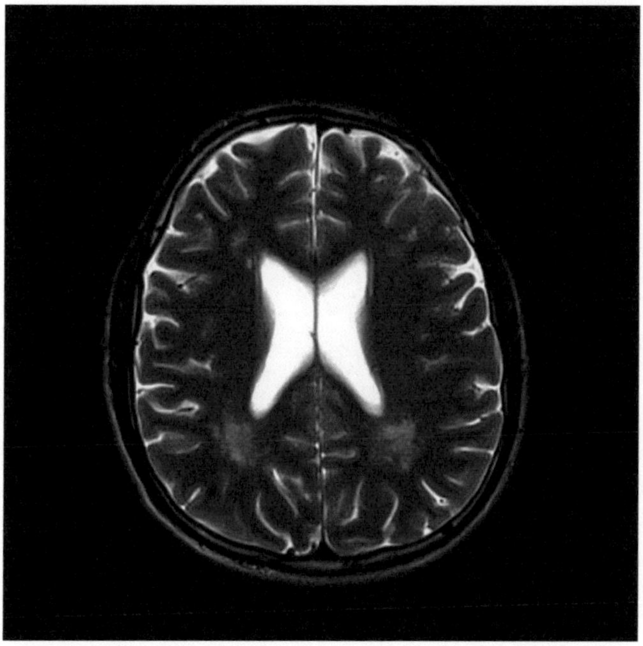

Fig. 2. HIVE. MRI (T2-w) transversal section: symmetric high signals in periventricular subcortical white matter, predominantly in parietal posterior areas (INBI Matei Bals collection, courtesy of Dr. M. Mardarescu)

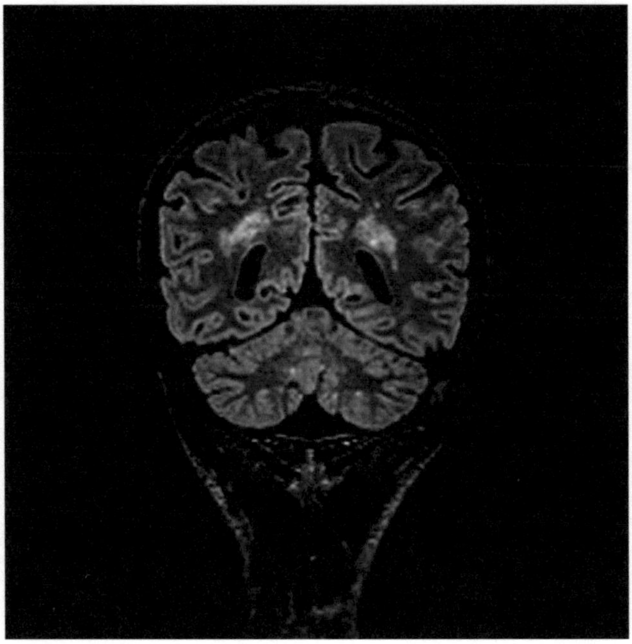

Fig. 3. HIVE. MRI (T2-w FLAIR) coronal section: symmetric high signals in periventricular white matter, predominantly in parietal posterior areas (INBI Matei Bals collection, courtesy of Dr. R. Draghicenoiu)

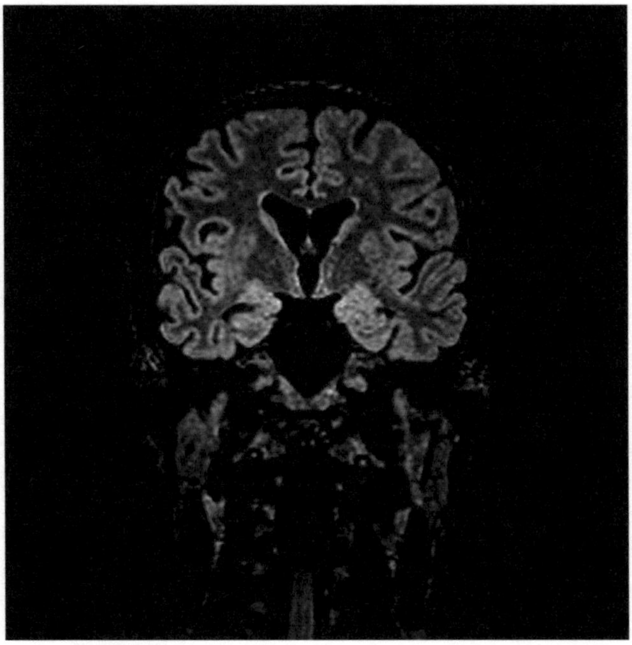

Fig. 4. HIVE. MRI (T2-w FLAIR) coronal section: mild ventriculomegaly with periventricular linear hypersignal and high signals in subcortical white matter (INBI Matei Bals collection, courtesy of Dr. R. Draghicenoiu)

Proton Magnetic Resonance Spectroscopy (MRS) is a functional imaging technique that allows measuring a specific set of brain metabolites concentrations noninvasively. The most commonly reported neurochemical spectra in the examination of HIV + patients are: *N* - acetyl aspartate (NAA) -a marker of neuronal integrity, myo-inositol (mI) a glial cell marker, Choline (Cho) a marker of cell turnover and creatine (Cr) a marker of energy metabolism. Choline is useful in examining the white matter abnormalities and the creatine spectra is often used as a reference peak because the Cr signal is relatively constant across subjects. Functional MRI studies are not yet widely available, but they may be useful in examining HIV associated CNS abnormalities before neurocognitive disorders can be detected by clinical or neuropsychological evaluation. (61). Altered metabolic function in HIV infected persons appears early in the course of disease progression and is demonstrable by an elevation in Cho, mI and occasionally Cr in frontal areas and in the basal ganglia even in the asymptomatic stages (62,63,64). Elevations of these metabolites are interpreted to be a marker of inflammation and of glial activation and astrocytosis. In more advanced stages of the disease has been observed a decrease of NAA, especially in the frontal and subcortical areas of the brain, signaling neuronal injury (65, 66,67). The decreased NA/Cr ratio is more important in younger persons, suggesting that in older individuals, the metabolic changes seen may be a combination of age and HIV infection. There are equivocal evidences of metabolites improvement in HAART-treated patients but this issue requires further studies.

Diffusion Magnetic Resonance Imaging (DTI) is a relatively new MRI technique that produces images of biological tissues weighted with the local microstructural characteristics of water diffusion, which is capable of showing connections between brain regions. Researchers have focused on two primary metrics: the mean diffusivity (MD) and fractional anisotropy (FA). Several studies suggest that DTI is sensitive in revealing subtle white-matter abnormalities in the HIV+ cohort. General reductions in FA and increases in MD are apparent in multiple white-matter regions, especially in the frontal white matter and the corpus calosum, as compared to healthy controls but continued research in this field must be done (68,69,70,71).

Single-photon emission computed tomography (SPECT) may reveal abnormalities in cerebral blood flow in frontal, temporal, and parietal areas of the brain, the severity of which was shown to be associated with severity of cognitive symptoms (72,73,74).

PET imaging: Several studies demonstrated hypermetabolism of glucose in the basal ganglia, thalamus, temporal and parietal lobes (75,76,77) early in the disease even in the asymptomatic stage (75). In more advanced stages of the disease it was observed a hypometabolism for cortical and subcortical gray matter (78). The use of a new PET ligand [11C]-PK11195 might provide a window into active areas of inflammatory processes in HIV infection. PET scanning may also be useful to exclude CNS lymphoma, which shows increased uptake, whereas the lesions of HAND do not.

There are several other MRI imaging modalities that have been used to examine HIV-associated CNS effects: perfusion MRI, magnetization transfer imaging, and postcontrast enhancement imaging but the studies available are limited.

6.3 Neuropsychological testing

The diagnosis of HAND implies exclusion of other causes of cognitive impairment by neurological examination and neuroimaging evaluations. Neuropsychological assessment is important to quantify and determine the specific pattern of the cognitive abnormality, to classify the severity of the deficits (to detect mild, early cognitive abnormalities) and to long term follow up.

The assessment needs to be comprehensive enough to assess abilities of attention, working memory, delayed recall, learning, verbal fluency, speed of information processing, abstraction/problem solving and motor functions. It is important to use demographically-corrected norms even for these screening tools (79).

European AIDS Clinical Society recommended screening for neurocognitive impairment.

Any HIV-infected person complaining of disturbances in his/her memory (comprehension, clarity or speed) should be evaluated extensively, including neurological examination, neuropsychological assessment, cerebrospinal exam and imaging of the brain.

Patients without such symptoms that should be targeted for screening:

- uncontrolled HIV infection (detectable plasma HIV RNA)
- use of antiretroviral agents with limited CNS penetration
- low CD4 nadir (<200 cells/mm^3)
- ongoing depression

Screening tool

- International HIV Dementia Scale (IHDS)

Assessment Methods:

S Letendre and co proposed a multi-step assessment of a HIV infected person susceptible for neurocognitive impairment consisting in:

Symptom Questionnaire: The Medical Outcomes Study HIV (MOS-HIV) Health Survey (table 2), The Patient's Assessment of Own Functioning Inventory PAOFI

Screening Tests: International HIV Dementia Scale, HIV Dementia Scale, Montreal Cognitive Assessment

Brief Neuropsychological Testing: ALLRT Brief Neurocognitive Screen, Grooved Pegboard, Action Fluency, Computerized Testing

Comprehensive Neuropsychological Testing: At least 5 cognitive abilities; At least 2 tests per ability

The most widely accepted neuropsychiatric screening techniques is the International HIV Dementia Scale (IHDS), although this scale is not enough sensitive for the assessment of early cognitive impairment. The scale consists of 4 subsets that target memory (e.g., recall, registration), psychomotor speed, constructional ability, and concentration.

A patient with a negative screening test may require more in-depth neuropsychological testing (80).

How much time during the past 4 weeks.....	All of the time	Most of the time	A good bit of the time	Some of the time	A little of the time	None of the time
Did you have difficulty reasoning and solving problems, e.g. making plans, making decisions, learning new things?	1	2	3	4	5	6
Did you forget things that happened recently, e.g., where you put things, appointments?	1	2	3	4	5	6
Did you have trouble keeping your attention on any activity for long?	1	2	3	4	5	6
Did you have difficulty doing activities involving concentration and thinking?	1	2	3	4	5	6

Knippels, et al. AIDS.2002; 16: 259-267

Table 2. MOS - HIV Cognitive Functional Status Scale

International HIV Dementia Scale (IHDS)

Memory-Registration: Give four words to recall (dog, hat, bean, red) – 1 second to say each. Then ask the patient all four words after you have said them.
Repeat words if the patient does not recall them all immediately. Tell the patient you will ask for recall of the words again a bit later.

1. Motor speed.
Have the patient tap the first two fingers of the non-dominant hand as widely and as quickly as possible.
4 = 15 in 5 seconds
3 = 11-14 in 5 seconds
2 = 7-10 in 5 seconds
1 = 3-6 in 5 seconds
0 = 0-2 in 5 seconds

2. Psychomotor speed.
Have the patient perform the following movements with the non-dominant hand as quickly as possible:

- Clench hand in fist on flat surface.
- Put hand flat on surface with palm down.
- Put hand perpendicular to flat surface on the side of the 5th digit.
- Demonstrate and have patient perform twice for practice.

4 = 4 sequences in 10 seconds
3 = 3 sequences in 10 seconds
2 = 2 sequences in 10 seconds
1 = 1 sequence in 10 seconds
0 = unable to perform

3. Memory-recall.
Ask the patient to recall the four words. For words not recalled, prompt with a semantic clue as follows: animal (dog); piece of clothing (hat); vegetable (bean); color (red).
Give 1 point for each word spontaneously recalled. Give 0.5 points for each correct answer after prompting
Maximum – 4 points.

Total International HIV Dementia Scale Score: This is the sum of the scores on items 1-3. The maximum possible score is 12 points.
A patient with a score of ≤ 10 should be evaluated further for possible dementia.

Sacktor NC; Wong M; Nakasujja N; Skolasky RL; Selnes OA; Musisi S; Robertson K; McArthur JC; Ronald A; Katabira E. AIDS 2005;19(13):1367-74.

In advancing disease, tests that explore the following abilities may be helpful:

- Motor ability : Finger Tapping Test, Grooved Pegboard Test
- Concentration: Continuous Performance Test, Trail Making Test A and B
- Processing :Trail Making Test A and B, Choice Reaction Time
- Memory/learning : Weschler Memory Scale, California Verbal Learning Test
- Abstraction: Wisconsin Card-Sorting Test
- Speech/language: Boston Naming Test, Verbal Fluency Test

In addition to the neuropsychological tests, it is also recommended to briefly assess the level of depressive complains using a validated psychiatric scale. The assessment should be complemented by an examination of activities of daily living (81) as this assessment serves to ascertain the presence of dementia versus milder stages of HAND (22,82).

Assessment of substance use history is of particular importance. The type of drugs, length of use, mode of use, and dosage should be recorded as they help to interpret the current level of neurocognitive abilities.

A brief assessment of medication adherence is recommended because it has been shown to be associated with severity of cognitive impairment in HIV-infection (83).

7. Differential diagnosis

Due to similar symptoms and signs, the differential diagnosis of HIV encephalopathy includes opportunistic infections as well as neoplastic etiology and encephalopathy due to reversible causes. We should also take into consideration HAART neurotoxicity and IRIS.

7.1 Opportunistic infections

Progressive multifocal leucoencephalopathy (PML) is the most common infiltrative brain lesion observed in patients with AIDS and is caused by a reactivation of the dormant JC virus,a DNA polyomavirus.The incidence of PML has not decreased after HAART introduction, being around 1-10% of AIDS patients.(84,85). The viral tropism for oligodendrocytes results in a progressive demyelinating disease and the symptoms depends on the afflicted areas. The common complaints are limb weakness (50% of cases), disturbance of speech, cognitive abnormalities(25 %), gait disorder (30%), seizures (10%) and visual impairments. The definitive diagnosis of PML is made by brain biopsy but due to its invasive character and occasional morbidity, it was replaced by newer techniques such as PCR for JC virus in the CSF and radiologic imaging.

PCR assays for the detection of JC virus DNA in the CSF are highly sensitive and specific (86) and could be used as a prognostic tool because it was observed that higher levels of JC in the CSF were correlated with lower survival rates. (87,88).

MRI is the modality of choice due to its higher sensitivity of lesion detection and superior contrast resolution compared to CT. Commonly, both PML and HIV encephalopathy displays nonenhancing lesions in the subcortical white matter, with little or no mass effect and hyperintense on T2-weighted and FLAIR magnetic resonance(89). But PML lesions are usually hypointense on T1-weighted images and become more hypointense as the disease progresses (89).Typical imaging findings are patchy areas, often bilateral and asymmetric, located predominantly just bellow the cortical ribbon, involving the arcuate (U) fibers and sometimes seen in brainstem and cerebellum (90).

Magnetization transfer (MT) imaging is a new type of MR imaging which appears to be much more sensitive than standard MRI for the demyelinating process seen in PML. The signal used in MT imaging alter the magnetization of the tissue - bound protons which in turn causes a decrease in the signal coming from the free protons, producing a change in signal intensity on the MR image. The result is expressed as the change in signal intensity compared to normal MR image and is called magnetization transfer ratio (MTR) .Studies(91,92) revealed that MTR in PML lesion is markedly reduced (22% to 26%) while in HIV encephalopathy has only mild reductions (38% to 40%), indicating that MT imaging could distinguish between them. Proton MR spectroscopy is another novel method which provides measurements of several neuromarkers, reflecting the neuronal viability. Only one study (93) compared the spectral changes in HIV encephalopathy with those in PML and found that the last one had a more profound decrease in NAA.

Although CNS tuberculosis and neurosyphilis are not opportunistic infections per se, they are discussed in this chapter due to their protean manifestations.

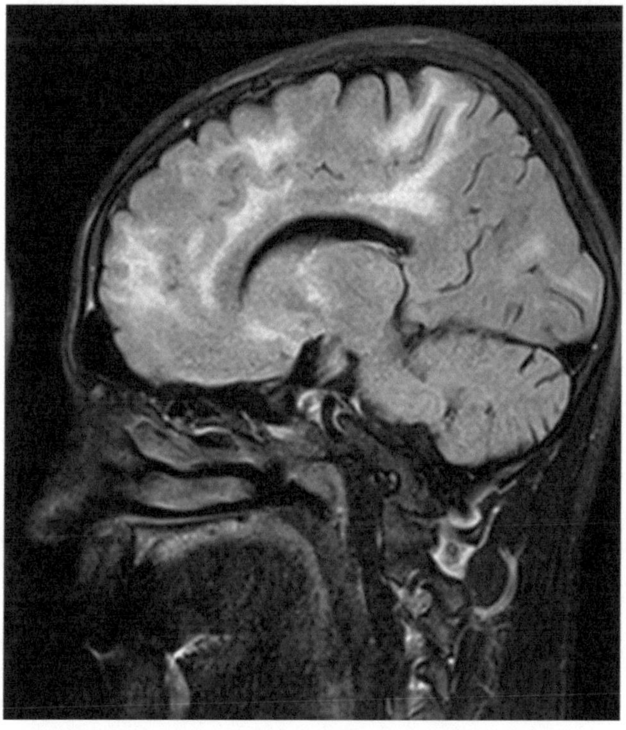

Fig. 5. PML: MRI (T2w FLAIR), sagital section: diffuse high signal changes in the subcortical white matter of the frontal, parietal and occipital lobes, suggesting U-fibres involvement, with no mass effect (INBI Matei Bals collection, courtesy of dr R. Ungurianu)

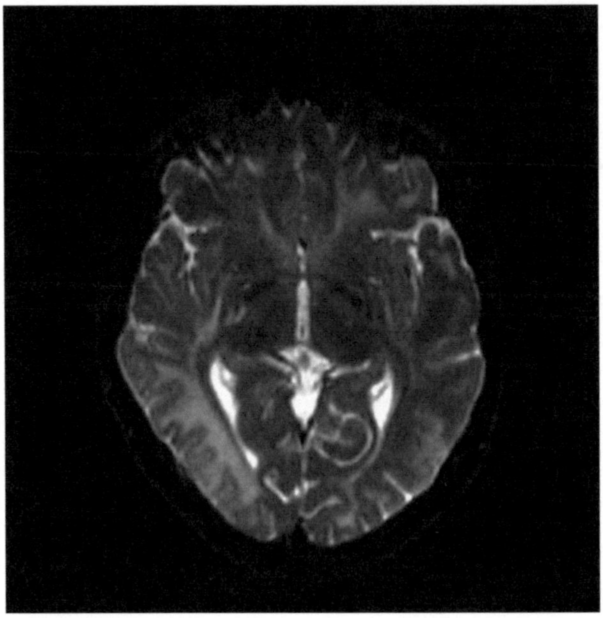

Fig. 6. PML: MRI (T2-w), transversal section: bilateral asymmetrical (predominantly on the right side) hyperintense signals in the subcortical white matter, just bellow the cortical ribbon (suggesting U-fibers involvement), without mass effect (INBI Matei Bals collection, courtesy of dr R. Ungurianu)

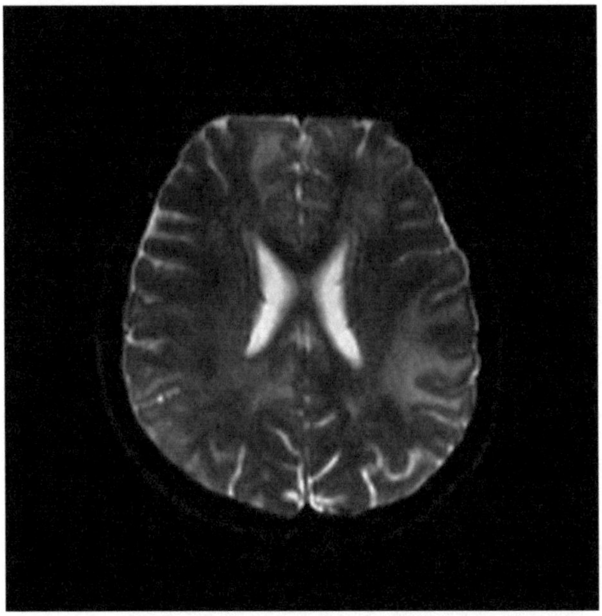

Fig. 7. PML: MRI transversal section (T2-w): bilateral asymmetrical, predominantly on left side, hyperintense signals in the subcortical white matter, just bellow the cortical ribbon (suggesting U-fibers involvement); no displacement of nervous substance, normal ventricles (INBI Matei Bals collection, courtesy of dr. R. Ungurianu)

Tuberculosis involves CNS in several ways including meningitis, cerebral abscess, tuberculoma and stroke due to vasospasm and thrombosis.

Besides typical presentations as meningitic syndrome, cases with atypical features are possible. Patients may present with a slowly progressive dementia characterized by personality changes, memory deficits and social withdrawal. Less common there is an encephalitic course manifested by seizures, stupor and coma.(94)

The diagnosis relies on CSF analysis which typically reveals low glycorahia, elevated protein and a lymphocytic pleocytosis. Although CSF culture for acid fast bacilli is the gold standard for diagnosis, it takes 6-8 weeks to obtain a result and the sensitivity is low. PCR testing of the CSF is a rapid method for the detection of M.tuberculosis but the sensitivity is only 60% [95]

Because CNS and pulmonary TB could have simultaneous onset, a chest radiograph may provide supportive evidence.

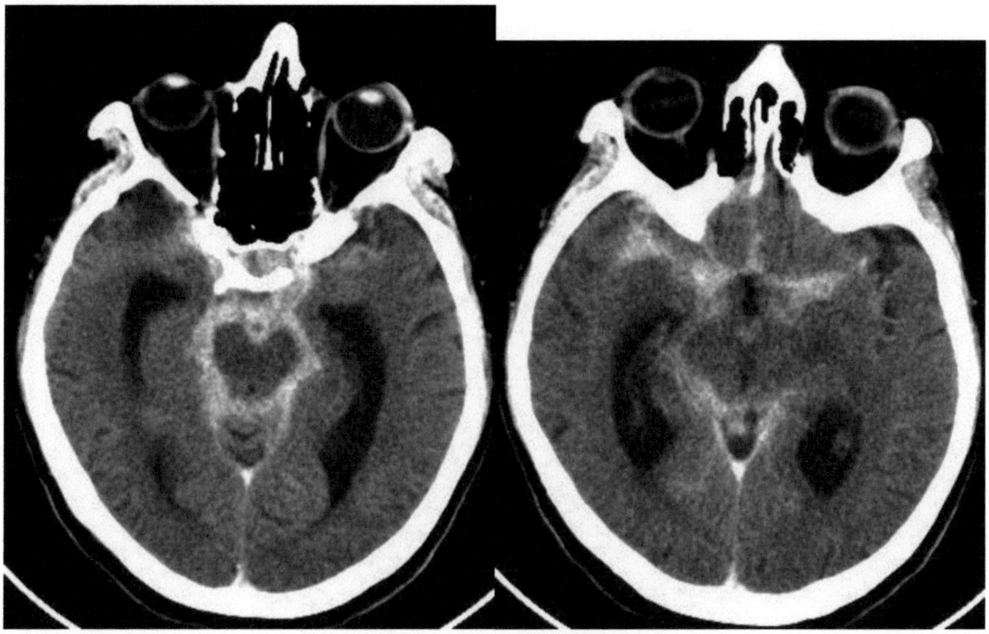

Fig. 8. Tuberculous meningo-encephalitis. CT (with contrast medium): Important enhancement in the basal cistern and meninges, in posterior and middle fossa, (cisterna magna, cisterna pontis, cisterna ambiens and suprachiasmatic cistern) with mild enlargement of the ventricles. Moderate cerebral edema - poor delineation between white matter and grey matter, with blurred appearance of cerebral sulcus (INBI Matei Bals collection, courtesy of dr V Molagic)

Neuroradiology plays an important role in diagnosis and the appearances take different forms:

- **intraparenchymal tuberculomas** appears as multiple lesions less than 1 cm that predominate at the gray-white matter interface and periventricular region; the lesions have little mass effect or edema (96).CT demonstrates the lesion poorly but shows the presence of basilar arachnoiditis, cerebral edema, infarction and the presence and course of hydrocephalus. On MRI , the aspect correlates with the evolutive phase: on T1W images the lesions are isointense to gray matter and may have a hyperintense rim; on T2W there is a hyperintensity and nodular enhancement for non-caseating granulomas. The lesions become hypointense on T2 with rim enhancement while caseation occurs. Healed tuberculomas may calcify or may progress to areas of encephalomalacia (97)

- **tuberculous abscesses** are larger in size compared to tuberculomas, presenting as solitary loculated masses with mass effect and oedema; the ring enhancement is usually thin and uniform. They appear as hypodense lesion on CT and of high T2 signal on MRI.(98)
- **tuberculous meningitis** - basilar meningitis is the most frequent form and is seen as leptomeningeal thickening and enhancement involving the basal cisterns, prepontine and ambient cisterns and suprasellar areas.(99). Hydrocephalus is a common finding and its association with basilar meningitis on CT and compatible clinical features is strongly suggestive of tuberculous meningitis.(100,101)

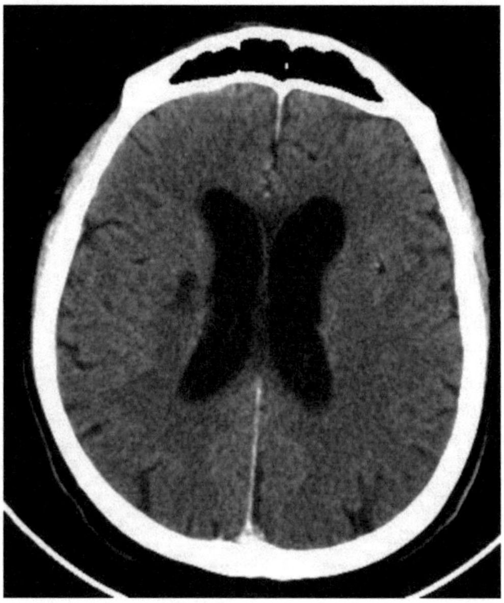

Fig. 9. Tuberculous meningo-encephalitis. CT (with contrast medium): Low-attenuating focal ischemic lesion in the fronto-parietal deep white matter in the proximity of right lateral ventricle (result from possible associated vasculitis) (INBI Matei Bals collection, courtesy of dr G Coltan)

CMV encephalitis- CMV reactivation in HIV patients emerges bellow a 50 CD4 T cells/mmc level (as opportunistic infection) and can lead to ocular manifestations (retinitis, vitritis), neurological (encephalitis), pulmonary (pneumonitis), digestive apparatus involvement (esophageal ulcers and colitis); hepato-splenomegaly, lymph nodes enlargement and fever. The diagnosis presumes a positive serology (IgG positive; rarely IgM positive).

Serial fundoscopies are indicated when a HIV patient with a poor immunological status complains about visual problems - showing a typical "cheese and ketchup" aspect of CMV retinitis. CMV viremia and blood pp65 antigen are positive. CMV PCR and pp65 antigen from CSF positive strengthen the diagnosis. Neuroimaging of CMV infection shows encephalitis (diffuse white matter impairment) and ventriculitis (ependymal enhancement).

CMV IRIS could be very harmful, with subsequent lost of sight and emphasizing of neurological signs.

Cerebral toxoplasmosis is an opportunistic parasitic infection in HIV infected patients, the most important neurological OI (opportunistic infections) in HAART era and it is due especially to a reactivation of a latent infection with Toxoplasma gondii. It appears bellow a level of 100 CD4 T cell/mmc with acute or subacute focal neurological deficits: paresis, sensory loss, aphasia; headache and a low degree of fever could be present; a chorioretinitis could accompany the neurological signs.

The serology must be positive (IgG antibodies) for proving reactivation. A negative result makes toxoplasmosis unlikely. Very rare, IgM antibodies are present and demonstrate acute illness.

The imaging exams are mandatory. MRI shows ring-enhancing mass(es) hyperintense lesions on T2W1/FLAIR, DWI; predilection for haemorrhages; decreased MR perfusion. There are solitary but typical multiple lesions.

CSF analysis may be contributory if PCR for toxoplasma is positive. A negative result never rules out the diagnostic.

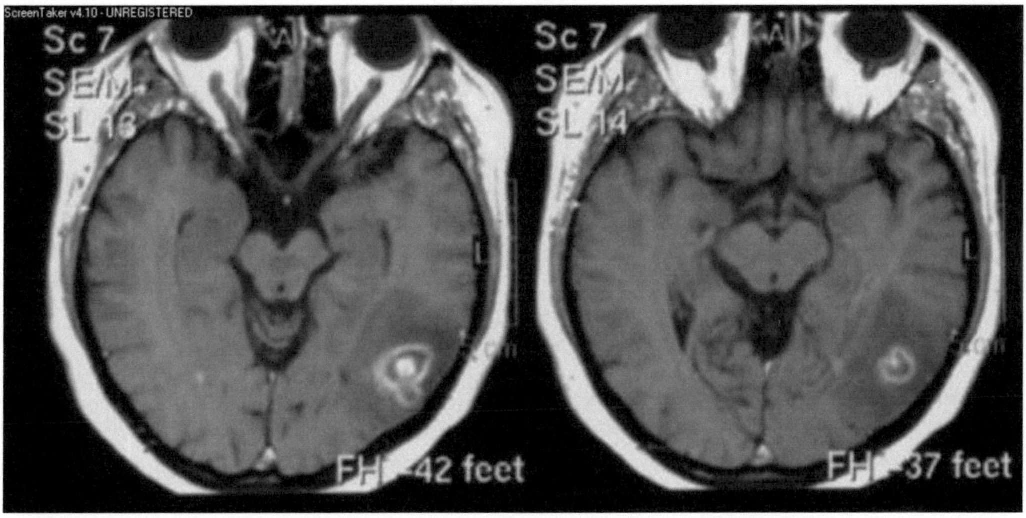

Fig. 10. Cerebral toxoplasmosis. MRI (T1-w with contrast medium) transversal sections: nodular lesion with annular peripheral enhancement (hypersignal) and surrounding edema (hyposignal); could produces mass effect (INBI Matei Bals collection)

A brain stereotactic biopsy can also be useful, especially when there is no clinical improvement in the first week of empirical antitoxoplasma treatment.

The fundoscopy is a necessary exam, especially for diagnose the association of a toxoplasmal chorioretinitis.

Toxoplasmosis IRIS is very uncommon.

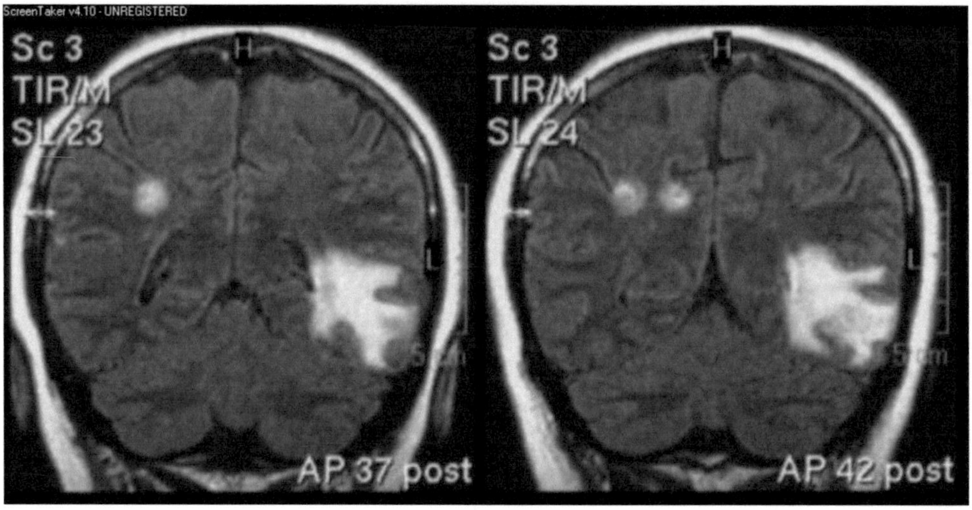

Fig. 11. Cerebral toxoplasmosis. MRI (T2-w FLAIR) coronal sections: several lesions, some nodular and one irregular with hypersignal - same patient as above (INBI Matei Bals collection)

Cryptococcosis is an opportunistic yeast infection with Cryptococcus neoformans, appearing lately during the HIV infection, below 100/mmc CD4 lymphocytes. It is an AIDS-defining illness. The CNS involvement is the most frequent manifestation (meningoencephalitis, rare cryptococcoma), but it could be accompanied by pulmonary symptoms (dry cough and chest pain) and skin lesions (moluscum-like appearance). Patients complain mainly of headaches and confusion, progressing in days, then gait impairment and cranial nerves signs due to the high CSF pressure; fever and meningeal signs could be absent. The lumbar puncture sets the diagnosis by highlighting the fungus: direct visualization by native preparation or with India ink stain, presence of Cryptococcus antigen, CSF culture positive; CSF has usually high pressure, low number of cells and mild raising in protein level. Relatively frequent the blood cultures are positive. Blood Cryptococcus antigen is positive (titer>1/8).

Imaging: The main manifestation, as a granulomatous meningitis has most often normal aspect on imaging exams, but a head CT scan or MRI are mandatory when there are even minimal neurological signs. There are some characteristic features in cryptococcal SNC infection: multiple T2 hyperintense small areas in basal ganglia, simetric nonenhancing cystic lesions - "gelatinous" pseudocysts within periventricular spaces, dilated Virchow-Robin spaces, mild ventricular dilatation with nodular meningeal enhancement; vasculitis and infarctions. Cryptococcomas are very rare and appear as isolated or multiple solid ring enhancing masses preferentially in choroid plexus.

In the course of IRIS, clinical signs are often atypical and characterized by extensive abscesses[8]

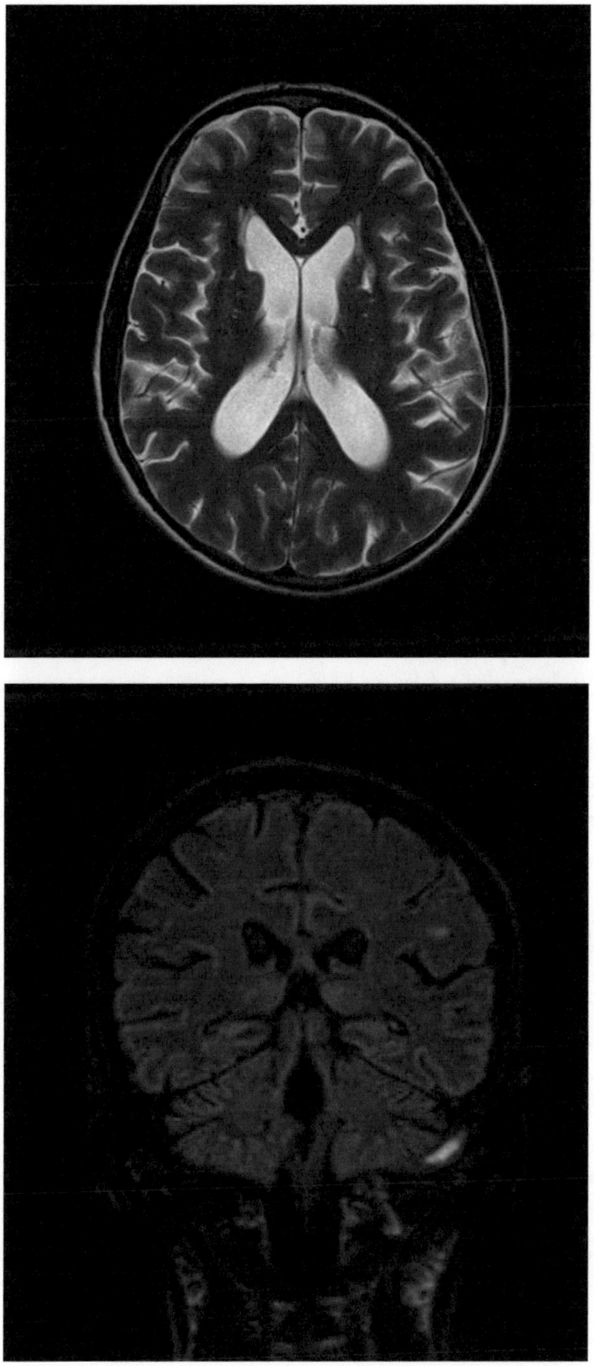

Fig. 12. Criptococcal meningitis (A) MRI (T2-w), transversal section: dilated Virchow-Robin spaces and mild ventricular dilatations; (B) MRI (T2-FLAIR), coronal section: hyperintense nodule and mild ventricular enlargement (INBI Matei Bals collection)

7.2 Neurosyphilis

Defines the infection of the CNS by Treponema pallidum (T.pallidum) Because T. pallidum and HIV have the same route of transmission and different forms of neurosyphilis could have similar clinical features with HIV encephalopathy, it is worthwiling mentioning. Neurosyphilis can be classified into early forms (asymptomatic, symptomatic meningitis, meningovascular syphilis) and late forms (general paresis and tabes dorsalis).

The early forms affect the meninges, CSF and vasculature while the late forms affect the brain and spinal cord.(102).Consequently, the clinical features for symptomatic meningitis consist in headache, nausea, vomiting and stiff neck associated with visual impairment ; for meningovascular syphilis the typical presentation is similar to an ischemic stroke with an acute or chronic onset in a young person. General paresis is a progressive dementia with deficits in memory and judgment and less often with psychiatric symptoms (depression, mania, psychosis). Tabes dorsalis is characterized by ataxia and attacks of severe pain.

There are described atypical forms of neurosyphilis, which mimic herpes encephalitis; the clinical presentation is dominated by cognitive changes with acute onset.(103)

Serologic tests are represented by non treponemal tests - Venereal Disease Research Laboratory (VDRL) and Rapid Plasma Reagin (RPR) test and treponemal test-fluorescent treponemal antibody absorption (FTA-ABS) or T.pallidum agglutination assay (TPPA). Usually, these tests are reactive in all patients with early neurosyphilis. However, non treponemal tests could be nonreactive in late forms of neurosyphilis. In this situation, if the clinical suspicion is high, a treponemal test should be done; in case of a nonreactive test, there is no indication for further evaluation. If the test is reactive, a lumbar puncture should be performed.

CSF examination is required for the diagnosis and should be done in every patient with compatible neurologic or ocular disease with known/unknown history of syphilis. CSF analysis reveals a lymphocytic pleocytosis (usually below 100 cells /microL), an elevated protein level and a reactive CSF VDRL, or a combination of these abnormalities. CSF VDRL is sensitive for the diagnosis but not specific. Therefore, in case of a negative CSF VDRL, a CSF-FTA-ABS should be performed.(104,105)

Neuroimaging shows different modifications for each stage;

- symptomatic meningitis –diffuse meningeal enhancement as well as enhancement of the CSF, cranial nerves and spinal root;-cerebral gummas appears as circumscribed masses with surrounding edema, located adjacent to the meninges and which extend into the cortex. On MRI , they are hypointense to isointense on T1W and hyperintense on T2W.
- meningovascular syphilis- single or multiple areas of infarction
- general paresis-cerebral atrophy
- atypical form (herpes encephalitis like)- on MRI the lesions have high signal on T2 and fluid attenuated-inversion recovery (FLAIR) and are unilateral or bilateral in medial temporal areas (103)

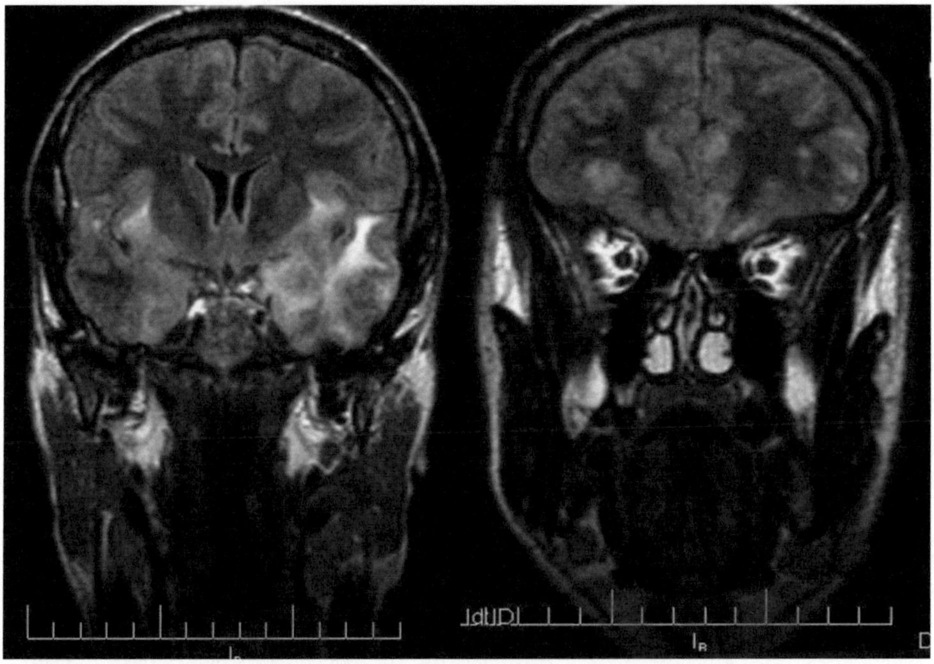

Fig. 13. Neurosyphilis. MRI (T2-w FLAIR) coronal section: bilateral diffuse hyperintensity signal in frontal and temporal areas, involving the subcortical white matter (Floreasca Emergency Clinical Hospital courtesy of dr C Predescu)

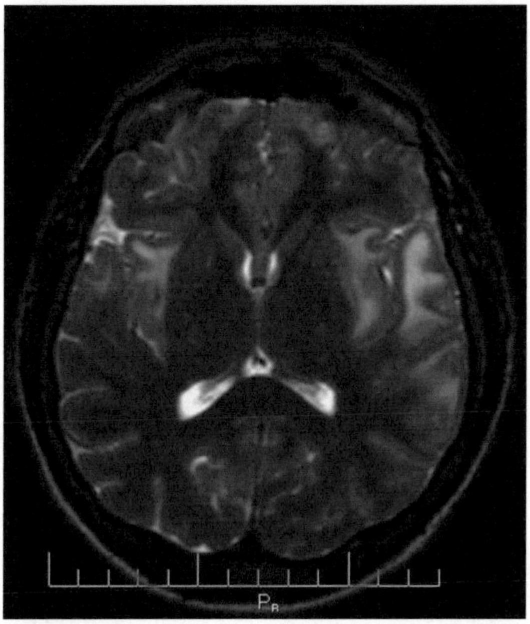

Fig. 14. Neurosyphilis MRI (T2-w) transversal section: bilateral hypointensity of the globus pallidus and putamen; disseminated temporal and insular high-signal lesions with subcortical topography (Floreasca Emergency Clinical Hospital, courtesy of dr C Predescu)

7.3 HAART neurotoxicity

There is a wide spectrum of CNS complications in patients with HIV, ranging from psychiatric syndromes to seizures and cognitive impairment. In some cases, these neuropsychiatric complications could be related with the antiretroviral drugs, especially for those which penetrate the CNS. For the clinician, it is important to distinguish between symptoms related to CNS complications of HIV infection and side effects of HAART.

The antiretrovirals most frequent associated with neuropsychiatric complications are nucleoside reverse transcriptase inhibitor (NRTI) and non nucleoside reverse transcriptase inhibitor (NNRTI).

NRTI

Zidovudine penetrate well the blood-brain barrier and therefore is a part of HAART regimens indicated for HAD. Moreover, Zidovudine has been found effective, at high doses, in slowing the progression of HAD . However, it was observed that up to 5% of patients who took Zidovudine for 1 year presented insomnia, agitation and confusion.(106)

In the past, there where some reports of psychiatric symptoms such as mania and depression, associated with Zidovudine treatment. If the treatment was discontinued, the manic symptoms disappeared.(107). In recent years, fewer psychiatric problems were reported, partly because nowadays Zidovudine is used in lower doses (600mg/day) compared to those used in pre HAART era (2000mg/day).

Other side effects reported were seizures, particularly in cases of overdose (108,109)

NNRTI

From this class of antiretrovirals, Efavirenz was the most frequent associated with CNS side effects including dizziness, headache, confusion, agitation, impaired concentration, amnesia,depersonalization, insomnia, hallucinations, abnormal or vivid dreams. These symptoms usually appear within the first month of treatment and decrease or even disappear spontaneously within 2 months.

Psychiatric adverse events associated with Efavirenz are less frequent than neurological ones, consisting in anxiety, depression and suicidal ideation.(110,111)

One of few studies investigating the neurotoxicity of Efavirenz on cognitive function showed that the treatment was associated with a higher risk of neurocognitive impairment, particularly on tasks requiring a higher attentional and executive load.(112)

Clinicians should carefully watch for changes in behavior, cognition and mood in HIV patients treated with Efavirenz and should advise their patients regarding CNS effects of therapy.

7.4 Neoplastic etiology

Primary CNS lymphoma (PCNSL) is the second most common cause of intracranial mass after toxoplasmosis. There are many possible presenting symptoms depending on the location and extent of the tumor. In general, half of the patients present with focal neurological deficits (seizures, aphasia, hemiparesis and localized weakness) and the other half present with non focal symptoms such as letharghy, headache, memory loss, altered mental status and personality changes. (113)

Neuroimaging plays a crucial role in the positive and differential diagnosis and MRI is more sensitive than CT.

MRI- typically, PCNSL lesions are solitary but in 50% of the cases multiple lesions could be seen; they are hypointense on both T1W and T2W imaging and the enhancement pattern is variable (homogeneous, heterogeneous or ring-like). PNCSL lesions can be located in the periventricular white matter, basal ganglia, corpus callosum and thalami. The most common location within the cerebral white matter is the frontal lobe followed by temporal, parietal and occipital lobes. Uncommon locations such as brain stem, cranial nerves, pineal gland and cavernous sinus are also encountered in AIDS patients. An important imaging characteristic which helps to differentiate PNCSL from toxoplasmosis is the tendency of extension toward the ependimal surface of the ventricular system.(98). PNCSL lesions often measure from 2 to 6 cm, have mass effect and are surrounded by perilesional edema.

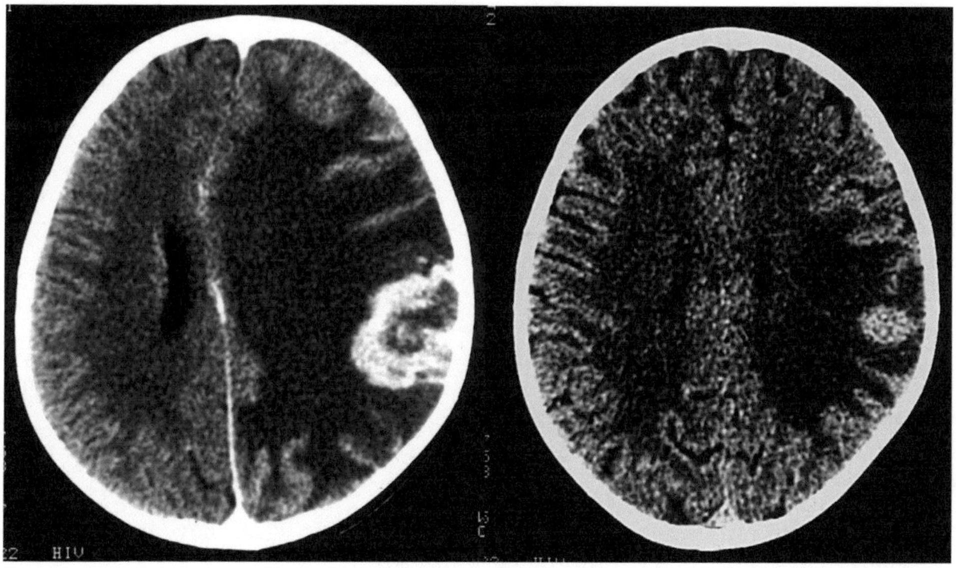

Fig. 15. Cerebral lymphoma: CT (with contrast medium), transverse section: solitary hyperintense lesion with annular enhancement and important perilesional edema with mass effect (A) at the diagnostic time and (B) after 4 months of treatment: important reduction of the lesion and remission of the mass effect (INBI Matei Bals and Fundeni Institute collections, courtesy of dr M Lazar)

Thallium 201 (201T1) SPECT (single -photon emission CT) could be an important diagnostic tool. PNCSL lesions typically show increased uptake of 201T1 on SPECT imaging, in contrast to infectious and inflammatory lesions. This differentiating pattern of uptake becomes more evident on delayed scans (at 3-4h).

PET (positron emission tomography) is useful for differential diagnosis because PNCSL lesions are more metabolically active than infectious lesions and take up F 18 fludeoxyglucose (FDG) during PET. Moreover, metabolic uptake in PNCSL lesions may not be affected by prior corticosteroid use.(114)

PCR detection of EBV DNA in CSF is limited by the risk of cerebral herniation in case of raised intracranial pressure.

7.5 Reversible encephalopathies

Complaints of cognitive impairment could be related to the coexistence of other medical conditions or substance abuse. Therefore, we should check for thyroid dysfunctions, anemia due to vitamin B12 deficiency, liver cirrhosis (portal encephalopathy), renal failure (uremia), infections (sepsis), intoxications (alcoholism, recreational drugs).

7.6 Immune reconstitution inflammatory syndrome (IRIS)

A paradoxical clinical deterioration can occur in HIV patients shortly after HAART initiation and is due to an abrupt increase in immune surveillance which leads to pathologic inflammatory reactions. IRIS can be clinically expressed as an worsening of manifestations of underlying (known) infection or an unmasking of a subclinical infection. Currently, there are no tested guidelines for the prevention or diagnosis of IRIS .Apart from clinical deterioration strictly related to HAART initiation, the diagnosis is suggested by a significant decrease in HIV RNA viral load and a rise in CD4 count.(17).

IRIS may actually worsen PML initially but a clinical improvement is possible in time. On neuroimaging there is a contrast enhancement atypical for non inflammatory PML lesions.(115,116)

8. Treatment

HAART- consists of multiple antiretroviral drugs from different classes which stop HIV replication by acting in several key points of its life cycle. Besides suppression of viral replication, HAART reduces the appearance of resistance and restores immune function, increasing the CD4 count.

ADJUVANT THERAPIES- consist of several small molecules which have been identified to possess anti-inflammatory and neuroprotective properties.

The introduction of HAART since 1996 has led to major improvements in medical morbidity and life expectancy in HIV patients. The prevalence of opportunistic infections markedly decreased and the progression to AIDS was prevented or at least delayed. There were also registered significant improvement in neurological outcomes with a marked decrease in the incidence of HAD.(117,118)

Pre-HAART era prevalence estimates were approximately 16% in AIDS cases (119), whereas more recent estimates are less than 5%.(3)

However, HAART alone cannot eradicate HAND. Moreover, studies of HAND in treated patients showed high persisting rates of mild-to-moderate neurocognitive impairment (120), suggesting that etiology of HAND could be multifactorial. Possible explanations for these observations are residual viral suppression in the CNS due to poor local penetration of some antiretroviral drugs, presence of drug-resistant viral strain and poor drug adherence. Other factors implicated are not HIV related and consist of possible neurotoxicity of antiretrovirals and coexisting illnesses such as cerebrovascular disease.(3)

Current recommendations on initiating or changing HAART are based on peripheral parameters such as CD4 count and plasma viral load and not on the status of infection in CNS.

Although the optimal treatment for HAND has not been established, several studies have shown that antiretrovirals with good CNS penetration might positively affect cognition. Better penetration in the CNS, estimated by CPE score (CNS penetration effectiveness) is associated with a lower CSF viral load. (2,120). Based upon concentrations in CSF, drug properties and the results of clinical studies, each antiretroviral is assigned with a CPE score, ranging from 1 (low penetration) to 2 -3 (intermediate) and 4 (best penetration/effectivenesss).

CPE score 1: Tenofovir, Zalcitabine, Nelfinavir, Ritonavir, Saquinavir/Ritonavir, Saquinavir, Tipranavir/Ritonavir, Enfuvirtide

CPE score 2: Didanosine, Lamivudine, Stavudine, Etravirine, Atazanavir/Ritonavir, Atazanavir, Fosamprenavir;

CPE score 3: Abacavir, Emtricitabine, Delavirdine, Efavirenz, Indinavir, Darunavir/Ritonavir, Fosamprenavir/Ritonavir, Lopinavir/Ritonavir, Maraviroc, Raltegravir

CPE score 4: Zidovudine, Nevirapine, Indinavir/Ritonavir

CPE rank is then calculated by adding up the scores for each antiretroviral drug in the regimen, according to CHARTER group score revised in 2010. (120)

In contrast, there are studies that failed to identify an association between a high CPE score and a better cognitive outcome. (112,121)

These controversial findings require further evaluation.

For the moment, EACS guidelines (version 5-4) recommend that, for patients who are not on treatment, the clinician should consider initiation an antiretroviral regimen in which at least 2 drugs penetrate CNS. Also for this category of patients, the risk for antiretroviral resistance should be considered (if prior virological failure exists).If the patient is already on treatment, changing the existing regimen with drugs which have better CNS penetration might be a solution. Whenever it is possible, genotyping of plasma and CSF HIV RNA should be done before changing the therapy.

Regarding adjuvant therapies, exploratory trials have focused on probable mechanisms of neurologic pathology. One study tested minocycline, which may have anti-inflammatory, antioxidant and antiapoptotic effects(122). Sellegiline was another tested compound due to its ability to block apoptotic cell death in chronic HIV brain infection.(123)

9. Conclusion

Despite HAART, cognitive impairment in HIV remains common. There are still unanswered questions regarding optimal timing and HAART regimen composition. Careful attention is needed to the treatment of cerebrovascular risk factors and co-morbidities.

10. References

[1] Valcour V, Sithinamsuwan P, Letendre S, Ances B: Pathogenesis of HIV in the Central Nervous System. CurrHIV/AIDS Rep. 2011;8 : 54-61

[2] Letendre S, Marquie-Beck J, Capparelli E, Best B, Clifford D, Collier A.C et al: Validation of the CNS Penetration-Effectiveness Rank for Quantifying Antiretroviral Penetration Into the Central Nervous System. Arch Neurol 2008;65: 65-70

[3] Heaton RK,Clifford DB,Franklin DR,et al. HIV-associated neurocognitive disorders persist in the era of potent antiretroviral therapy: CHARTER Study. Neurology 2010;75:2087-2096

[4] Duiculescu D, Ene L, Burlacu R, Marin C, Tardei G, Marcotte T, Ellis R, Everall I, Achim C. Neurocognitive Impairment in a Romanian Cohort of Children and Young Adults Infected with HIV-1 Clade F. 16th CROI 2009: P477

[5] Ances B: HIV-Associated Neurocognitive Disorders in the Era of Highly Active Antiretroviral Therapies http://www.medscape.com/viewarticle/581024

[6] Heaton RK, Franklin DR, Ellis RJ et al. HIV-associated neurocognitive disorders before and during the era of combination antiretroviral therapy: differences in rates, nature, and predictors. J. Neurovirol. 2011; 17(1):3–16 Epub 2010 Dec 21.

[7] Duiculescu D, Ene L, Radoi R, Ruta S, Achim CL. High prevalence and particular aspects of HIV- related neurological complications in a Romanian cohort of HIV-1 infected children and young adults .WEPDB 03 - IAS Sydney 2007

[8] Hoffmann C, Rockstroh JK. HIV 2009. Medizin Fokus Verlag, Hamburg, 2009; ISBN: 978-3-941727-02-1: 562-570

[9] Ellis R, Heaton R, S Letendre S et al. Higher CD4 Nadir is Associated with Reduced Rates of HIV-associated Neurocognitive Disorders in the CHARTER Study: Potential Implications for Early Treatment Initiation. 17th CROI 2010, Abstract 429

[10] Letendre S, McClernon D, Ellis R et al. Persistent HIV in the central nervous system during treatment is associated with worse ART penetration and cognitive impairment [abstract 484b]16th CROI 2009

[11] Letendre S, FitzSimons C, Ellis R et al. Correlates of CSF Viral Loads in 1221 Volunteers of the CHARTER Cohort. Abstract 172, 17th CROI 2010

[12] Xia C, Luo D, Yu X, Jiang S, Liu S. HIV-associated dementia in the era of highly active antiretroviral therapy (HAART). Microbes and Infection 13 (2011) 419-25

[13] Hoffmann C, Rockstroh JK. HIV 2011. Medizin Fokus Verlag, Hamburg, 2011; ISBN: 978-3-941727-08-3; 623-629

[14] Diesing TS, Swindells S, Gelbard H, Gendelman HE. HIV-1-associated dementia: a basic science and clinical perspective. AIDS Read. 2002; 12(8):358-68

[15] Osborn AG, Salzman KL, Katzman G et al. Diagnosting Imaging Brain 2004;8: 560-640. 1st ed. Salt Lake City: Amirsys; ISBN: 0-7216-2905-9

[16] Munteanu D, Arama V, Mihailescu R et al. Inflammatory markers and metabolic syndrome in HIV-positive adults undergoing highly active antiretroviral therapy 21th ECCMID& 27th ECC 2011: P 2189

[17] Venkataramana A, Pardo CA, Mc Arthur JC,et al. Immune reconstitution inflammatory syndrome in the CNS of HIV-infected patients. Neurology 2006;67:383-388

[18] Kumar AM, Borodowski L, Fernandez B, Gonzalez L, Kumar M. Human immunodeficiency virus type 1 RNA levels in different regions of human brain: quantification using real-time reverse transcriptase-polymerase chain reaction. J Neurovirol 2007;13(3):210-224

[19] American Academy of Neurology AIDS Task Force. Nomenclature and research case definitions for neurologic manifestations of Human Immunodeficiency Virus-type 1(HIV-1) infection. Neurology 1991; 41:778–785

[20] Marder K, Albert S, Dooneief G, Stern Y, Ramachandran G, Todak G, et al. Clinical confirmation of the American Academy of Neurology algorithm for HIV-1 associated cognitive/motor disorder. Neurology 1996; 47:1247–1253

[21] Sacktor N,Tarwater PM, Skolasky RL, Mc Arthur JC, Selnes OA, Becker J, Cohen B,Miller EN: CSF antiretroviral drug penetrance and the treatment of HIV associated psychomotor slowing. Neurology 2001; 57:542-544

[22] Antinori A, Arendt G, Becker JT,et al : Updated research nosology for HIV- associated neurocognitive disorders. Neurology 2007; 69 (18): 1789-1799

[23] Van Gorp WG, Satz P, Hinkin C, Evans G, Miller EN: The neuropsychological aspects of HIV-1 spectrum disease. Psychiatr Med 1989;7 (2):59-78

[24] Cummings JL: Subcortical dementia. Neuropsychology, neuropsychiatry and pathophysiology. Br J Psychiatr 1986; 149: 682-697

[25] Cummings JL, Benson DF : Subcortical dementia. Review of an emerging concept. Arch Neurol 1984 ; 41(8) :874-879

[26] Sacktor N, Bacellar H, Hoover D et al: Psychomotor slowing in HIV infection : a predictor of dementia, AIDS and death. J Neurovirol 1996; 2 (6): 404-410

[27] Dunlop O, Bjorklund R, Bruun JN et al: Early psychomotor slowing predicts the development of HIV dementia and autopsy-verified HIV encephalitis. Acta Neurol Scand 2002; 105 (4) : 270-275

[28] Hardy DJ , Castellon SA , Hinkin CH . Perceptual span deficits in adults with HIV . J Int Neuropsychol Soc 2004 ; 10 (1) : 135 –140 .

[29] Gonzalez R , Vassileva J , Bechara A , et al . The influence of executive functions, sensation seeking, and HIV serostatus on the risky sexual practices of substance-dependent individuals . J Int Neuropsychol Soc 2005 ; 11 (2) :121–131

[30] Chang L , Speck O , Miller EN , et al . Neural correlates of attention and working memory deficits in HIV patients . Neurology 2001 ; 57 (6) : 1001 –1007

[31] Paul Woods S , Morgan EE , Dawson M , Cobb Scott J , Grant I . Action (verb) fluency predicts dependence in instrumental activities of daily living in persons infected with HIV-1 . J Clin Exp Neuropsychol 2006 ; 28 (6) : 1030 –1042

[32] Cohen RA , Boland R , Paul R , et al . Neurocognitive performance enhanced by highly active antiretroviral therapy in HIV-infected women . AIDS 2001 ; 15 (3) : 341 -345
[33] Stern Y, McDermott MP, Albert S, Palumbo D, Selnes OA, McArthur J, et al. Factors associated with incident Human Immunodeficiency Virus-dementia. Arch Neurol 2001; 58:473–479
[34] Ances BM, Ellis RJ. Dementia and neurocognitive disorders due to HIV-1 infection. Semin Neurol. 2007;27:86-92
[35] Marshall DW , Brey RL , Cahill WT , Houk RW , Zajac RA , Boswell RN . Spectrum of cerebrospinal fluid findings in various stages of human immunodeficiency virus infection . Arch Neurol 1988 ; 45 (9) : 954 -958 .
[36] De Gans J, Tiessens G, Portegies P, Troost D; Predominance of polymorphonuclear leukocytes in cerebrospinal fluid of AIDS patients with cytomegalovirus related polyradiculo(myelo)pathy.International Conference on AIDS. *Int Conf AIDS.* 1989 Jun 4-9; 5: 244 (abstract no. M.B.P.134
[37] Cysique LA, Brew BJ, Halman M, et al. Undetectable cerebrospinal fluid HIV RNA and beta-2 microglobulin do not indicate inactive AIDS dementia complex in highly active antiretroviral therapy-treated patients. J Acquir Immune Defic Syndr. 2005;39:426-429.
[38] Gisslen M, Hagberg L, Brew BJ, Cinque P, Price RW, Rosengren L. Elevated cerebrospinal fluid neurofilament light protein concentrations predict the development of AIDS dementia complex. J Infect Dis. 2007;195:1774-1778.
[39] Brew BJ , Bhalla RB , Paul M , et al . Cerebrospinal fluid beta 2-microglobulin in patients with AIDS dementia complex: an expanded series including response to zidovudine treatment . AIDS 1992 ; 6 (5) : 461 -465
[40] Brew BJ , Bhalla RB , Paul M , et al . Cerebrospinal fluid neopterin in human immunodeficiency virus type 1 infection . Ann Neurol 1990 ; 28 (4) : 556 -560
[41] Abdulle S , Hagberg L , Svennerholm B , Fuchs D , Gisslen M . Continuing intrathecal immunoactivation despite two years of effective antiretroviral therapy against HIV-1 infection . AIDS 2002 ; 16 (16) : 2145 - 2149 .
[42] Abdulle S , Mellgren A , Brew BJ , et al . Cerebrospinal fluid neurofilament protein (NFL) - a marker of AIDS dementia complex . J Neurol 2006 ; 254 (8) : 1026 -1032 .
[43] Gisslen M , Rosengren L , Hagberg L , Deeks SG , Price RW . Cerebrospinal fluid signs of neuronal damage after antiretroviral treatment interruption in HIV-1 infection . AIDS Res Ther 2005 ; 18: 2-6
[44] Mellgren A, Price RW, Hagberg L, Rosengren L, Brew BJ, Gisslen M. Antiretroviral treatment reduces increased CSF neurofilament protein (NFL) in HIV-1 infection. Neurology 2007;69:1536–1541.
[45] McArthur JC , McClernon DR , Cronin MF , et al . Relationship between human immunodeficiency virus-associated dementia and viral load in cerebrospinal fluid and brain . Ann Neurol 1997 ; 42 (5) : 689 - 698 .
[46] Brew BJ, Pemberton L, Cunningham P , Law MG . Levels of human immunodeficiency virus type 1 RNA in cerebrospinal fluid correlate with AIDS dementia stage . J Infect Dis 1997 ; 175 (4) : 963 -966

[47] Ellis RJ , Hsia K , Spector SA , et al . Cerebrospinal fluid human immunodeficiency virus type 1 RNA levels are elevated in neurocognitively impaired individuals with acquired immunodeficiency syndrome. HIV Neurobehavioral Research Center Group . Ann Neurol 1997 ; 42 (5) : 679 -688

[48] Ellis RJ , Gamst AC , Capparelli E , et al . Cerebrospinal fluid HIV RNA originates from both local CNS and systemic sources . Neurology 2000 ; 54 (4) : 927 - 936

[49] Cysique LA , Maruff P , Brew BJ . Variable benefit in neuropsychological function in HIV infected HAART-treated patients . Neurology 2006 ; 66 (9) : 1447 - 1450 .

[50] Sevigny JJ , Albert SM , McDermott MP , et al . Evaluation of HIV RNA and markers of immune activation as predictors of HIV-associated dementia . Neurology 2004 ; 63 (11) : 2084 -2090

[51] Shiramizu B , Lau E , Tamamoto A , Uniatowski J , Troelstrup D . Feasibility assessment of cerebrospinal fluid from HIV-1-infected children for HIV proviral DNA and monocyte chemoattractant protein 1 alleles . J Investig Med 2006 ; 54 (8) : 468 - 472

[52] .Hawkins CP , McLaughlin JE , Kendall BE , McDonald WI . Pathological findings correlated with MRI in HIV infection . Neuroradiology1993 ; 35 (4) : 264 - 268

[53] Aylward EH , Henderer JD , McArthur JC , Brettschneider PD , Harris GJ , Barta PE , Pearlson GD . Reduced basal ganglia volume in HIV-1-associated dementia: results from quantitative neuroimaging . Neurology, 1993 43 (10) : 2099 - 2104

[54] Jernigan TL , Archibald S , Hesselink JR , Atkinson JH , Velin RA , McCutchan JA , Chandler J , Grant I . Magnetic resonance imaging morphometric analysis of cerebral volume loss in human immunodeficiency virus infection. The HNRC Group . Arch Neurol , 1993 ;50 (3) : 250 - 255

[55] Hall M , Whaley R , Robertson K , Hamby S , Wilkins J , Hall C . The correlation between neuropsychological and neuroanatomic changes over time in asymptomatic and symptomatic HIV-1-infected individuals . Neurology 1996 . 46 (6) : 1697 - 1702

[56] Raininko R , Elovaara I , Virta A , Valanne L , Haltia M , Valle SL . Radiological study of the brain at various stages of human immunodeficiency virus infection: early development of brain atrophy. Neuroradiology,1992;34(3):190-196

[57] McArthur JC , Kumar AJ , Johnson DW , Selnes OA , Becker JT , Herman C , Cohen BA , Saah. Incidental white matter hyperintensities on magnetic resonance imaging in HIV-1 infection. Multicenter AIDS Cohort Study . J Acquir Immune Defic Syndr 1990 ; (3) : 252 - 259 .

[58] Pomara N,Crandall dt, Choi SJ, Johnson G, Lim KO: White matter abnormalities in HIV-1 infection: a diffusion tensor imaging study. Psychiatry Res,2001; 106(1):15-24

[59] Archibald S, Masliah E, Fennema-Notestine C,Marcotte T, Ellis R, Mc Cutchan J, Heaton R, Grant I, Mallory M, Miller A, Jernigan T: Correlation of in vivo neuroimaging abnormalities with postmortem human immunodeficiency virus encephalitis and dendritic loss. Arch Neurol 2004;61:369-376

[60] Valcour VG, Sithinamsuwan P, Nidhinandana S, Thitivichianlert S, Ratto-Kim S, Apateerapong W, Shiramizu BT, Desouza MS, Chitpatima ST, Watt G, Chuenchitra T, Robertson KR, Paul RH, McArthur JC, Kim JH, Shikuma CM: Neuropsychological abnormalities in patients with dementia in CRF 01_AE HIV-1 infection.Neurology 2007;68(7):525-527

[61] Ernst T, Chang L, Jovicich J et al: Abnormal brain activation on functional MRI in cognitively asymptomatic HIV patients. Neurology 2002;59(9):1343-1349

[62] Chang L, Lee PL, Yiannoutsos CT, Ernst T, Marra CM, Richards T et al: A multicenter in vivo proton-MRS study of HIV-associated dementia and its relationship to age. Neuroimage 2004;23(4): 1336-1347

[63] Chang L, Ernst T, Leonido-Yee M, Walot I, Singer E : Cerebral metabolite abnormalities correlate with clinical severity of HIV-1 cognitive motor complex. Neurology 1999; 52(1):100-108

[64] Tarrasow E, Wiercinska-Drapalo A, Jaroszewicz J, Orzechowska-Bobkiewicz A, Dzienis W, Prokopowicz D, Walecki J : Antiretroviral theraphy and its influence on the stage of brain damage in patients with HIV-1H MRS evaluation. MedSciMonit 2004;10(suppl3):101-106

[65] Pfefferbaum A, Adalsteinsson E, Sullivan E : Cortical NAA deficits in HIV infection without dementia: Influence of alcoholism comorbidity. Neuropsychopharmacology 2005; 30:1392-1399

[66] Sacktor N, Skolasky R, Ernst T, Mao X, Selnes O, Pomper M, Chang L, Zhong K, Shungu D, Marder K, Shibata D, Schiffito G, Bobo L, Barker P : A multicenter study of two magnetic resonance spectroscopy techniques in individuals with HIV dementia. J of Magn Reson Imag 2005:21:325-333

[67] Taylor M, Schweinsburg B, Alhassoon O, Gongvatana A, Brown G,Young-Cassey C, Lettendre S, Grant I, Group.H. Effects of human immunodeficiency virus and methamphetamine on cerebral metabolites measured with magnetic resonance spectroscopy. J Neurovirol 2007;13(2): 150-159

[68] Ragin AB , Storey P , Cohen BA ,Epstein LG , Edelman RR . Whole brain diffusion tensor imaging in HIV-associated cognitive impairment . AJNR Am J Neuroradiol 2004 ; 25 (2) : 195 – 200

[69] Ragin AB , Wu Y , Storey P , Cohen BA , Edelman RR , Epstein LG . Diffusion tensor imaging of subcortical brain injury in patients infected with human immunodeficiency virus . J Neurovirol 2005; 11 (3) : 292 – 298

[70] Wu Y , Storey P , Cohen BA , Epstein LG , Edelman RR , Ragin AB . Diffusion alterations in corpus callosum of patients with HIV . AJNR Am J Neuroradiol 2006 ; 27 (3) : 656 –660

[71] Tate DF, Zhang S, Sampat M, Conley J, Russel T, Kertesz K, Paul RH, Coop K, Laidlaw DH, Guttmann CRC, Navia B, Tashima K, and Flanigan T (submitted). Altered fractional anisotropy and tractography metrics in the corpus callosum is associated with measures of HIV infection disease burden and cognitive performance. Submitted to Journal of Neurovirology 2009

[72] Tozzi V , Narciso P , Galgani S , Sette P , Balestra P , Gerace C , Pau FM , Pigorini F , Volpini V ,Camporiondo MP , et al . Effects of zidovudine in 30 patients with mild to end-stage AIDSdementia complex . AIDS 1993;7 (5) : 683 - 692

[73] Ernst T , Itti E , Itti L , Chang L . Changes in cerebral metabolism are detected prior to perfusion changes in early HIV-CMC: A coregistered (1)H MRS and SPECT study . J Magn Reson Imaging 2000 ;12 (6) : 859 - 865

[74] Chang L , Ernst T , Leonido-Yee M , Speck O . Perfusion MRI detects rCBF abnormalities in early stages of HIV-cognitive motor complex . Neurology 2000; 54 (2) : 389 - 396 .

[75] Hinkin CH , van Gorp WG , Mandelkern MA , Gee M , Satz P , Holston S , Marcotte TD , Evans G , Paz DH , Ropchan JR , et al . Cerebral metabolic change in patients with AIDS: report of a six-month follow-up using positron-emission tomography . J Neuropsychiatry Clin Neurosci, 1995; 7 (2) : 180 - 187

[76] Rottenberg DA , Sidtis JJ , Strother SC , Schaper KA , Anderson JR , Nelson MJ , Price RW . Abnormal cerebral glucose metabolism in HIV-1 seropositive subjects with and without dementia . J Nucl Med1996 ; 37 (7) : 1133 - 1141

[77] Rottenberg DA , Moeller JR , Strother SC , Sidtis JJ , Navia BA , Dhawan V , Ginos JZ , Price RW . The metabolic pathology of the AIDS dementia complex . Ann Neurol 1987 ; 22 (6) : 700 - 706

[78] O'Doherty MJ , Barrington SF , Campbell M , Lowe J , Bradbeer CS . PET scanning and the human immunodeficiency virus-positive patient . J Nucl Med1997 ; 38 (10) : 1575 - 1583

[79] Morgan EE , Woods SP , Scott JC , et al . Predictive validity of demographically adjusted normative standards for the HIV dementia scale . J Clin Exp Neuropsychol 2007 ; 20 : 1 - 8

[80] Valcour V, Paul R, Chiao S, Wendelken LA, Miller B. Screening for cognitive impairment in human immunodeficiency virus. *Clin Infect Dis*. Oct 2011;53(8):836-42

[81] Heaton R , Marcotte TD , Rivera Mindt M , et al . The impact of HIV-associated neuropsychological impairment on everyday functioning . J Int Neuropsychol Soc 2004 ; 10 : 317 - 31 .

[82] Cherner M , Cysique L , Heaton RK , et al . Neuropathologic confirmation of definitional criteria for human immunodeficiency virus-associated neurocognitive disorders . J Neurovirol 2007 ; 13 : 23 -28

[83] Hinkin CH , Hardy DJ , Mason KI , et al . Medication adherence in HIV-infected adults: effect of patient age, cognitive status and substance . AIDS 2004 ; 18 : S19 - S25

[84] Berger JR, Major EO: Progressive multifocal leukoencephalopathy. Semin Neurol 1999; 19:193-200

[85] Welch K, Morse A, and the Adult Spectrum of Disease Project in New Orleans: The clinical profile of end- stage AIDS in the era of highly active antiretroviral theraphy. AIDS Patient Care and STDs 2002; 16:75-81

[86] Antinori A, Ammassari A, De Luca A, Cingolani A, Murri R, Scoppettuolo G, et al. Diagnosis of AIDS-related focal brain lesions: a decision making analysis based on clinical and neuroradiologic characteristics combined with polymerase chain reaction assays in CSF. Neurology 1997;48: 687-694

[87] De Luca A, Giancola ML, Ammassari A,et al : The effect of potent antiretroviral theraphy and JC virus load in cerebrospinal fluid on clinical outcome of patients with AIDS-associated progressive multifocal leukoencephalopathy. J Infect Dis 2000;182:1077-1083
[88] Garcia de Viedma D, Diaz Infantes M, Miralles P, et al: JC virus load in progressive multifocal leucoencephalopathy: analysis of the correlation between the viral burden in cerebrospinal fluid, patient survival, and the volume of neurological lesions. Clin Infect Dis 2002; 34:1568-1575
[89] Post MJ, Yiannoutsos C, Simpson D, et al: Progressive multifocal leucoencephalopathy in AIDS: are there any MRI findings useful to patient management and predictive of patient survival ? AJNR Am J Neuroradiol 1999;20: 1896-1906
[90] Kastrup O, Maschke M, Diener HC,et al: Progressive multifocal leucoencephalopathy limited to the brain stem. Neuroradiology2002;44:227-229
[91] Dousset V, Armand JP, Lacoste D, et al: Magnetization transfer study of HIV encephalitis and progressive multifocal leucoencephalopathy. AJNR Am J Neuroradiol 1997;18:895-901
[92] Ernst T, Chang L, Witt M, et al: : Progressive multifocal leucoencephalopathy and human immunodeficiency virus-associated white matter lesions in AIDS: : magnetization transfer MR imaging. Radiology 1999;210:539-543
[93] Simone IL, Federico F, Tortorella C, et al: Localised ^{1} H-MR spectroscopy for metabolic characterization of diffuse and focal brain lesions in patients infected with HIV. JNeurol Neurosurg Psychiatry1998;64:516-523
[94] Udani PM, Dastur DK. Tuberculous encephalopathy with and without meningitis.Clinical features and pathological correlations. JNeurol Sci1970; 10: 541
[95] Bonington A, Strang JI,Klapper PE, et al. Use of Roche AMPLICOR Mycobacterium tuberculous meningitis. JClinMicrobiol 1998;36:1251
[96] Hansman ,Whiteman ML. Neuroimaging of central nervous system tuberculosis in HIV-infected patients. Neuroimaging Clin N Am1997;7:199-214
[97] Bowen BC, Post MJD. Intracranial infection.In: Atlas SW,editor.Magnetic resonance imaging of the brain and spine.New York:Raven Press,1991:501-38
[98] Sibtain NA,Chinn RJS. Imaging of the central nervous system in HIV infection. Imaging2002,14:48-59
[99] Gupta RK,Gupta S, Singh D, Sharma D,Kohli A, Gujral RB. MR imaging and angiography in tuberculous meningitis. Neuroradiology 1994;36:87-92
[100] Bhargava S, Gupta AK, Tandon PN. Tuberculous meningitis-a CT study. Br J Radiol 1982;55:189
[101] Ozates M, Kemaloglu S, Gurkan F et al. CT of the brain in tuberculous meningitis.A review of 289 patients. Acta Radiol 2000;41:13
[102] Marra CM. Update on neurosyphilis. Curr Infect Dis Rep.2009b;11:127-134
[103] Bash S, Harthout GM, Cohen S. Mesiotemporal T2-weighted hyperintensity: neurosyphilis mimicking herpes encephalitis. AJNR Am J Neuroradiol2001;22: 314

[104] Hart G.Syphilis tests in diagnostic and therapeutic decision making. Ann Intern Med 1986; 104:368
[105] Jaffe HW, Larsen SA, Peters M, et al. Tests for treponemal antibody in CSF. Arch Intern Med 1978;138:252
[106] Rachlis A, Fanning MM. Zidovudine toxicity. Clinical features and management.Drug Safety 1993,8:312-320
[107] Maxwell S, Scheftner WA, Kessler HA, Busch K. Manic syndrome associated with zidovudine treatment. JAMA 1988,259:3406-3407
[108] Hagler DN, Frame PT. Azidothymidine neurotoxicity. Lancet 1986,2;1392-1393
[109] D'Silva M, Leibowitz D, Flaherty JP. Seizure associated with zidovudine. Lancet 1995,346: 452-452
[110] Colebunders R, Verdonck K.Reply to Gonzalez and Everall: Lest we forget: neuropsychiatry and the new generation anti HIV drugs. AIDS 1999,13:869-869
[111] Moyle G . Efavirenz: practicalities,considerations and new issues. Int J Clin Pract Suppl 1999,103:30-34
[112] Ciccarelli N,Fabbiani M, Di Giambenedetto S,et al. Neurology 2011;76:1403-1409
[113] Rosenblum ML, Levy RM, Bredesen DE. Primary central nervous system lymphoma in patients with AIDS. Ann Neurol. 1988;23:S13-S16
[114] Rosenfeld SS, Hoffmann JM, Coleman RE,et al. Studies of primary central nervous system lymphoma with fluorine-18-fluorodeoxyglucose positron emission tomography. J Nucl Med.1992;3:532-536
[115] Hoffmann C,Horst HA, Albrecht H, Schlote W. Progressive multifocal leucoencephalopathy with unusual inflammatory response during antiretroviral treatment. J Neurol Neurosurg Psychiatry 2003,74:1142-1144
[116] Du Pasquier RA, Koralnik IJ. Inflammatory reaction in progressive multifocal leucoencephalopathy : harmful or beneficial? J Neurovirol 2003,9 Suppl 1:25-31
[117] Sacktor N, Lyles RH, Skolasky R, Kleeberger C, Selnes OA, Miller EN,et al. HIV-associated neurologic disease incidence changes: multicenter AIDS Cohort Study, 1990-1998. Neurology 2001;56:257-260
[118] Mc Arthur JC, HooverDR, Bacellar H, et al. Dementia in AIDS patients: incidence and risk factors. Multicenter AIDS Cohort Study. Neurology 1993,43:2245-2252
[119] Robertson KR, Smurzynski M, Parsons TD, et al. The prevalence and incidence of neurocognitive impairment in the HAART era. AIDS 2007;21:1915-1921
[120] Letendre S,Ellis R, Ances B, Mc Cutchan J. Neurologic complications of HIV disease and their treatment. Top HIV Med 2010; 18:45-55
[121] Marra CM, Zhao Y, Clifford DB, Letendre S, Evans S, Henry K,et al. Impact of combination antiretroviral therapy on cerebrospinal fluid HIV RNA and neurocognitive performance. AIDS 2009;23:1359-1366
[122] Zink MC, Uhrlaub J, De Witt J, et al. Neuroprotective and anti-human immunodeficiency virus activity of minocycline. JAMA.2005; 293:2003-2011

[123] Sacktor N, Schifitto G, Mc Dermott MP, Marder K, Mc Arthur JC, Kierbutz K. Transdermal selegiline in HIV-associated cognitive impairment: pilot, placebo-controlled study. Neurology.2000;54:233-235

3

Central Nervous System Involvement in Lyme Disease – Making the Diagnosis and Choosing the Correct Treatment

Ruxandra Calin[1,2], Adriana Hristea[1,2] and Radu Tanasescu[2,3]
[1]*Professor Dr. Matei Bals National Institute of Infectious Diseases, Bucharest,*
[2]*Carol Davila University of Medicine and Pharmacy Bucharest,*
[3]*Department of Neurology, Colentina Hospital, Bucharest,*
Romania

1. Introduction

Lyme disease is a tick-borne systemic illness caused by three pathogenic species of the spirochete *Borrelia burgdorferi sensu lato* (*B. burgdorferi sensu stricto, B. afzelii* and *B. garinii*). They are flagellated bacteria close to *Treponema pallidum*, the ethiologic agent of syphilis. All three pathogenic species occur in Europe, *Ixodes ricinus* being the tick responsible for their transmission in this area. Two of the Borrelia species (*B. afzelii* and *B. garinii*) have been identified in Asia. *B. burgdorferi* is the sole cause of the disease in the United States. Although in United States the proportion of neuroborreliosis among Lyme disease manifestations is of about 8%, in Europe the incidence of this form of disease is more elevated 16-46% (1).

Lyme disease has a broad spectrum of clinical manifestations, and variable degrees of severity due, in part, to differences in the infecting species. In France, for example, neurologic manifestations of Lyme disease are frequent due to the endemic presence of *B. garinii* (2). Historically, the first case of neuroborreliosis in medical literature was described in 1922 in Lyon: meningoradiculitis, preceded by a tick bite and migratory erithema, in a patient who presented a false positive syphilis serology. Meningoraticulitis remains even today the most frequent form of neurolyme, even though the known spectrum of disease can be very broad, varying from mild impairment to severe, cognitive or even psychiatric manifestations. Phenomenology-based assertions that "Lyme disease can do anything" in the nervous system or that Lyme disease is the new "grand imitator", make difficult the task of differentiating between true nervous system disorders and the effects of extra-neurologic disease on behavior and cognitive function.

In this section the neurologic manifestations of Lyme disease, with special emphasis on Lyme meningitis, encephalomyelitis will be reviewed. The definition of a controversial entity - Lyme encephalopathy - will be discussed. Much of the confusion and controversy surrounding Lyme disease relates to misunderstandings about what does and does not constitute evidence of nervous system infection. Emphasis on several nonspecific symptoms in early studies (3,4) led to sometimes erroneous conclusions regarding symptoms specific for Lyme disease. This misunderstanding was one of the elements that contributed to debatable attitudes regarding which individuals required treatment for Lyme disease, what constituted effective treatment, and how to define cure (5).

In order to have an accurate understanding of nervous system Lyme disease the true scope of nervous system disorders attributable to Lyme disease and their corresponding pathophysiologic mechanisms, need to be better defined.

2. Epidemiological background

Epidemiological context is essential to establishing the diagnosis of Lyme disease. Even so, it is not always easily highlighted.

Following the infestation of a tick during a meal on an infected mammal, Borrelia will develop inside the acarian and will accidentally be transmitted to a human host. Transmission will mostly occur in a humid environment (forest, field, even garden). The risk of transmission is proportional to the duration of tick attachment: at least 12 hours are necessary in order for the Borrelia to reach the salivary glands of the tick. The bite of Ixodes ricinus is painless and the larva tick measures up to 1 mm. Consequently tick bites are discovered in only 26-38% patients (6,7).

Few studies have looked into the different clinical patterns seen with different Borrelia species. Strle et al has shown in a study of 33 european patients in which Borrelia could be isolated in culture, that B. garinii was mostly associated with meningitis symptoms (61% for B. garinii versus 10% for B. afzelii, p=0,009) and painful radicular symptoms (65% versus 0%, p<0.001), while neurocognitiv impairment seemed more frequent in patients infected with B. afzelii, even though statistical significance was not proven (8).

There are two age incidence peaks: in childhood and between 50-60 years of age. Males are 1,5 times more often infected than females. The first manifestations of the diseases develop most often in spring-autumn, especially in June - November (6,7).

The early, localized phase, occurring a few days to one month after the tick bite consists in migratory erythema. The diameter of the lesion can range from a few millimeters to tens of centimeters. It is mostly annular, but can be polymorphe and can be easily mistaken for the local inflammatory reaction at the site of the bite or can remain unperceived (9). Consequently migratory erythema is noted in less than half of the patients (18-46%) (9). Associated symptoms and signs during this early, localized, stage may include: fatigue, malaise, lethargy, mild headache, mild neck stiffness, myalgias, arthralgias and/or regional lymphadenopathy.

3. Clinical spectrum of neuroborreliosis

Neuroborreliosis is found either in the context of an early disseminated disease or during late, chronic Lyme disease. The clinical features of nervous system Lyme disease, although proteiform?, have certain characteristics. Clinical features of Lyme disease may be a result of direct bacterial infection (particularly in the early stages of disease) or a consequence of the immune response leading to symptoms in different organs.

Just as in neurosyphilis, nervous system involvement begins during early disseminated Lyme disease, when spread of the spirochetes can result in meningeal seeding (10). As in syphilis, untreated Borrelia infection probably subsides in some patients but becomes chronic in others. Also as in syphilis, appropriate antimicrobial treatment results in microbiologic cure in the overwhelming majority of patients, regardless of the duration of the infection.

Neurologic features of **early disseminated Lyme**, developing at weeks to months after tick bite disease may include:

- Lymphocytic meningitis
- Unilateral or bilateral cranial nerve palsies (especially of the facial nerve)
- Radiculopathy
- Peripheral neuropathy
- Mononeuropathy multiplex
- Cerebellar ataxia (rarely)
- Encephalomyelitis (rarely)

They can occur in the absence of any prior features of Lyme disease. The classic triad of acute neurologic abnormalities is meningitis, cranial neuropathy, and motor or sensory radiculoneuropathy, although each of these findings may occur alone (5).

Although the facial nerve is the most commonly affected cranial nerve, other nerves such as the abducens nerve may be involved. Lyme disease is one of the few causes of bilateral cranial nerve palsies. Other causes include tuberculosis, sarcoidosis, and trauma.

The neurologic manifestations of **late Lyme disease** are different from those in early disseminated disease. They occur month to years after tick bite and in the absence of any prior features of Lyme disease and only about 25 percent of patients with erythema migrans recall the tick bite that transmitted Lyme disease (6, 7). In the United States, a mild neurologic syndrome, called Lyme encephalopathy, has been reported, manifested primarily by subtle cognitive disturbances (11,12). In the United States and Europe, a chronic axonal polyneuropathy may develop, manifested primarily as spinal radicular pain or distal paresthesias (7,11,12). In Europe, B. garinii may rarely cause chronic encephalomyelitis, characterized by spastic paraparesis, cranial neuropathy, or cognitive impairment with marked intrathecal antibody production to the spirochete (7).

It is unknown whether the time course of these syndromes is related to differences in spirochetal strain, inoculum size, or host response. However, the syndromes associated with abrupt onset typically occur early in infection (within the first few months), whereas those that are more indolent and protracted often present later in the course (eg, many months after initial infection) (5). Consideration of the clinical findings of nervous system Lyme disease is divided into disorders of the peripheral versus central nervous systems. In both, the predominant mechanism appears to be multifocal inflammatory involvement of the affected structure, be it patchy peripheral nerve involvement or, rarely, patchy inflammation of the central nervous system.

Regardless of the clinical syndrome, a frequently found accompanying feature of disseminated disease is radicular pain, reported in 38% to up to 86% of patients with neuroborreliosis (6,7,9). Headache is also found in 18-43%, neck stiffness is almost exlusively found in children, while arthralgias are described in only 1-18% of patients and myalgias are rarely found, in up to 13% patients with neuroborreliosis (6,7). Fever is noted in 10% of patients. Other very rare manifestations are: myocarditis with atriventricular block (1%), atrophic acrodermatitis (dermatologic features of chronic diseases, found in less than 1% of patients with neuroborreliosis, in large cohorts) and chorioretinitis (6,7,9).

4. Acute meningoradiculitis and meningitis

The two largest European studies published to date, on a total of 187 patients (Hansen et al, Danmark) and 330 patients (Oschmann et al, Germany), reported meningoradiculitis as the predominant form of neuroborreliosis (with an incidence of 67% and 85% respectively) (6,7). The delay between the tick bite and the neurologic syndrome is, in average, 3 weeks, but can extend to more than three months (6). The typical, but non compulsory, sequence is: migratory erythema at 3 days after the bite, sensitive radiculitis 3 weeks after, than paresis in the two following weeks, with or without the apparition of new radicular impairment (6). In the European literature, involvement is said to parallel the site of the tick bite (14); this has not been addressed systematically in the United States. Pain is often a prominent element, the hallmark of the syndrome. It can be described as severe, "burn", "tear" or painful paresthesias, more accentuated at night and preventing sleep (9). Pain is not always confined to strict radicular topography, is accompanied by hypo/disesthesia, local or diffuse and is not easily alleviated by usual painkillers, including opiods (9). Only antibiotic treatment by ceftriaxone can lead to a resolution of the symptoms. This disorder can mimic a mechanical radiculopathy (eg, sciatica) with radicular pain in one or several dermatomes, accompanied by corresponding sensory, motor and reflex changes, but the presence of such deficits is not constant, even in the presence of subjective complaints. Lyme disease should be considered in patients in endemic areas presenting in spring through autumn with severe limb or truncal radicular pain without an apparent mechanical precipitant (5). In European neuroborreliosis, the term Garin-Bujadoux-Bannwarth syndrome (or Bannwarth syndrome) has been applied to the constellation of painful radiculoneuritis, often accompanied by meningitis with minimal headache and sometimes with cranial neuropathy (15).

In more than 50% of cases meningoradiculitis are accompanied by cranial nerves involvement (7). The spectrum of Lyme cranial neuropathies will not be detailes here, but facial nerve involvement represents about 80-90 percent of all Lyme disease-associated cranial neuropathies (6). Since facial nerve palsy is uncommon in children, Lyme disease should be strongly considered as the cause of facial nerve palsy affecting a child who has been in an endemic area. In adults in endemic areas, during spring through fall, a significant percentage of facial nerve palsies are attributable to Lyme disease. In one study in an endemic region, one quarter of cases of facial nerve palsy in the summer were likely due to Lyme disease, based upon serologies (16). Involvement can be bilateral, with onset being either simultaneous or in rapid succession. Because bilateral facial nerve palsies are generally uncommon, such cases should bring Lyme disease to mind in patients with potential recent exposure. The differential diagnosis of bilateral facial nerve palsies is limited and includes sarcoidosis, Guillain-Barré syndrome, HIV infection and other basilar meningitides (5).

Cerebrospinal fluid analysis is essential to the diagnosis of meningoradiculitis, but the findings are non specific. Most often there is increased cellularity, with lymphocytic predominance, similar to viral meningitis. Hyperproteinorahia (frequently around 1g/l, but can be normal or as elevated as 5g/l) and IgG oligoclonal bands can be found in 70% of cases (7). When accompanied by peripheric involvement, axonal damage can by proven by EMG. MRI can show enhancement of spinal or cranial nerve roots. Usually though the clinical picture and the lumbar puncture are sufficient for guiding the diagnosis (9).

The clinical spectrum can include several atypical forms as: ataxic sensitive neuropathy with meningitis, multiple neuropathy with meningitis or motor polyradiculoneuritis with meningitis (9).

Isolated meningitis represents only 4-5% of neuroborreliosis and is more frequently found in children (6,7). In this setting, headache is rarely severe and the meningitic syndrome, if present, is never as serious as in purulent meningitis. Fever is reported in 4-10% of patients with isolated meningitis and migratory erythema in only 17% of cases (7).

Due to their quiet clinical appearance, these acute meningitis forms can remain undiagnosed and progress to chronic infection. The term "chronic" is used when the duration of symptoms extends beyond 6 months, in which case other organic symptoms, such as weight loss, can be present (7,9).

CSF study in isolated meningitis has the same features as in meningoradiculitis. Pleiocytosis is around 200/mm3 and the presence of oligoclonal bands is less frequent (around only 22% of cases) (7). Hypoglycorahia can be an important finding, raising the need for a differential diagnosis with tuberculosis. In this context of nonspecific findings, the essential diagnostic tool is the intrathecal anti-Borrelia antibody index (17), which will be described later in this section.

Interestingly, certain tick species are able to transmit both tick-borne encephalitis (TBE) and Lyme borreliosis. Therefore, it is possible that a patient can simultaneously be infected with the TBE-virus and Borrelia burgdorferi-spirochete as a result of a single tick bite. Although this is a rare event, its possibility has to be taken into account, since only neuroborreliosis beneficiates from a specific treatment

Benign intracranial hypertension – A pseudotumor cerebri-like picture (benign intracranial hypertension) occurs with increased frequency in children with Lyme disease (18,19). Virtually all of the reported cases have had inflammatory cerebrospinal fluid, suggesting that the increased intracranial pressure is a result of meningitis, in contradistinction to the usual picture of pseudotumor with a normal cerebrospinal fluid profile. Regardless of the mechanism, the symptoms and potential consequences are identical, including compression of cranial nerves with a particular threat to the optic nerves and vision (5).

5. Acute myelitis

In the two large European cohort studies mentioned above acute myelitis are reported in 4-5% of cases (6,7). They are associated in 35% of cases with a cranial radiculopathy and in 59% of cases with spinal neuropathy. Fever is present in 6% of cases. The medullar syndrome includes: paraparesis (75% of cases), proprioceptive ataxia (35% of cases), urinary dysfunction (20% of cases) (7). Although reported in a majority of cases, CSF pleyocytosis is not a constant finding. There are only 12 published cases describing a medullar MRI (20). By the time this localization is proven, it usually involves more than three metamers. The localization is most often cervical, high thoracic or cervico-thoracic, but the exact pattern can be variable (most cited: transverse myelitis and predominantly posterior myelitis) (20). Sometimes, when myelitis is not proven on MRI, leptomeningeal enhancement, coupled with clinical data, will orient towards the diagnosis.

6. Acute encephalitis

Acute encephalitis and meningoencephalitis represents only 0,5-8% of neurolyme in Europe (6,7). Headache is present in two thirds of cases. In 40-50% of patients radicular pain, cranial neuropathies (mostly VI and VII), as well as fever, are part of the clinical picture (7). On the other hand, in 57 % of cases encephalitis presents as acute neuropsychiatric disease: cognitive of memory impairment, disorientation, depression or sleep disorder. In 21% of cases cerebral ataxia has been described. An asymmetric extrapyramidal syndrome is present in 21% of patients and hemiparesis in 7% of cases (7). The consciousness level is rarely and only mildly impaired.

CSF analysis shows lymphocytic pleyocytosis than can be modest, of only a few cells. Proteinorahia is less often elevated and can be normal. The presence of IgG oligoclonal bands in CSF is proven in up to 55% of cases (7).

Noteworthy, the electroencephalogram (EEG) is abnormal in all patients: a moderate slowing with generalized slow waves with or without spikes is most often found. In 14% of patients slow theta-delta waves can be found (7). Seizures are present in up to 4% of patients. The cerebral CT is normal in most cases, as is the MRI. Hypersignal T2 temporal or brainstem lesions have been described (7).

7. Acute optic neuropathy

This is an extremely rare manifestation of Lyme disease, which can be circumscribed to the spectrum of neuroborreliosis. In a study of 440 patients with optic neuropathy, Sibony et al found the presence of Lyme disease in only 2 patients (21). There are only 2 other cases of isolated Lyme optic neuropathy described in literature. Nine other cases of associations between optic neuropathy and other neurologic features of Lyme disease have been reported. In the majority of these cases a positive intratechal anti-Borrelia antibody index was found, accompanied in less than half of the cases by CSF pleyocytosis. The antibiotic treatment led to the amelioration of visual symptoms, even when a delay of a few months existed between the clinical onset and the initiation of treatment (22,23). Lyme disease as a cause of optic neuropathy may be underdiagnosed.

8. Cerebrovascular disease

Presenting as both acute and chronic manifestations, cerebrovascular disease is rare, around 1% of neurolyme cases (7). Ischemic disease, transitory or not, seems to be more frequent, preceded by symptoms of progressive encephalopathy with headache, cognitive impairment and behavioral changes or cranial neuropathy (7). In a recently described case of ischemic neuroborreliosis the patient complained for two years of acustic impairment, for which no etiology was found (24). Ischemic lesions seem to be more frequently localized in the basal ganglia, the vertebrobassilar system or the subcortical regions. Diffuse or local stenosis can be proven on angio MRI (7,24). In this context CSF study will show a lymphocytic pleyocytosis with hyperproteinorahia and oligoclonal bands.

Hemorrhagic vascular lesions have been described in only a few case-reports: 4 cases of subarachnoid hemorrhage, 3 cerebral and 1 medullary, 2 cases of intracerebral hematomas and one atypical case associating myelitis and meningeal hemorrhage (20). One pathology study showed an important lymphocytic perivascular infiltrate, rich in T lymphocytes, which could provide a possible explanation for a presumptive vascular damage leading to ischemic or hemorrhagic consequences (25).

9. Chronic encephalomyelitis

The chronic forms of neuroborreliosis are rare and are preceded by acute unrecognized and untreated Lyme diseases. They represent 4-6% of neurolyme cases in Europe (6,7). The clinical spectrum can range from a progressive myelopathy to an encephalitic form manifested by seizures, focal deficit or cerebellar syndrome (9). Without treatment, there is no remission in the majority of cases. Medullar syndromes are most frequent (74-100%), associated with proprioceptive ataxia (63-100%), urinary dysfunction (37-62%) and/or para/tetraparesis (63-100%) (6). The chronic encephalitic form is rarer: cerebellar syndrome (26%), cognitive impairment/psychiatric symptoms (16%), hemiparesis (11%) (6).

Like the other nervous system forms of Lyme, this chronic encephalomyelitis is frequently accompanied by cranial neuropathy (32-75%): II, VI, VII, VIII usually implicated. Unlike acute encephalitis, chronic encephalomyelitis can involve the optic nerve (6,9). Also, neurosensorial hearing loss is described in 6 patients with chronic Lyme disease in the study of Hansen et al.

CSF analysis shows constantly a hyperproteinorahia (in average of 3,5g/l, but potentially as elevated as 10g/l), associated with lymphocytic pleiocytosis (7). In 70% of cases cerebral MRI is abnormal, showing subcortical or brainstem inflammatory lesions. Meningeal enhancement can also be found, sometimes as the sole finding. Rarely, lesions can be mistaken for multiple sclerosis (1).

10. Lyme encephalopathy – A controversial entity

The notion of Lyme encephalopathy is mostly exclusively found in American medical literature. The term was labeled in early studies that found that many patients with Lyme disease described fatigue, cognitive slowing, and memory difficulty (3). However, these symptoms are nonspecific and are frequent concomitants of many inflammatory disorders. They are not, in isolation, diagnostic of either Lyme disease or brain infection. In fact, the term "encephalopathy" was used to describe this state, since this term is most often used to indicate alterations in brain function due to non-neurologic causes. Subsequent work demonstrated that only in rare instances were these symptoms associated with brain infection (ie, encephalitis). In such cases, the diagnosis was readily confirmed by cerebrospinal fluid abnormalities and brain MRI findings (3,12,26). According to experts, in the absence of such objective evidence of brain infection, these symptoms should **not** be considered evidence of nervous system infection with B. burgdorferi.

Clinically, most often cited are: memory impairment (anterograde or retrograde), attention deficit, sleeping disorders (30%) and profound asthenia (70%) (27). Depression and/or irritability can be associated. Half of patients complain of headache. The neurologic exam in usually normal or signs of chronic axonal polyneuropathy can sometimes be found. Recently five case of dementia, with important impairment of mnesic and executive functions, have been reported in which a positive intratechal anti-Borrelia antibody index was found, in the absence of any other etiologic explanation (9).

In those instances where nervous system infection can be demonstrated, standard antimicrobial therapy is effective. Multiple studies have shown that prolonged antimicrobial treatment offers such patients no lasting benefit but carries significant risk (28,29,30).

Post Lyme disease syndrome versus chronic Lyme disease — A particular challenge has been the sizable population of individuals labeled as having "chronic Lyme disease" on the basis of nonspecific symptoms including persistent musculoskeletal pain, cognitive problems, and fatigue (31). In a minority of patients, these symptoms have followed microbiologically successful treatment of Lyme disease, a condition termed "post Lyme disease syndrome". However, all objective evidence indicates that these individuals, while suffering from debilitating symptoms, do not have chronic infection with B. burgdorferi and that antibiotic treatment is **not** beneficial (30). In its typical usage, “chronic Lyme disease” includes the post-Lyme disease syndrome, as well as illnesses and symptom complexes for which there is no convincing scientific evidence of any relationship to B. burgdorferi infection (5) and that are common enough in general population. The relationship between neuroborreliosis and cognitive impairment still remains to be proven and analyzed in prospective studies.

11. Approach to diagnostic confirmation

The diagnosis of central nervous system Lyme disease rests on three elements:

- Possible exposure to Ixodes ticks, the only species capable of disease transmission
- Objective evidence of central nervous system Lyme disease
- Laboratory testing (positive Lyme serologies with positive cerebrospinal fluid [CSF] Lyme antibodies) which supports the diagnosis

A positive blood Lyme serology does not always imply that the patient has an active Lyme disease. This serology shows that the patient has been in contact, at some time point, with the *B. burgdorferi sensu lato* (9). It does not mean that the microorganism has developed any pathogenic effect. In the general, healthy population the prevalence of positive Borrelia serology ranges between 3,3%-6%, depending of the study. In this context positive blood Lyme serology allows only an orientation for the diagnosis (32).

Moreover the different laboratory techniques, with different reference values and variable intra-patient, inter-kit and inter-laboratory reproducibility, can sometimes be misleading.

In order to prevent these serologic diagnostic pitfalls, the US Centers for Disease Control and Prevention, recommends the "two-tier strategy", which is uses a sensitive enzyme-linked immunosorbent assay (ELISA) followed by a Western blot (5). An immunofluorescent assay (IFA) may be substituted for the ELISA. If the ELISA is positive or equivocal, then the same serum sample should be tested by Western blot (IgM and IgG immunoblots if early disease is suspected; IgG Western blot alone if late disease is suspected). If the ELISA is negative, the sample needs no further testing.

With the exception of the first four to six weeks of infection, when the specific immune response may not yet have developed sufficiently to provide a measurable antibody response, serologic testing using the two-tier approach for antibodies to B. burgdorferi is highly sensitive and specific for the detection of antibodies.

In patients with suspected central nervous system Lyme disease (ie, Lyme meningitis or encephalomyelitis), testing the CSF for **intrathecal production of antibodies to B. burgdorferi** is useful for establishing the diagnosis. This test is not applicable if involvement is limited to the peripheral nervous system. Even in central nervous system disease, the sensitivity remains unclear. A negative test for Lyme antibodies in the CSF does not exclude central nervous system Lyme disease. Rare cases with negative blood tests and positive CSF have been described, this possibly being due to very recent exposure (33). However such cases should be interpreted with caution.

As in other infections, in nervous system Lyme disease, specific B cells may migrate to the central nervous system and proliferate locally, resulting in intrathecal production of antibodies to B. burgdorferi. However, even in the absence of nervous system Lyme disease, a substantial proportion of B. burgdorferi-specific antibodies diffuse from the serum to the CSF. Therefore, the presence of B. burgdorferi-specific antibodies in CSF does not itself establish the presence of central nervous system Lyme disease or prove that there is local production of antibodies (5).

CSF B. burgdorferi antibody measurement is highly specific for nervous system Lyme disease, with cross-reactions occurring primarily in neurosyphilis (5). However, neurosyphilis usually results in production of reaginic antibodies in the CSF, such as those measured in the venereal disease research laboratory (VDRL) test, which is not the case for Lyme disease. Thus, differentiating between these two spirochetal infections is generally easy.

Determination of test sensitivity is far more challenging, primarily because the studies that have addressed this issue have used quite different patient populations (17,34,35). In Europe, sensitivity for detecting anti-Borrelia antibodies in CSF is reportedly over 90 percent (33). Similarly, in some studies of Lyme meningitis from the United States, sensitivity was approximately 90 percent (36). However, in a more heterogeneous population of patients from the US, sensitivity was lower (34). In a patient with a clinical picture suggesting Lyme disease, a positive study from a reputable laboratory should be viewed as significant evidence in favor of the diagnosis (36). However, negative CSF studies should not eliminate neurologic Lyme disease from consideration if clinical circumstances support the diagnosis.

The existing consensus is that the most appropriate test that allows with a specificity of more than 95% to attribute a neurologic syndrome to Lyme disease is the **intrathecal anti-**

Borrelia antibody index. This index has a sensitivity of 75%, which is superior to culture and PCR. It implies that a blood and CSF sample be collected at the same time (17). A reference laboratory must indicate if the index is positive (in favor of neuroborreliosis), negative or intermediary. An European consensus exist for the utilization of this index in terms of specificity and sensitivity, in order to prevent inter-laboratory variables (17,33,37).

In clinical practice, the first exam to be performed is Lyme blood serology. If positive or if negative in the presence of a highly evocative neurologic syndrome, lumbar puncture should be performed in order to determinate Lyme CSF serology and the intrathecal anti-Borrelia antibody index (17). In children, in the presence of facial paralysis with positive blood Lyme serology, lumbar puncture is not necessary (9). The usefulness of the intrathecal anti-Borrelia index in uniquely peripheral forms of Lyme disease, has not yet been established.

Although CSF or serum B. burgdorferi antibody concentrations typically decline after treatment, these antibodies may persist for 10 or more years following successful treatment (38,39,40). Thus, determination of active neuroborreliosis requires combining these results with less specific measures of active central nervous system inflammation (ie, a CSF pleocytosis and/or elevated protein).

As in other infections in which there is a prominent antibody response, when nervous system Lyme disease has been present long enough for the B cell response to mature, there are often increases not only in specific anti-B. burgdorferi antibodies but also in nonspecific immunoglobulin concentrations. Consequently IgG synthesis rate or IgG index can be elevated, and, particularly in patients in Europe with central nervous system Lyme disease, oligoclonal bands can be seen in the CSF (40). The frequency with which these findings are found has varied widely among series. The important point is that oligoclonal bands and increased IgG synthesis occur in infections including central nervous system Lyme disease, and do not support a differential diagnosis with multiple sclerosis.

Other diagnostic tests have been proposed, but are seldom used.

Polymerase chain reaction — The polymerase chain reaction (PCR) for B. burgdorferi can be performed on CSF, although it has low sensitivity (41) probably reflecting the very low number of organisms typically present in spinal fluid. Between this low sensitivity, and a tendency for some laboratories to have difficulty avoiding false positives, the positive and negative predictive values both tend to be low, rendering this test of marginal utility. For that reason, PCR is not recommended for routine testing of CSF in Lyme disease

CXCL13 — Although elevated concentrations of CXCL13, the chemokine B lymphocyte chemoattractant, are not unique to active nervous system Lyme disease, when combined with other diagnostic information, they might serve as a marker of disease activity or response to treatment (42). Like patients with neurosyphilis (43), patients with acute untreated nervous system Lyme disease and a CSF pleocytosis have elevated CSF concentrations of CXCL13 (44). Among 17 such patients, concentrations of CXCL13 were proportionately greater in CSF than in serum and were highly elevated in all CSF samples compared with the CSF of 178 controls without nervous system Lyme disease (mean 15,149 pg/mL versus 247 pg/mL) (44). Five patients who had received at least two weeks of treatment for nervous system Lyme disease did not have substantially elevated CXCL13 concentrations (mean 202 pg/mL), whereas five patients who had been treated for less than two weeks had slightly elevated CXCL13 concentrations (mean 1412 pg/mL). Among the 178 controls, seven had an elevated CXCL13 concentration, five with CNS lymphoma and two with bacterial meningitis. Relapsing-remitting multiple sclerosis has also been reported to cause elevated levels of CXCL13 in the CSF (45).

These observations, coupled with polymerase chain reaction-based findings in patients with early nervous system Lyme disease (10), and the frequent description of increased immunoglobulin production including the presence of oligoclonal bands in CSF of neuroborreliosis patients, suggest that the spirochetes invade the central nervous system very early in infection and elicit a vigorous innate immunity-triggered B cell response, leading to prolonged antibody production.

12. Treatment, evolution an reinfection

Three antibiotic regimens have shown their efficacy in neuroborreliosis. In Europe Ceftriaxone iv 2g/day for 21-28 days remains of first intention. The Infectious Diseases Society of America and the American Academy of Neurology recommend a treatment duration of only 14 days, due to the lack of supporting evidence that a one month treatment is superior to a shorter, two weeks, regimen. In Europe, other options include Peniciline G 18-24 MUI/day and Doxycycline 200 mg/day for an equal 21-28 days. Peniciline G is not recommended by the American Guidelines for neurologic Lyme disease. Resolution of symptoms under treatment can be rapid (within the first 48h) or delayed, after the first two weeks of antibiotic therapy. 90% of acute forms improve under treatment versus 40-50% of chronic forms (6). Facial paralysis or myelitis can persist as residual neurologic impairment after the end of treatment (9). As noted above, follow-up be serologic testing is of no use, as antibodies can still be detected after cure, even though they do not provide any kind of protection for reinfection.

One single study proved the efficacy of a single dose flash therapy of 200mg of Doxycycline in the 72h that follow a tick bite in endemic areas (46). Taking into account the scare data available, the potential for adverse effects and cross resistance, the Lyme consensus conference of 2006 recommends the use of this strategy only in endemic areas and only if the infecting tick has remained attached for more than 48 hours (47).

13. References

[1] Blanc F; Gebly. Neurologic and psychiatric manifestations of Lyme disease Med Mal Infect. 2007 Jul-Aug;37(7-8):435-45. Epub 2007 Mar 9

[2] Tranchant C, Warter JM. Lyme borreliosis, Rev Neurol (Paris). 2003 Jan;159(1):23-30

[3] Halperin JJ, Krupp LB, Golightly MG, Volkman DJ, Lyme borreliosis-associated encephalopathy. Neurology. 1990;40(9):1340

[4] Halperin, JJ, Heyes, MP, Keller, TL, Whitman, M. Neuroborreliosis - encephalopathy vs encephalitis. Proceedings of the Vth International Conference on Lyme Borreliosis, Arlington, Virginia, May 1992. Abstr. 1. 1992:1.

[5] Halperin JJ, Nervous system Lyme disease, 2011 UpToDate, Inc, Last update juin 10, 2011

[6] Hansen K, Lebech AM. The clinical and epidemiological profile of Lyme neuroborreliosis in Denmark 1985-1990. A prospective study of 187 patients with Borrelia burgdorferi specific intrathecal antibody production Brain. 1992 Apr;115 (Pt 2):399-423
[7] Oschmann P, Dorndorf W, Hornig C, Schäfer C, Wellensiek HJ, Pflughaupt KW. Stages and syndromes of neuroborreliosis. J Neurol. 1998 May;245(5):262-72.
[8] Strle F, Ruzić-Sabljić E, Cimperman J, Lotric-Furlan S, Maraspin V. Comparison of findings for patients with Borrelia garinii andBorrelia afzelii isolated from cerebrospinal fluid, Clin Infect Dis. 2006 Sep 15;43(6):704-10. Epub 2006 Aug 8
[9] De Seze J, Blanc F, Lyme neuroborreliosis: epidemiology, diagnosis and treatment, Lettre Infectiologue, XXVI (3) Mai-Juin 2011, 88-94
[10] Luft BJ, Steinman CR, Neimark HC, et al. Invasion of the central nervous system by Borrelia burgdorferi in acute disseminated infection. JAMA 1992; 267:1364.
[11] Logigian EL, Kaplan RF, Steere AC. Chronic neurologic manifestations of Lyme disease. N Engl J Med 1990; 323:1438.
[12] Halperin JJ, Luft BJ, Anand AK, et al. Lyme neuroborreliosis: central nervous system manifestations. Neurology 1989; 39:753.
[13] Logigian EL, Steere AC. Clinical and electrophysiologic findings in chronic neuropathy of Lyme disease. Neurology 1992; 42:303.
[14] Rupprecht TA, Koedel U, Fingerle V, Pfister HW. The pathogenesis of lyme neuroborreliosis: from infection to inflammation. Mol Med 2008; 14:205.
[15] Stanek G, Strle F, Lyme disease: European perspective. Infect Dis Clin North Am. 2008;22(2):327
[16] Halperin JJ, Golightly M. Lyme borreliosis in Bell's palsy. Long Island Neuroborreliosis Collaborative Study Group. Neurology 1992; 42:1268.
[17] Blanc F, Jaulhac B, Fleury M, de Seze J, de Martino SJ, Remy V, Blaison G, Hansmann Y,Christmann D, Tranchant C Relevance of the antibody index to diagnose Lymeneuroborreliosis among seropositive patients, Neurology. 2007 Sep 4;69(10):953-8.
[18] Rothermel H, Hedges TR 3rd, Steere AC Optic neuropathy in children with Lyme disease. Pediatrics. 2001;108(2):477
[19] Belman AL, Iyer M, Coyle PK, Dattwyler R Neurologic manifestations in children with North American Lyme disease, Neurology. 1993;43(12):2609
[20] Blanc F, Froelich S, Vuillemet F, Carré S, Baldauf E, de Martino S, Jaulhac B, Maitrot D,Tranchant C, de Seze J., Acute myelitis and Lyme disease, Rev Neurol (Paris). 2007 Nov;163(11):1039-47
[21] Sibony P, Halperin J, Coyle PK, Patel K. Reactive Lyme serology in optic neuritis, J Neuroophthalmol. 2005 Jun;25(2):71-82
[22] Krim E, Guehl D, Burbaud P, Lagueny A., Retrobulbar optic neuritis: a complication of Lyme disease? J Neurol Neurosurg Psychiatry. 2007 Dec;78(12):1409-10
[23] Blanc F, Ballonzoli L, Marcel C, De Martino S, Jaulhac B, de Seze J. Lyme optic neuritis, J Neurol Sci. 2010 Aug 15;295(1-2):117-9. Epub 2010 Jun
[24] Sparsa L, Blanc F, Lauer V, Cretin B, Marescaux C, Wolff V Recurrent ischemic strokes revealing Lymemeningovascularitis Rev Neurol (Paris). 2009 Mar;165(3):273-7. Epub 2008 Aug 28

[25] Oksi J, Kalimo H, Marttila RJ, Marjamäki M, Sonninen P, Nikoskelainen J, Viljanen MK,Inflammatory brain changes in Lyme borreliosis. A report on three patients and review of literature. Brain. 1996 Dec;119 (Pt 6):2143-54
[26] Krupp LB, Masur D, Schwartz J, Coyle PK, Langenbach LJ, Fernquist SK, Jandorf L, Halperin JJ, Cognitive functioning in late Lyme borreliosis Arch Neurol. 1991;48(11):1125
[27] Logigian EL, Kaplan RF, Steere AC. Chronic neurologic manifestations of Lyme disease. N Engl J Med 1990; 323:1438
[28] Klempner MS, Hu LT, Evans J, et al. Two controlled trials of antibiotic treatment in patients with persistent symptoms and a history of Lyme disease. N Engl J Med 2001; 345:85.
[29] Fallon BA, Keilp JG, Corbera KM, et al. A randomized, placebo-controlled trial of repeated IV antibiotic therapy for Lyme encephalopathy. Neurology 2008; 70:992.
[30] Halperin JJ. Prolonged Lyme disease treatment: enough is enough. Neurology 2008; 70:986.
[31] Feder HM Jr, Johnson BJ, O'Connell S, et al. A critical appraisal of "chronic Lyme disease". N Engl J Med 2007; 357:1422.
[32] Blanc F. Epidemiology of Lyme borreliosis and neuroborreliosis in France Rev Neurol (Paris). 2009 Aug-Sep;165(8-9):694-701. Epub 2009 May 17
[33] Stiernstedt GT, Granström M, Hederstedt B, Sköldenberg B. Diagnosis of spirochetal meningitis by enzyme-linked immunosorbent assay and indirect immunofluorescence assay in serum and cerebrospinal fluid. J Clin Microbiol 1985; 21:819.
[34] Steere AC, Berardi VP, Weeks KE, et al. Evaluation of the intrathecal antibody response to Borrelia burgdorferi as a diagnostic test for Lyme neuroborreliosis. J Infect Dis 1990; 161:1203.
[35] Ljøstad U, Skarpaas T, Mygland A. Clinical usefulness of intrathecal antibody testing in acute Lyme neuroborreliosis. Eur J Neurol 2007; 14:873.
[36] Halperin JJ, Volkman DJ, Wu P. Central nervous system abnormalities in Lyme neuroborreliosis. Neurology 1991; 41:1571.
[37] Pícha D, Moravcová L, Zdárský E, Benes J. Clinical comparison of immunoblot and antibody index for detection of intrathecal synthesis of specific antibodies in Lymeneuroborreliosis Eur J Clin Microbiol Infect Dis. 2000 Oct;19(10):805-6.
[38] Baig S, Olsson T, Hansen K, Link H. Anti-Borrelia burgdorferi antibody response over the course of Lyme neuroborreliosis. Infect Immun 1991; 59:1050.
[39] Lakos A. CSF findings in Lyme meningitis. J Infect 1992; 25:155.
[40] Hansen K, Cruz M, Link H. Oligoclonal Borrelia burgdorferi-specific IgG antibodies in cerebrospinal fluid in Lyme neuroborreliosis. J Infect Dis 1990; 161:1194.
[41] Nocton JJ, Bloom BJ, Rutledge BJ, et al. Detection of Borrelia burgdorferi DNA by polymerase chain reaction in cerebrospinal fluid in Lyme neuroborreliosis. J Infect Dis 1996; 174:623.
[42] Tumani H, Cadavid D. Are high CSF levels of CXCL13 helpful for diagnosis of Lyme neuroborreliosis? Neurology 2011; 76:1034.
[43] Marra CM, Tantalo LC, Sahi SK, et al. CXCL13 as a cerebrospinal fluid marker for neurosyphilis in HIV-infected patients with syphilis. Sex Transm Dis 2010; 37:283.

[44] Schmidt C, Plate A, Angele B, et al. A prospective study on the role of CXCL13 in Lyme neuroborreliosis. Neurology 2011; 76:1051.
[45] Rupprecht TA, Pfister HW, Angele B, et al. The chemokine CXCL13 (BLC): a putative diagnostic marker for neuroborreliosis. Neurology 2005; 65:448.
[46] Nadelman RB, Nowakowski J, Fish D, Falco RC, Freeman K, McKenna D, Welch P, Marcus R, Agüero-Rosenfeld ME, Dennis DT, Wormser GP; Tick Bite Study Group Prophylaxis with single-dose doxycycline for the prevention of Lymedisease after an Ixodes scapularis tick bite. N Engl J Med. 2001 Jul 12;345(2):79-84
[47] Clavelou P.Consensus conference on Lyme borreliosis.Presse Med. 2008 Dec;37(12):1707-8. Epub 2008 Nov 1

4

Mechanisms of Cell Death in the Transmissible Spongiform Encephalopathies

Fiona Lane*, James Alibhai*, Jean C. Manson and Andrew C. Gill†
The Roslin Institute and R(D)SVS, University of Edinburgh, Easter Bush Veterinary Centre, Roslin, Edinburgh UK

1. Introduction

The transmissible spongiform encephalopathies (TSEs) constitute a family of fatal, neurodegenerative diseases, including scrapie in sheep, chronic wasting disease (CWD) in deer and elk, bovine spongiform encephalopathy (BSE) and a range of human disorders, such as Creutzfeldt-Jakob disease (CJD), kuru and fatal familial insomnia. The archetypal TSE disease is scrapie of sheep and goats, which has been present in the UK flock for over 200 years as a result of both horizontal and vertical transmission. The most prevalent TSE disease of humans is sporadic Creutzfeldt-Jakob disease (spCJD), which affects 1-3 individuals per million worldwide. A new form of CJD, known as variant CJD (vCJD), was diagnosed in humans in the mid 1990s and it is likely that vCJD was contracted by consumption of contaminated beef, since this disease is indistinguishable from BSE on transmission to a panel of mice (Bruce et al., 1997). To date, there have been 175 cases of vCJD in the UK and a further 49 cases across 11 other countries (www.eurocjd.ed.ac.uk, data correct as of Aug 2011).

During pathogenesis of TSE disease the principal molecular event is the conformational rearrangement of a normal, host protein called the prion protein. The normal form of the prion protein, PrP^{C}, misfolds to a form known as PrP^{Sc}. PrP^{Sc} is insoluble and partially resistant to digestion by proteolytic enzymes that would usually recycle incorrectly folded proteins. PrP^{Sc} therefore accumulates in proteinaceous aggregates, including plaques and fibrils. The prion protein is ubiquitously expressed, but is most abundant in the central nervous system (CNS). Hence accumulation of PrP^{Sc} occurs principally in the brain, but peripheral lymphoreticular tissues can also accumulate proteinaceous deposits. The prion hypothesis suggests that PrP^{Sc} is the infectious agent in TSE diseases and that it catalytically causes nascent PrP^{C} molecules also to misfold (Prusiner, 1998). TSEs exist as discrete strains of disease, which can be stably passaged in suitable hosts resulting in differences in incubation time, clinical signs and pathology. It is suggested that PrP^{Sc} exists in different conformations, which encode the information necessary to transmit each disease and cause the strain-specific pathology (Prusiner, 1998). As a result of the critical involvement of the prion protein in TSEs, these disorders are also known as prion diseases.

---

*These authors contributed equally to this work
†Corresponding Author

At clinical end point of TSE disease, there is characteristic vacuolation in various areas of the brain, the exact locations of which depends on the infecting strain. Loss of neurons can also be detected at late stages of disease as can alterations in membrane morphology. Several excellent reviews cover neuropathology of animal (Jeffrey et al., 2011) and human (Kovacs & Budka, 2009) diseases that is evident on post mortem examination. In general, there are good correlations between disease, neurodegeneration and prion protein aggregation in many TSE diseases, which has led to suggestions that PrP^{Sc}-containing aggregates are directly toxic to neurons. *In vitro* studies largely support this conjecture, but the evidence *in vivo* is less convincing. Even assuming that a misfolded form of the prion protein is responsible for neurotoxicity, the mechanisms that initiate the cascade leading to neuronal loss are unknown. It is also unknown whether loss of function of PrP^{C}, as it is sequestered from the cell surface into proteinaceous aggregates, plays a role in rendering neurons susceptible to degeneration. Reactive astrocytosis is evident during the clinical phase and whilst time course studies have also suggested that astrocytes are activated at earlier stages, it is not known to what these cells are responding. In this chapter we review briefly the state of knowledge of the processes leading the neurodegeneration in TSE diseases, with a particular focus on the earliest detectable events.

2. Early morphological events in TSE-induced neuronal loss

In both prion diseases and other neurodegenerative disorders, the mechanisms leading to neurodegeneration remain particularly poorly understood. As mentioned above, the clinical phase of a variety of natural prion diseases has been studied, which has produced descriptions of the targeting of pathology, including the localisation of PrP^{Sc} deposits and of characteristic vacuolation and spongiform alterations. Substantial neuronal loss occurs by terminal endpoint, but it has become clear that loss of neurons is a relatively late development in the progression of pathology. In common with other neurodegenerative diseases, at later time points there are characteristic abnormalities in a range of normal neuronal molecular processes; this includes defects in ion homeostasis, aberrant mitochondrial morphologies and function, increased production of reactive oxygen species, endoplasmic reticulum stress and reduced proteasome function. Many of these homeostatic defects are thought to drive each other and it is therefore not clear which, if any, is the initiating factor. Thus, gross defects in several biochemical pathways represent the end stages of disease, but to determine causal mechanisms, it is necessary to describe in molecular and morphological detail the earliest stages of the neurodegenerative process. In naturally-contracted diseases, such descriptive studies are frequently not possible because (i) it is difficult to diagnose disease in advance of clinical signs (ii) outbred animals and humans can show significant variability in specific responses to disease and (iii) it is often impossible to know how and when individuals became infected. To remedy this situation, much use has been made of rodents as models of prion disease; C57BL/6 mice infected with the ME7 murine scrapie strain is the experimental system that has been studied in the greatest detail. There are clear advantages in using experimental prion diseases as a model, since the disease begins and ends at defined points (inoculation and death) and the homogeneity afforded by inbreeding produces standardised results. One caveat to murine models is that it appears that not all aspects of TSE disease in rodents are replicated in natural disease of large animals (Jeffrey et al., 2011). Nevertheless, some key findings from study of ME7 infection of mice are depicted graphically in Figure 1 and discussed below.

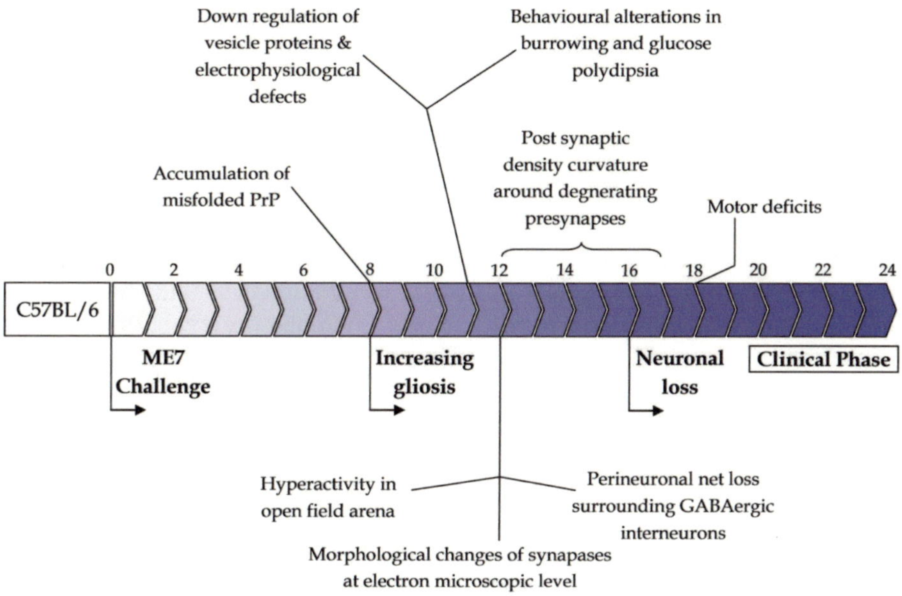

Fig. 1. Schematic timeline, in weeks, of pathological and behavioural events during infection of C57BL/6 mice with the mouse-passaged prion stain ME7. Information contained in this figure has been abstracted from multiple publications, referenced in section 2.

2.1 Synaptic degeneration precedes neuronal loss in prion disease

Recent studies of the pathogenesis of the ME7 strain of murine scrapie have allowed the identification of synaptic deficits within the hippocampus of C57BL/6 mice that occur well before neuronal loss can be observed (Betmouni et al., 1999, Cunningham et al., 2003, Guenther et al., 2001, Jeffrey et al., 2000). From roughly half way though the incubation period, synaptic deficits can be characterised at a molecular level by a loss of integral synaptic vesicle proteins and reduced synaptophysin staining (Cunningham, et al., 2003, Cunningham et al., 2005, Gray et al., 2009). Importantly, molecular changes appear to correlate with functional deficits, since electrophysiological abnormalities have also been observed within a similar timeframe (Chiti et al., 2006). At week 12, an accumulation of electron rich material within the pre-synapse in the CA1 region of the hippocampus was observed by use of electron microscopy, specifically between CA3 pre-synapses and CA1 post-synaptic densities within the Schaffer-Collateral pathway (Siskova et al., 2009). As the disease progressed, a distinct curvature of the post-synaptic densities around the degenerating pre-synapses could be visualised (Siskova, et al., 2009), potentially an attempt to maximise synaptic transmission. In addition, a loss of perineuronal nets surrounding GABAergic interneurons of the hippocampus coincided with a reduction in synaptic plasticity at early time-points (week 11/12) (Franklin et al., 2008). Early synaptic changes are a feature of other strains of murine disease, suggesting that these events may be early pathological markers of a TSE infection (Siso et al., 2002), at least in rodents. Synaptic dysfunction also appears to be a consistent, early pathological sign in many other neurodegenerative diseases, but there are suggestions that the exact morphological changes seen may differ depending on whether the insults to synapses are caused by processes leading to intra- or extra-cellular protein deposits. In addition, synaptic dysfunction in prion diseases differs from that seen during Wallerian degeneration in the periphery, in which axons are dissected or otherwise compromised and presynapses retract (Gillingwater et al., 2003). In prion diseases, loss of synapses appears to be followed by a retraction of the dendritic spine, but whether loss of any given synapse impacts on neighbouring synapses and ultimately on the respective cell body remains to be determined.

The early loss of synapses in prion disease must occur in response to a disease-associated molecular event or biochemical pathway. It is possible that this event may be the beginnings of the misfolded protein cascade, since in C57BL/6 mice infected with ME7 scrapie the accumulation of PrP^{Sc} can be detected at week 8, before the first observable signs of synaptic defects. The first deposits of abnormal PrP accumulate in the dentate gyrus of the hippocampus, subsequently spreading to encompass the CA3 sub-region of the hippocampus (Gray, et al., 2009). This suggests a progression of PrP^{Sc} formation along the Mossy-Fibre pathway, connecting the dentate gyrus and CA3 field, and a subsequent pathological dysfunction of CA3 neurons leading to degeneration of CA3 pyramidal cell pre-synapses in the CA1 region along the Schaffer-Collateral pathway. In the majority of prion diseases that have been studied in detail, PrP^{Sc} accumulation is one of the earliest detectable pathological signs and precedes, or is concurrent with, cellular or synaptic changes. These results suggest a causative correlation between the initial signs of PrP conversion and synaptic dysfunction. This raises the question of whether neurodegenerative processes are also similar in other prion disease models, particularly those that have small quantities of misfolded PrP present at the clinical end point (Barron et al., 2007). In the majority of cases, time course studies of such disease models have not been performed in sufficient detail to dissect the earliest pathological events. It is clear, nevertheless, that synaptic dysfunction and degeneration occur well before neuronal loss is observed in TSEs.

2.2 The role of glia in prion disease-induced neurodegeneration

Although neuronal death in TSEs is the most widely recognised pathological manifestation at a cellular level, alterations in non-neuronal cells are also apparent occurring alongside the first obvious signs of PrP^{Sc} accumulation in the brain. Reactive astrogliosis, exemplified by up regulation of *Gfap*, can be seen in various areas of the brain (Betmouni et al., 1996, Cunningham, et al., 2003). An increased understanding of astrocytes suggests that these cells have an integral role in maintaining homeostatic functions within the CNS (Butt et al., 1994, Chang Ling & Stone, 1991, Ransom et al., 2003, Robinson & Dreher, 1989, Slezak & Pfrieger, 2003). Astrocytic processes come into close contact with synapses (Bushong et al., 2004, Grosche et al., 1999) forming a 'tripartite' between the pre and post synaptic elements and the fine astrocytic processes (Araque et al., 2009). Astrocytes can undergo excitatory mediated release of chemical neurotransmitters as a result of increases of intracellular Ca^{2+} concentrations in the astrocyte cytoplasm (Kreft et al., 2009). Reactive astrogliosis is thought to play a neuroprotective role during acute brain injuries, for example during cerebral ischemia (Pekny et al., 2008), but it is not clear whether the activation of astrocytes is also neuroprotective during chronic infections, such as TSE diseases.

Microglia also exhibit an activated morphology prior to and concurrent with neurodegeneration, however, this doesn't appear to represent the classic inflammation one may expect during infection with classical pathogens (Perry et al., 2002). Instead, a concept of 'microglial priming' is thought to occur. Activated microglia produce an anti-inflammatory phenotype in response to ongoing TSE pathology, but subsequent systemic insults can elicit a rapid inflammatory response, initially by increases in IL-1β (Perry et al., 2007, Perry et al., 2003). Since the microglial response is not associated with classic inflammation, the role that these cells play in neurodegenerative disease remains unknown. It has been hypothesised that microglia have a neurotoxic role in neurodegeneration (Block et al., 2007) but other studies suggest microglia could be neuroprotective (Solito et al., 2010). There are also suggestions that microglia are not involved in the neurodegenerative process at all, but that degeneration is a neuron-autonomous process, at least at early stages (Perry & O'Connor, 2010). For both astrocytes and microglia, it remains unknown what these cells are responding to and whether this response aids or is detrimental to neuronal health. However, their activation at around the time that PrP^{Sc} deposition can first be observed suggests that they respond to the ongoing conversion process, to the accumulation of PrP^{Sc} itself or to the changes that PrP conversion and/or PrP^{Sc} deposition elicits in cellular mechanisms or synaptic morphology, plasticity and function. Mice in which PrP^{C} expression is restricted to astrocytes are susceptible to TSE infection (Raeber et al., 1997) suggesting that these cells are important in replication of PrP^{Sc} as well as in responding to its presence. In many studies using the ME7 murine scrapie strain, there exists strong correlations between the initial accumulation of PrP^{Sc} and neurodegeneration suggesting a key role for misfolded PrP in the mechanism of neuronal degeneration. This raises the key question of whether abnormal PrP isoforms are neurotoxic and, if so, what their molecular structures are.

3. Molecular mechanisms underlying degeneration of neurons

Prion protein deficient mice are resistant to TSE infection (Bueler et al., 1993, Manson et al., 1994b), demonstrating that PrP^{C} is required for disease. However, it is unclear what property of PrP is important for pathology: whether the PrP^{Sc} that accumulates during disease is actually toxic to neurons directly, whether the loss of PrP^{C} plays a role in rendering neurons susceptible to toxic insults (either involving PrP^{Sc} or not) or whether the ongoing process of agent replication compromises normal neuronal homeostasis. Although PrP^{Sc} accumulation appears to precede neuronal loss in ME7 scrapie, there are reasons to suggest that the accumulation of misfolded PrP is not responsible for neurotoxicity directly. For example (i) neurons which lack PrP^{C} do not degenerate in the presence of infected graft tissue rich in PrP^{Sc} (Brandner et al., 1996) and (ii) a variety of models exist in which levels of PrP^{Sc} and neuronal loss are poorly correlated (Barron, et al., 2007, Baumann et al., 2007, Chiesa et al., 1998, Flechsig et al., 2003, Hegde et al., 1998, Lasmezas et al., 1997, Li et al., 2007, Ma et al., 2002, Muramoto et al., 1997, Piccardo et al., 2007, Shmerling et al., 1998). But if classical PrP^{Sc} is not neurotoxic, then what is the toxic species?

3.1 Neurotoxicity of different aberrantly folded PrP isoforms

Considerable morphological heterogeneity can be observed in the protein deposited *in vivo* and recombinant PrP (recPrP) also exhibits conformational flexibility *in vitro*. There are also reports of aberrant cell biological behaviour of PrP^{C} at various stages of its cellular life-cycle, as depicted in figure 2, and these factors make pinpointing the neurotoxic entity rather challenging. Recent studies seem to support the idea that relatively small, (pre-fibrillar?) oligomeric protein species are highly neurotoxic (Bucciantini et al., 2002, Caughey &

Lansbury, 2003, Novitskaya et al., 2006, Simoneau et al., 2007, Zhang et al., 2010) and this appears true not just for prion diseases but also for other neurodegenerative protein misfolding diseases, further suggesting that common mechanisms of neurodegeneration may exist. RecPrP preparations have been used to investigate what the mechanisms underlying neuronal death may be, but *in vitro* studies such as these come with their own set of limitations. Nevertheless, a consensus from several studies suggests that oligomeric protein assemblies physically disrupt cellular membranes affecting the calcium levels within the cell (Sanghera et al., 2008, Simoneau, et al., 2007, Zhang, et al., 2010). This may occur by the insertion of oligomers into the phospholipid membrane (Kayed et al., 2004) and, since the plasma membrane is accessible to both intracellular and extracellular proteins, perturbation of the membrane may provide a mechanistic link between protein misfolding diseases that are associated with either intra- or extracellular deposits. An alternative theory is that functional structures, composed of oligomeric proteins, form within the lipid bilayer. These structures appear to act as relatively porous ion channels, affecting the cellular membrane potential and ionic homeostasis, leading to apoptosis (Quist et al., 2005).

In contrast to oligomers, fibrillar aggregates of recPrP have shown variable toxicity *in vitro*: some researchers have found that fibrils are not toxic to cells (Simoneau, et al., 2007), suggesting that fibril formation *in vivo* is a protective mechanism or an "end-point" in the misfolding pathway (Caughey & Lansbury, 2003, Silveira et al., 2005). Conversely, other studies have shown fibrils to be just as toxic as oligomers (Novitskaya, et al., 2006), but since protein preparations are generally not extensively characterised prior to incubation with cells *in vitro,* it is possible that differences in protein structure may account for these inconsistencies. Although fibrils are typically perceived to be rather inert, it is also conceivable that smaller species could fragment from fibrillar aggregates, which may then possess the neurotoxic properties of oligomers (Tanaka et al., 2006). A study using Aβ fibrils showed that interaction of the fibrils with lipids led to fragmentation, forming oligomers which were highly toxic (Martins et al., 2008). Thus the toxicity of amyloid fibrils may be inversely proportional to their stability. However, Novitskaya *et al.* showed that fibrils composed of recPrP caused cells to aggregate and subsequently undergo apoptosis, an effect that wasn't seen for oligomers in the same experiments (Novitskaya, et al., 2006). This aggregation was reduced when PrP^{C} was down-regulated, suggesting a role for PrP^{C} in mediating toxicity. There have also been recent reports that PrP^{C} is required for the toxicity exhibited by a range of molecular species (Resenberger et al., 2011a).

PrP^{C} is expressed heavily at synapses and the misfolding process may initiate in and around the synaptic cleft. This localises all relevant molecular species in the compartment in which the first morphological changes are detected, but this is still someway short of proving that abnormal PrP is neurotoxic. Through ongoing studies in our laboratories, we are endeavouring to dissect the relationship between PrP^{Sc}, infectivity, neurotoxicity and mechanisms of neurodegeneration (Barron, et al., 2007, Bradford et al., 2009, Cancellotti et al., 2010, Cancellotti et al., 2005, Manson et al., 2001, Piccardo, et al., 2007, Tuzi et al., 2008, Tuzi et al., 2004). Through the use of several unique models of prion disease in mice, we are beginning to accumulate evidence suggesting that the levels of infectivity are not always dependent on the quantity of misfolded PrP present (Barron, et al., 2007, Piccardo, et al., 2007). In conjunction with studies on the neurotoxicity of misfolded recombinant prion proteins, this leads to the theory that specific subpopulations of PrP conformations represent either the infectious or neurotoxic agents of TSEs (Weissmann, 1991). The role of PrP^C in neuronal toxicity is still controversial and prompts the question of whether a reduction in the levels of PrP^C on the cell surface, as it is converted into PrP^{Sc}, is a critical factor in prion disease-specific neurodegeneration.

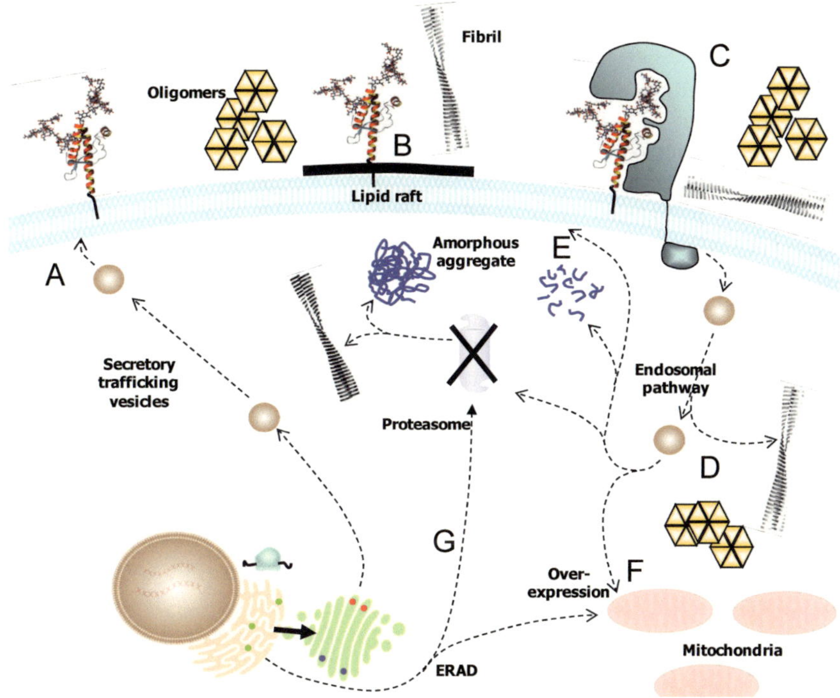

Fig. 2. Normal cell biology and putative misfolding pathways of PrP leading to toxicity. The prion protein is expressed in the secretory pathway and, after transiting the endoplasmic reticulum and Golgi apparatus, the protein is trafficked to the cell surface (A). Here it resides in specialised microdomains known as lipid rafts (B) but must move out of these domains to undergo endocytosis (C), presumably mediated by a cell surface receptor. After endocytosis PrP^C is routed on the endosomal pathway (D). Both the cell surface and the endosomal pathway have emerged as candidate locations for prion protein misfolding to intra- and/or extra-cellular oligomers or fibrils. After trafficking through endosomes, a proportion of the protein can be degraded, whilst some of it is routed back to the cell surface (E). Over-expression of PrP^C results in its localisation in mitochondria (F) whilst blockade of proteasome function leads to cytoplasmic accumulation (G). Both processes may follow retrograde transport of PrP from the ER by endoplasmic reticulum associated degradation (ERAD) processes.

3.2 Does loss of PrP^C function play a role in neurodegeneration?

The failure to infect prion protein knockout mice demonstrated conclusively that PrP^C is needed to sustain prion disease (Bueler, et al., 1993, Manson, et al., 1994b). These animals were also expected to inform on PrP function, but initial observations suggested that knockout mice developed normally (Bueler et al., 1992, Manson et al., 1994a). More in depth studies have highlighted a range of subtle and not so subtle alterations, including abnormal circadian rhythms (Tobler et al., 1996), defects in long term potentiation (Curtis et al., 2003, Maglio et al., 2006) and abnormalities of mitochondrial numbers and morphologies (Miele et al., 2002). From additional studies, primarily in cells lacking PrP^C, there have been suggestions that PrP^C has roles in copper binding and trafficking (Brown et al., 1997), the response to reactive oxygen species (Brown et al., 1999), neuritogenesis (Graner et al., 2000, Lopes et al., 2005) and calcium homeostasis (Colling et al., 1996, Fuhrmann et al., 2006, Herms et al., 2001). A key recent finding in PrP^C knockout mice was defects in the maintenance of the myelin sheath surrounding peripheral nerves, a phenotype that appeared specifically to result from depletion of PrP^C from neurons (Bremer et al., 2010). Thus, prion protein knockout mice have a range of physiological phenotypes primarily related to neuronal functions and this has led to a consensus that PrP^C is a neuroprotective molecule, although it is not clear how, specifically, this neuroprotection is manifest (Resenberger et al., 2011b). A thorough review of prion protein function is beyond the scope of this chapter but, in the context of TSE disease, a key question is whether the loss of a neuroprotective function of PrP^C plays a role in neurodegenerative mechanisms. Some intriguing observations came from experiments in which tissue from PrP-expressing mice was grafted into the brains of PrP knockout mice. After intracerebral prion infection, the grafted tissue developed pathology typical of prion disease, including PrP^{Sc} deposition, neuronal loss and vacuolation (Brandner, et al., 1996). However, despite PrP^{Sc} spreading from the grafted tissue into the surrounding brain area, no loss of PrP-null neurons was observed. These data strongly suggest that PrP^{Sc} is not neurotoxic in the absence of PrP^C expression in neurons, results that were backed up by experiments in which PrP^C expression in neurons was conditionally turned off in mice during an ongoing prion infection (Mallucci et al., 2003). Further evidence comes from infection of PrP^C-$GPI^{-/-}$ mice (discussed further below), which do not express PrP^C on the surface of neurons or indeed any neural cells (Chesebro et al., 2005). In $GPI^{-/-}$ mice, significant levels of PrP^{Sc} accumulated during disease but neuronal loss was not observed. These lines of evidence suggest that PrP^C loss does not play a role in neurotoxicity and actually suggests the contrary - that normal neuronal PrP^C expression is required for neurotoxicity (Resenberger, et al., 2011a).

Contradictory evidence comes from studies in PrP^C-null mice transgenically expressing hamster PrP^C exclusively on astrocytes; these mice were capable of supporting hamster-passaged prion disease and developed clinical signs, indicating that neuronal PrP^C was not necessary for neuronal degeneration (Raeber et al., 1997). In the same studies, astrocytic hamster PrP^C was expressed in mice in addition to wild type murine PrP^C and these mice propagated hamster prion infectivity but did not develop disease, suggesting a role for mouse PrP^C in protecting neurons from the toxicity of PrP^{Sc}. There are also several studies demonstrating that the toxicity of prion-related polypeptides is independent of the expression of PrP^C on neurons. Hence, the role of PrP^C in neurotoxicity is not clear and further understandings of how misfolded proteins can lead to synaptic degeneration and/or neurodegeneration will require a closer relationship between *in vivo* and *in vitro* studies. It seems likely that the initiation and progression of pathology leading from synaptopathy to neuronal loss requires a combination of (i) interaction of PrP^{Sc} with the synaptic membrane/vesicle membranes (ii) ongoing PrP^{Sc} propagation (iii) loss of PrP^C function and (iv) extracellular toxic PrP^{Sc} deposits. Since misfolding of PrP is required for the pathology associated with TSE disease, understanding the factors that aid this process will also aid our understanding of neurotoxicity and neuronal loss.

4. The mechanisms of prion protein misfolding leading to neuronal loss

The prion protein is an obligatory component of TSE disease and its misfolding appears central to disease pathogenesis. Understanding how protein misfolding leads to pathology is of crucial importance but it is extremely challenging to study mechanistic aspects of protein folding and misfolding *in vivo*, hence *in vitro* studies have contributed almost all knowledge that currently exists in this area. This has involved solving and/or modelling structures of normal and aberrant forms of PrP and modelling the structural transition. The normal form of the protein has been investigated by use of recombinant prion proteins expressed in prokaryotic systems and refolded *in vitro*. The atomic level structures of such isoforms have been defined by both nuclear magnetic resonance (NMR) spectroscopy, for a range of different prion proteins e.g. (Calzolai et al., 2005, Christen et al., 2008, Gossert et al., 2005, Lysek et al., 2005, Perez et al., 2010, Wuthrich & Riek, 2001), and X-ray crystallography for sheep (Eghiaian et al., 2004, Haire et al., 2004) human (Antonyuk et al., 2009, Knaus et al., 2001, Lee et al., 2010) and rabbit proteins (Khan et al., 2010). These studies found that the C-terminal region of PrP has globular structure (depicted in Fig 3) and NMR investigations of native PrP^C purified from cattle brains confirmed these structural assignments (Hornemann et al., 2004).

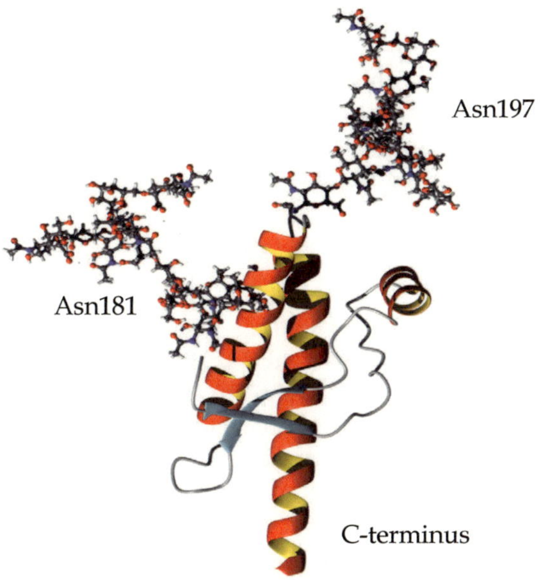

Fig. 3. The tertiary structure of PrP^C with two average sized N-linked glycans added at the two N-linked consensus sites (human numbering), to scale, demonstrating the contribution that these moieties make to the total volume of the prion protein

By contrast, the N-terminal region appears dynamically disordered. This domain incorporates 4-5 glycine-rich octapeptide repeats, which bind copper ions *in vitro* (Nadal et al., 2009, Pauly & Harris, 1998, Whittal et al., 2000, Wong et al., 2000a) and possibly *in vivo* (Brown, et al., 1997, Waggoner et al., 2000) and the region also mediates the binding of PrP^C to polyanionic compounds (Brimacombe et al., 1999). Although the N-terminal domain has been reported to be flexibly disordered, there have also been several reports of polyproline

II structure in this region (Blanch et al., 2004, Gill et al., 2000, Taubner et al., 2010). The N-terminal region is present in the majority of PrP^{Sc} in diseased brains (Hope et al., 1986), but it seems to be dispensable for disease-specific misfolding, since transgenic mice expressing protein lacking the N-terminal domain are fully susceptible to disease (Fischer et al., 1996). The globular C-terminal region incorporates two consensus sites for N-linked glycosylation, a single disulphide bond and a glycosylphosphatidyl inositol (GPI) membrane anchor is appended to the extreme C-terminus. After conversion of PrP^{C} to PrP^{Sc}, the C-terminal domain is resistant to protease digestion, indicating that it is this section of the protein that undergoes conformational change during prion protein misfolding.

By contrast to PrP^{C}, atomic level detail of PrP^{Sc} tertiary structure is lacking, which is a result of the insolubility of PrP^{Sc}-containing aggregates and the heterogeneity of morphologies of these aggregates. The structure of PrP^{Sc} has been probed by use of several low resolution techniques and Fourier-transform infra red (FT-IR) spectroscopic analysis suggests that the transition from PrP^{C} to PrP^{Sc} is associated with a partial increase in β-sheet structure (Caughey et al., 1991). Initially it was proposed that the second and third α-helices are not misfolded and theoretical structures followed, the most detailed of which is based upon empirical structural investigations by electron crystallography (Govaerts et al., 2004, Wille et al., 2002). However, recent data from hydrogen/deuterium-exchange experiments in conjunction with mass spectrometry has cast doubt on the existence of α-helical sections in PrP^{Sc} (Smirnovas et al., 2011). Instead, H/D exchange rates in PrP^{Sc} appear consistent with formation of β-sheet across the entire C-terminal domain, a result that challenges conventional wisdom of PrP^{Sc} structure. The problems associated with solving the structure of PrP^{Sc} appear insurmountable, at least at the present time and we are more likely to derive useful information from reasonable models of PrP^{Sc}.

4.1 Misfolding of PrP can be modelled *in vitro*

The structural transition from PrP^{C} to PrP^{Sc} can be mimicked *in vitro* by a variety of techniques and this has allowed various determinants of protein misfolding to be investigated. By mixing together PrP^{Sc} and recPrP expressed in mammalian cell lines to result in newly protease resistant PrP (PrP^{Res}) the group of Byron Caughey showed that PrP^{Sc} can auto-catalytically seed the conformational conversion of recPrP (Kocisko et al., 1994). This technique was termed the cell free conversion assay (CFCA) and it was subsequently shown to mimic many aspects of disease seen *in vivo*, including species barriers (Kirby et al., 2003, Kocisko et al., 1995) and the inhibitory effects of specific chemicals (Caughey et al., 1998, Demaimay et al., 2000, Demaimay et al., 1998). Quantifying conversion efficiency allows insights into mechanistic aspects of conversion: for example, there are two distinct phases of prion protein conversion - binding followed by conformational alteration (Horiuchi & Caughey, 1999) - and single amino acid substitutions were shown to dramatically affect the efficiency of conversion of the substrate (Bossers et al., 1997, Eiden et al., 2011, Kirby et al., 2010, Kirby et al., 2006). Furthermore, use of microsomes containing PrP^{Sc} and PrP^{C} in CFCA reactions indicated that the two proteins must be in the same vesicle for conversion to take place (Baron et al., 2002).

More recently, a second generation of *in vitro* prion misfolding assays has arisen, principally in response to the need for improved prion diagnostics. By the use of exogenous sources of energy to agitate the classical CFCA reaction, coupled with replenishment of the substrate, conversion efficiencies can be dramatically enhanced. Conversion reactions driven by sonication or shaking have been developed and include methods known as protein misfolding cyclic amplification (PMCA) (Saa et al., 2006, Saborio et al., 2001), quaking induced conversion (QuIC) (Atarashi et al., 2011, Atarashi et al., 2008) and amyloid seeding assay (ASA) (Colby et al., 2007). The PMCA technique has also been shown to be capable of creating prion infectivity *de novo* from PrP^{C} substrate in the absence of a PrP^{Sc} seed (Castilla et al., 2005). The protocols for CFCA, PMCA or QuIC assays differ in detail but generic principles underlie all such assays, as depicted in figure 4. In all cases a catalytic seed of PrP^{Sc} causes misfolding of a substrate, and this phenomenon firmly establishes that auto-catalytic, templated misfolding is a generic process in prion diseases. In addition to sources of physical energy, believed to aid fragmentation of large fibrils thereby generating fresh seed, many of the prion amplification techniques also require facilitation with other factors to amplify both infectivity and misfolded protein (Deleault et al., 2007, Wang et al., 2010). In this context, it is notable that several techniques exist to misfold recPrP in the absence of a physiological seed. Pathways leading to fibrils (Baskakov et al., 2002, Stohr et al., 2011) or oligomers (Rezaei, 2008, Tahiri-Alaoui et al., 2004, Tahiri-Alaoui et al., 2006) have been described, where misfolding is promoted by partially denaturing conditions. These processes occur comparatively rapidly and generally do not replicate features of disease, such as species barriers (Makarava et al., 2007) or polymorphic control of susceptibility (Baskakov et al., 2005, Kirby, et al., 2010), and also do not appear to generate *bona fide* prion infectivity (Legname et al., 2004, Makarava et al., 2010). These lines of evidence argue for a role for molecular cofactors in disease-specific prion protein misfolding (Birkmann & Riesner, 2008, Gill et al., 2010, Graham et al., 2010). Identifying these co-factors *in vivo* will allow significant progress in the prevention of disease transmission.

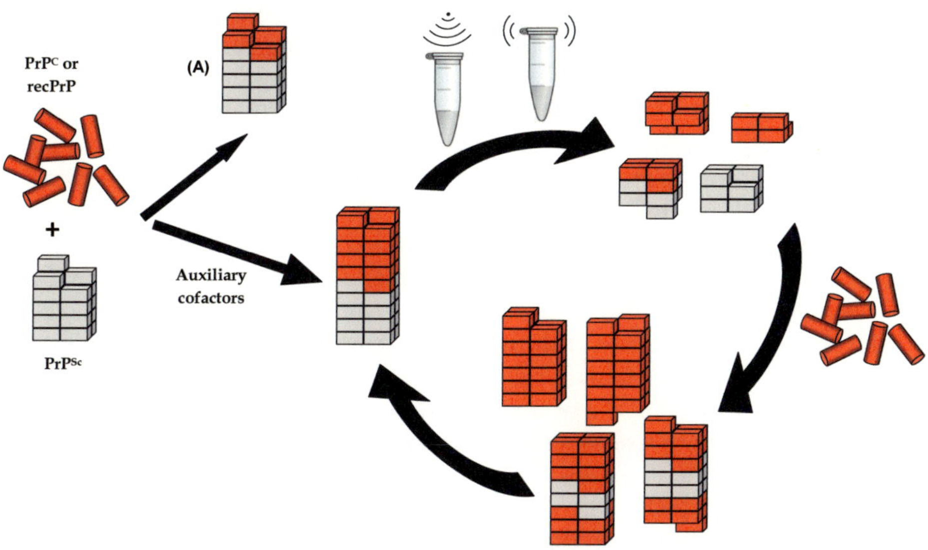

Fig. 4. Schematic pathways for seeded conversion of normal PrP to a protease-resistant isoform. In the absence of auxiliary cofactors, conversion is inefficient and only a small amount of available substrate is converted (A). This pathway is exemplified by the classic CFCA. By addition of auxiliary cofactors, conversion efficiency can be improved and periodic shaking (QuIC) or sonication (PMCA), coupled with replenishment of substrate, allows cyclic conversion leading to amplification of PrP^{Res}

4.2 Factors contributing to prion protein misfolding

Dramatic breakthroughs in the search for determinants of the prion protein misfolding process have been made in recent years. Deleault *et al* used the PMCA technique to amplify PrP^C that had been highly purified from brain tissue to which polyanionic species (RNA or glycosaminoglycans) were added. This mixture was sufficient to allow amplification of abnormal PrP when seeded with PrP^{Sc}, but also allowed the generation of abnormal PrP *de novo* in the absence of a catalytic seed. Crucially, the newly-synthesised abnormal PrP was shown to cause a TSE-like disease after inoculation to wild type animals. These data imply that purified PrP^C (along with lipids that co-purified with the protein) in addition to a polyanionic cofactor are the minimal requirements for creation of prion infectivity (Deleault, et al., 2007). Various researchers have since replicated or extended this work (Barria et al., 2009, Edgeworth et al., 2010, Weber et al., 2007), culminating in the publication of a study describing prion infectivity, created *de novo,* from bacterially-expressed recPrP supplemented with just synthetic lipid and total RNA extracted from murine liver (Wang, et al., 2010). What are the identities of molecules playing the roles of cofactors *in vivo*?

One approach to determine *in vivo* cofactors is to investigate the aggregates present in prion-infected animals for molecules that may have played a role in their formation. Other than PrP, various proteinaceous molecules appear specifically enriched in infectious prion fibrils (Giorgi et al., 2009, Moore et al., 2010, Petrakis et al., 2009) and recent data from our laboratory suggest that at least one such protein can enhance prion protein conversion efficiency (Graham et al., 2011). The most likely places for PrP^C to encounter PrP^{Sc} and for conversion to take place are on the cell surface or within the endocytic pathway and it would appear reasonable to expect cofactors to reside in these locations. Results from experiments in cell lines supporting either location as a site for conversion have been published (Borchelt et al., 1992, Hooper, 2011). Recent data from our laboratories (Graham, et al., 2010, Graham, et al., 2011) and others (Abid et al., 2010), suggest that the plasma membrane is a more likely source of cofactors modulating prion protein misfolding. It is plausible that specific compositions of lipid can modulate prion protein structure thereby creating conditions for strain specific misfolding. Misfolding in or around the plasma membrane would facilitate toxic mechanisms that involve disturbances in membrane permeability. There are also various properties intrinsic to the prion protein that exert an influence on misfolding and which therefore may impact on neuronal toxicity of the resulting aggregates. Amino acid substitutions in the prion protein affect susceptibility of animals to prion disease and mutations in the human *PRNP* gene (encoding the prion protein) appear to be a direct cause of familial prion diseases. In general, those amino acid substitutions associated with resistance to prion disease in animals appear to decrease the stability of recombinant prion proteins *in vitro* (Bujdoso et al., 2005, Kirby, et al., 2010, Paludi et al., 2007, Thackray et al., 2004) potentially leading to differing levels of cellular toxicity. By contrast, there is conflicting data on the ability of mutations associated with human familial disease to affect the structure and stability of PrP^C (e.g. (Apetri et al., 2004, Bae et al., 2009, Inouye et al., 2000, Rossetti et al., 2011, van der Kamp & Daggett, 2010, Vanik & Surewicz, 2002, Yin et al., 2007)) and there is a lack of clear data suggesting that human mutations confer increased neurotoxicity upon misfolded PrP. It seems likely that the effects of individual amino acid changes depend on the specific substitution as well as the position within the sequence of PrP^C and potentially the species that the amino acid change is in.

PrP^C undergoes various post translational modifications *in vivo* and many have been investigated for their impact on prion protein misfolding. In transgenic mice that express prion protein lacking the C-terminal signal sequence, the GPI anchor is not attached ($GPI^{-/-}$) and this results in secretion of PrP^C into the extracellular milieu. When $GPI^{-/-}$ mice are infected with a prion disease there is dramatic accumulation of large amyloid plaques composed of anchorless PrP but no evidence of neurodegeneration (Chesebro, et al., 2005). The reasons for this are unclear but presumably result from the lack of association of PrP^C with the plasma membrane (Caughey et al., 2009), however, preventing GPI anchor addition also inhibits glycosylation of PrP^C and this may be a compounding factor in the lack of pathology/disease. Nevertheless, as mentioned earlier, these results further indicate that large aggregates composed of prion protein are not neurotoxic *per se*.

N-linked glycosylation of PrP^C occurs at two sites in the C-terminal region of the protein (Rudd et al., 2002) and a variety of techniques have been used to study the effect of glycosylation on prion protein misfolding. *In vitro* studies suggest that glycosylation of PrP^C affects its interaction with PrP^{Sc} (Priola & Lawson, 2001), but that glycosylation is not required for strain properties (Nishina et al., 2006, Piro et al., 2009). Initial reports from studies in cell lines suggested that removing prion glycosylation produced spontaneously misfolded protein (Lehmann & Harris, 1997), however, this may have been a result of over-expression, since more recent studies have shown that blocking glycosylation of endogenously expressed PrP^C does not produce this phenotype (Cancellotti, et al., 2005). In some cases, studies have been hampered by the folding and trafficking abnormalities that can occur when PrP^C is expressed without glycosylation (Cancellotti, et al., 2005, DeArmond et al., 1997) depending on the specific mutations used to prevent glycosylation (Capellari et al., 2000, Ikeda et al., 2008, Salamat et al., 2011, Wong et al., 2000b). Neuendorf *et al* selected deglycosylating mutations that retained authentic PrP^C cellular trafficking and mice in which these proteins were over-expressed were susceptible to both scrapie and BSE (Neuendorf et al., 2004). However, in some cases, incubation times were shorter than with wild type mice, which is probably an artefact of over-expression. In our laboratories we have produced gene-targeted mice lacking prion protein glycosylation (Cancellotti, et al., 2005) and analysis of these mice confirm that glycosylation is important for efficient trafficking of PrP^C, but that glycosylation is not always required to sustain prion infection after intracranial inoculation (Tuzi, et al., 2008). Intra-cranial infection of these mice with multiple prion strains indicates dramatically different requirements for occupation of each of the glycosylation sites of host PrP for infection. However, since disease outcomes are significantly modulated following peripheral infection of glycosylation-deficient, gene-targeted mice, our data also suggest that glycosylation of PrP is important for either peripheral replication of PrP^{Sc} or for trafficking of the infection to the CNS (Cancellotti, et al., 2010). The glycans present at either site are highly heterogeneous (Ritchie et al., 2002, Rudd et al., 1999, Stimson et al., 1999); at least 60 different glycan moieties can be present on the protein and genetic removal of glycosylation does not distinguish between individual glycan structures. Thus, it is unclear whether any individual carbohydrate chains render the prion protein particularly susceptible to misfolding.

In summary, although we know the structure of PrP^C to atomic resolution and we can model the conversion to PrP^{Sc} *in vitro,* the details of how this process takes place *in vivo* are still unknown. Although various factors are known to affect the way that PrP^C may misfold, the only factor absolutely known to direct this process is exogenous PrP^{Sc}. It is assumed that the PrP^{Sc} catalysed misfolding of PrP^{C} results in a species that is neurotoxic, but it remains possible that loss of PrP^{C} is an important process in mediating neurotoxicity. Once neurotoxicity results, it appears clear that synaptic dysfunction is one of the first pathological alterations that can be detected. Approaches that integrate studies of protein misfolding, *in vitro* toxicity and *in vivo* toxicity are required to allow us to address the many unknowns of neuronal loss in prion disease

5. Acknowledgements

The authors would like to thank Drs Sandra McCutcheon and James F. Graham for constructive comments on the manuscript. FML and JA are supported by Doctoral Training Account scholarships from the BBSRC, UK. JCM and ACG acknowledge funding from a BBSRC Institute Programme Grant, the Department of Health, UK and the MRC, UK.

6. References

Abid, K., Morales, R. & Soto, C. (2010). Cellular factors implicated in prion replication. *FEBS Lett*, Vol. 584, No. 11, pp. 2409-14

Antonyuk, S. V., Trevitt, C. R., Strange, R. W., Jackson, G. S., Sangar, D., Batchelor, M., Cooper, S., Fraser, C., Jones, S., Georgiou, T., Khalili-Shirazi, A., Clarke, A. R., Hasnain, S. S. & Collinge, J. (2009). Crystal structure of human prion protein bound to a therapeutic antibody. *Proc Natl Acad Sci U S A*, Vol. 106, No. 8, pp. 2554-8

Apetri, A. C., Surewicz, K. & Surewicz, W. K. (2004). The effect of disease-associated mutations on the folding pathway of human prion protein. *J Biol Chem*, Vol. 279, No. 17, pp. 18008-14

Araque, A., Perea, G. & Navarrete, M. (2009). Tripartite synapses: astrocytes process and control synaptic information. *Tr Neurosci*, Vol. 32, No. 8, pp. 421-431

Atarashi, R., Satoh, K., Sano, K., Fuse, T., Yamaguchi, N., Ishibashi, D., Matsubara, T., Nakagaki, T., Yamanaka, H., Shirabe, S., Yamada, M., Mizusawa, H., Kitamoto, T., Klug, G., McGlade, A., Collins, S. J. & Nishida, N. (2011). Ultrasensitive human prion detection in cerebrospinal fluid by real-time quaking-induced conversion. *Nat Med*, Vol. 17, No. 2, pp. 175-8

Atarashi, R., Wilham, J. M., Christensen, L., Hughson, A. G., Moore, R. A., Johnson, L. M., Onwubiko, H. A., Priola, S. A. & Caughey, B. (2008). Simplified ultrasensitive prion detection by recombinant PrP conversion with shaking. *Nat Methods*, Vol. 5, No. 3, pp. 211-2

Bae, S. H., Legname, G., Serban, A., Prusiner, S. B., Wright, P. E. & Dyson, H. J. (2009). Prion proteins with pathogenic and protective mutations show similar structure and dynamics. *Biochemistry*, Vol. 48, No. 34, pp. 8120-8

Baron, G. S., Wehrly, K., Dorward, D. W., Chesebro, B. & Caughey, B. (2002). Conversion of raft associated prion protein to the protease-resistant state requires insertion of PrP-res (PrP(Sc)) into contiguous membranes. *Embo J*, Vol. 21, No. 5, pp. 1031-40

Barria, M. A., Mukherjee, A., Gonzalez-Romero, D., Morales, R. & Soto, C. (2009). *De novo* generation of infectious prions *in vitro* produces a new disease phenotype. *PLoS Pathog*, Vol. 5, No. 5, pp. e1000421

Barron, R. M., Campbell, S. L., King, D., Bellon, A., Chapman, K. E., Williamson, R. A. & Manson, J. C. (2007). High titers of transmissible spongiform encephalopathy infectivity associated with extremely low levels of PrP^{Sc} *in vivo*. *J Biol Chem*, Vol. 282, No. 49, pp. 35878-86

Baskakov, I., Disterer, P., Breydo, L., Shaw, M., Gill, A., James, W. & Tahiri-Alaoui, A. (2005). The presence of valine at residue 129 in human prion protein accelerates amyloid formation. *FEBS Lett*, Vol. 579, No. 12, pp. 2589-96

Baskakov, I. V., Legname, G., Baldwin, M. A., Prusiner, S. B. & Cohen, F. E. (2002). Pathway complexity of prion protein assembly into amyloid. *J Biol Chem*, Vol. 277, No. 24, pp. 21140-8

Baumann, F., Tolnay, M., Brabeck, C., Pahnke, J., Kloz, U., Niemann, H. H., Heikenwalder, M., Rulicke, T., Burkle, A. & Aguzzi, A. (2007). Lethal recessive myelin toxicity of prion protein lacking its central domain. *Embo J*, Vol. 26, No. 2, pp. 538-47

Betmouni, S., Deacon, R. M. J., Rawlins, J. N. P. & Ferry, V. H. (1999). Behavioral consequences of prion disease targeted to the hippocampus in a mouse model of scrapie. *Psychobiology*, Vol. 27, No. 1, pp. 63-71

Betmouni, S., Perry, V. H. & Gordon, J. L. (1996). Evidence for an early inflammatory response in the central nervous system of mice with scrapie. *Neuroscience*, Vol. 74, No. 1, pp. 1-5

Birkmann, E. & Riesner, D. (2008). Prion infection: seeded fibrillization or more? *Prion*, Vol. 2, No. 2, pp. 67-72

Blanch, E. W., Gill, A. C., Rhie, A. G., Hope, J., Hecht, L., Nielsen, K. & Barron, L. D. (2004). Raman optical activity demonstrates poly(L-proline) II helix in the N-terminal region of the ovine prion protein: implications for function and misfunction. *J Mol Biol*, Vol. 343, No. 2, pp. 467-76

Block, M. L., Zecca, L. & Hong, J. S. (2007). Microglia-mediated neurotoxicity: uncovering the molecular mechanisms. *Nat Rev Neurosci*, Vol. 8, No. 1, pp. 57-69

Borchelt, D. R., Taraboulos, A. & Prusiner, S. B. (1992). Evidence for synthesis of scrapie prion proteins in the endocytic pathway. *J Biol Chem*, Vol. 267, No. 23, pp. 16188-99

Bossers, A., Belt, P., Raymond, G. J., Caughey, B., de Vries, R. & Smits, M. A. (1997). Scrapie susceptibility-linked polymorphisms modulate the *in vitro* conversion of sheep prion protein to protease-resistant forms. *Proc Natl Acad Sci U S A*, Vol. 94, No. 10, pp. 4931-6

Bradford, B. M., Tuzi, N. L., Feltri, M. L., McCorquodale, C., Cancellotti, E. & Manson, J. C. (2009). Dramatic reduction of PrP^{C} level and glycosylation in peripheral nerves following PrP knock-out from Schwann cells does not prevent transmissible spongiform encephalopathy neuroinvasion. *J Neurosci*, Vol. 29, No. 49, pp. 15445-54

Brandner, S., Isenmann, S., Raeber, A., Fischer, M., Sailer, A., Kobayashi, Y., Marino, S., Weissmann, C. & Aguzzi, A. (1996). Normal host prion protein necessary for scrapie-induced neurotoxicity. *Nature*, Vol. 379, No. 6563, pp. 339-43

Bremer, J., Baumann, F., Tiberi, C., Wessig, C., Fischer, H., Schwarz, P., Steele, A. D., Toyka, K. V., Nave, K. A., Weis, J. & Aguzzi, A. (2010). Axonal prion protein is required for peripheral myelin maintenance. *Nat Neurosci*, Vol. 13, No. 3, pp. 310-8

Brimacombe, D. B., Bennett, A. D., Wusteman, F. S., Gill, A. C., Dann, J. C. & Bostock, C. J. (1999). Characterization and polyanion-binding properties of purified recombinant prion protein. *Biochem J*, Vol. 342, No. 3, pp. 605-13

Brown, D. R., Qin, K., Herms, J. W., Madlung, A., Manson, J., Strome, R., Fraser, P. E., Kruck, T., von Bohlen, A., Schulz-Schaeffer, W., Giese, A., Westaway, D. & Kretzschmar, H. (1997). The cellular prion protein binds copper *in vivo*. *Nature*, Vol. 390, No. 6661, pp. 684-7

Brown, D. R., Wong, B. S., Hafiz, F., Clive, C., Haswell, S. J. & Jones, I. M. (1999). Normal prion protein has an activity like that of superoxide dismutase. *Biochem J*, Vol. 344, No. 1, pp. 1-5

Bruce, M. E., Will, R. G., Ironside, J. W., McConnell, I., Drummond, D., Suttie, A., McCardle, L., Chree, A., Hope, J., Birkett, C., Cousens, S., Fraser, H. & Bostock, C. J. (1997). Transmissions to mice indicate that 'new variant' CJD is caused by the BSE agent. *Nature*, Vol. 389, No. 6650, pp. 498-501

Bucciantini, M., Giannoni, E., Chiti, F., Baroni, F., Formigli, L., Zurdo, J., Taddei, N., Ramponi, G., Dobson, C. M. & Stefani, M. (2002). Inherent toxicity of aggregates implies a common mechanism for protein misfolding diseases. *Nature*, Vol. 416, No. 6880, pp. 507-11

Bueler, H., Aguzzi, A., Sailer, A., Greiner, R. A., Autenried, P., Aguet, M. & Weissmann, C. (1993). Mice devoid of PrP are resistant to scrapie. *Cell*, Vol. 73, No. 7, pp. 1339-47

Bueler, H., Fischer, M., Lang, Y., Bluethmann, H., Lipp, H. P., DeArmond, S. J., Prusiner, S. B., Aguet, M. & Weissmann, C. (1992). Normal development and behaviour of mice lacking the neuronal cell-surface PrP protein. *Nature*, Vol. 356, No. 6370, pp. 577-82

Bujdoso, R., Burke, D. F. & Thackray, A. M. (2005). Structural differences between allelic variants of the ovine prion protein revealed by molecular dynamics simulations. *Proteins*, Vol. 61, No. 4, pp. 840-9

Bushong, E. A., Marton, M. E. & Ellisman, M. H. (2004). Maturation of astrocyte morphology and the establishment of astrocyte domains during postnatal hippocampal development. *Int J Dev Neurosci*, Vol. 22, No. 2, pp. 73-86

Butt, A. M., Colquhoun, K., Tutton, M. & Berry, M. (1994). Three-dimensional morphology of astrocytes and oligodendrocytes in the intact mouse optic nerve. *J Neurocytol*, Vol. 23, No. 8, pp. 469-85

Calzolai, L., Lysek, D. A., Perez, D. R., Guntert, P. & Wuthrich, K. (2005). Prion protein NMR structures of chickens, turtles, and frogs. *Proc Natl Acad Sci U S A*, Vol. 102, No. 3, pp. 651-5

Cancellotti, E., Bradford, B. M., Tuzi, N. L., Hickey, R. D., Brown, D., Brown, K. L., Barron, R. M., Kisielewski, D., Piccardo, P. & Manson, J. C. (2010). Glycosylation of PrP^{C} determines timing of neuroinvasion and targeting in the brain following transmissible spongiform encephalopathy infection by a peripheral route. *J Virol*, Vol. 84, No. 7, pp. 3464-75

Cancellotti, E., Wiseman, F., Tuzi, N. L., Baybutt, H., Monaghan, P., Aitchison, L., Simpson, J. & Manson, J. C. (2005). Altered glycosylated PrP proteins can have different neuronal trafficking in brain but do not acquire scrapie-like properties. *J Biol Chem*, Vol. 280, No. 52, pp. 42909-18

Capellari, S., Zaidi, S. I., Long, A. C., Kwon, E. E. & Petersen, R. B. (2000). The Thr183Ala Mutation, Not the Loss of the First Glycosylation Site, Alters the Physical Properties of the Prion Protein. *J Alzheimers Dis*, Vol. 2, No. 1, pp. 27-35

Castilla, J., Saa, P., Hetz, C. & Soto, C. (2005). *In vitro* generation of infectious scrapie prions. *Cell*, Vol. 121, No. 2, pp. 195-206

Caughey, B., Baron, G. S., Chesebro, B. & Jeffrey, M. (2009). Getting a grip on prions: oligomers, amyloids, and pathological membrane interactions. *Annu Rev Biochem*, Vol. 78, pp. 177-204

Caughey, B. & Lansbury, P. T. (2003). Protofibrils, pores, fibrils, and neurodegeneration: separating the responsible protein aggregates from the innocent bystanders. *Annu Rev Neurosci*, Vol. 26, pp. 267-98

Caughey, B. W., Dong, A., Bhat, K. S., Ernst, D., Hayes, S. F. & Caughey, W. S. (1991). Secondary structure analysis of the scrapie-associated protein PrP 27-30 in water by infrared spectroscopy. *Biochemistry*, Vol. 30, No. 31, pp. 7672-80

Caughey, W. S., Raymond, L. D., Horiuchi, M. & Caughey, B. (1998). Inhibition of protease-resistant prion protein formation by porphyrins and phthalocyanines. *Proc Natl Acad Sci U S A*, Vol. 95, No. 21, pp. 12117-22

Chang Ling, T. & Stone, J. (1991). Factors determining the morphology and distribution of astrocytes in the cat retina: a 'contact-spacing' model of astrocyte interaction. *J Comp Neurol*, Vol. 303, No. 3, pp. 387-99

Chesebro, B., Trifilo, M., Race, R., Meade-White, K., Teng, C., LaCasse, R., Raymond, L., Favara, C., Baron, G., Priola, S., Caughey, B., Masliah, E. & Oldstone, M. (2005). Anchorless prion protein results in infectious amyloid disease without clinical scrapie. *Science*, Vol. 308, No. 5727, pp. 1435-9

Chiesa, R., Piccardo, P., Ghetti, B. & Harris, D. A. (1998). Neurological illness in transgenic mice expressing a prion protein with an insertional mutation. *Neuron*, Vol. 21, No. 6, pp. 1339-51

Chiti, Z., Knutsen, O. M., Betmouni, S. & Greene, J. R. (2006). An integrated, temporal study of the behavioural, electrophysiological and neuropathological consequences of murine prion disease. *Neurobiol Dis*, Vol. 22, No. 2, pp. 363-73

Christen, B., Perez, D. R., Hornemann, S. & Wuthrich, K. (2008). NMR structure of the bank vole prion protein at 20 degrees C contains a structured loop of residues 165-171. *J Mol Biol*, Vol. 383, No. 2, pp. 306-12

Colby, D. W., Zhang, Q., Wang, S., Groth, D., Legname, G., Riesner, D. & Prusiner, S. B. (2007). Prion detection by an amyloid seeding assay. *Proc Natl Acad Sci U S A*, Vol. 104, No. 52, pp. 20914-9

Colling, S. B., Collinge, J. & Jefferys, J. G. (1996). Hippocampal slices from prion protein null mice: disrupted Ca(2+)-activated K+ currents. *Neurosci Lett*, Vol. 209, No. 1, pp. 49-52

Cunningham, C., Deacon, R., Wells, H., Boche, D., Waters, S., Diniz, C. P., Scott, H., Rawlins, J. N. & Perry, V. H. (2003). Synaptic changes characterize early behavioural signs in the ME7 model of murine prion disease. *Eur J Neurosci*, Vol. 17, No. 10, pp. 2147-55

Cunningham, C., Wilcockson, D. C., Campion, S., Lunnon, K. & Perry, V. H. (2005). Central and systemic endotoxin challenges exacerbate the local inflammatory response and increase neuronal death during chronic neurodegeneration. *J Neurosci*, Vol. 25, No. 40, pp. 9275-84

Curtis, J., Errington, M., Bliss, T., Voss, K. & MacLeod, N. (2003). Age-dependent loss of PTP and LTP in the hippocampus of PrP-null mice. *Neurobiol Dis*, Vol. 13, No. 1, pp. 55-62

DeArmond, S. J., Sanchez, H., Yehiely, F., Qiu, Y., Ninchak-Casey, A., Daggett, V., Camerino, A. P., Cayetano, J., Rogers, M., Groth, D., Torchia, M., Tremblay, P., Scott, M. R., Cohen, F. E. & Prusiner, S. B. (1997). Selective neuronal targeting in prion disease. *Neuron*, Vol. 19, No. 6, pp. 1337-48

Deleault, N. R., Harris, B. T., Rees, J. R. & Supattapone, S. (2007). Formation of native prions from minimal components *in vitro*. *Proc Natl Acad Sci U S A*, Vol. 104, No. 23, pp. 9741-6

Demaimay, R., Chesebro, B. & Caughey, B. (2000). Inhibition of formation of protease-resistant prion protein by Trypan Blue, Sirius Red and other Congo Red analogs. *Arch Virol Suppl*, Vol. No. 16, pp. 277-83

Demaimay, R., Harper, J., Gordon, H., Weaver, D., Chesebro, B. & Caughey, B. (1998). Structural aspects of Congo red as an inhibitor of protease-resistant prion protein formation. *J Neurochem*, Vol. 71, No. 6, pp. 2534-41

Edgeworth, J. A., Gros, N., Alden, J., Joiner, S., Wadsworth, J. D., Linehan, J., Brandner, S., Jackson, G. S., Weissmann, C. & Collinge, J. (2010). Spontaneous generation of mammalian prions. *Proc Natl Acad Sci U S A*, Vol. 107, No. 32, pp. 14402-6

Eghiaian, F., Grosclaude, J., Lesceu, S., Debey, P., Doublet, B., Treguer, E., Rezaei, H. & Knossow, M. (2004). Insight into the PrP^{C}-->PrP^{Sc} conversion from the structures of antibody-bound ovine prion scrapie-susceptibility variants. *Proc Natl Acad Sci U S A*, Vol. 101, No. 28, pp. 10254-9

Eiden, M., Soto, E. O., Mettenleiter, T. C. & Groschup, M. H. (2011). Effects of polymorphisms in ovine and caprine prion protein alleles on cell-free conversion. *Vet Res*, Vol. 42, No. 1, pp. 30

Fischer, M., Rulicke, T., Raeber, A., Sailer, A., Moser, M., Oesch, B., Brandner, S., Aguzzi, A. & Weissmann, C. (1996). Prion protein (PrP) with amino-proximal deletions restoring susceptibility of PrP knockout mice to scrapie. *Embo J*, Vol. 15, No. 6, pp. 1255-64

Flechsig, E., Hegyi, I., Leimeroth, R., Zuniga, A., Rossi, D., Cozzio, A., Schwarz, P., Rulicke, T., Gotz, J., Aguzzi, A. & Weissmann, C. (2003). Expression of truncated PrP targeted to Purkinje cells of PrP knockout mice causes Purkinje cell death and ataxia. *Embo J*, Vol. 22, No. 12, pp. 3095-101

Franklin, S. L., Love, S., Greene, J. R. & Betmouni, S. (2008). Loss of Perineuronal Net in ME7 Prion Disease. *J Neuropathol Exp Neurol*, Vol. 67, No. 3, pp. 189-99

Fuhrmann, M., Bittner, T., Mitteregger, G., Haider, N., Moosmang, S., Kretzschmar, H. & Herms, J. (2006). Loss of the cellular prion protein affects the Ca2+ homeostasis in hippocampal CA1 neurons. *J Neurochem*, Vol. 98, No. 6, pp. 1876-85

Gill, A. C., Agarwal, S., Pinheiro, T. J. & Graham, J. F. (2010). Structural requirements for efficient prion protein conversion: cofactors may promote a conversion-competent structure for PrP(C). *Prion*, Vol. 4, No. 4, pp. 235-42

Gill, A. C., Ritchie, M. A., Hunt, L. G., Steane, S. E., Davies, K. G., Bocking, S. P., Rhie, A. G., Bennett, A. D. & Hope, J. (2000). Post-translational hydroxylation at the N-terminus of the prion protein reveals presence of PPII structure in vivo. *Embo J*, Vol. 19, No. 20, pp. 5324-31

Gillingwater, T. H., Ingham, C. A., Coleman, M. P. & Ribchester, R. R. (2003). Ultrastructural correlates of synapse withdrawal at axotomized neuromuscular junctions in mutant and transgenic mice expressing the Wld gene. *Journal of Anatomy*, Vol. 203, No. 3, pp. 265-276

Giorgi, A., Di Francesco, L., Principe, S., Mignogna, G., Sennels, L., Mancone, C., Alonzi, T., Sbriccoli, M., De Pascalis, A., Rappsilber, J., Cardone, F., Pocchiari, M., Maras, B. & Schinina, M. E. (2009). Proteomic profiling of PrP27-30-enriched preparations extracted from the brain of hamsters with experimental scrapie. *Proteomics*, Vol. 9, No. 15, pp. 3802-14

Gossert, A. D., Bonjour, S., Lysek, D. A., Fiorito, F. & Wuthrich, K. (2005). Prion protein NMR structures of elk and of mouse/elk hybrids. *Proc Natl Acad Sci U S A*, Vol. 102, No. 3, pp. 646-50

Govaerts, C., Wille, H., Prusiner, S. B. & Cohen, F. E. (2004). Evidence for assembly of prions with left-handed beta-helices into trimers. *Proc Natl Acad Sci U S A*, Vol. 101, No. 22, pp. 8342-7

Graham, J. F., Agarwal, S., Kurian, D., Kirby, L., Pinheiro, T. J. & Gill, A. C. (2010). Low density subcellular fractions enhance disease-specific prion protein misfolding. *J Biol Chem*, Vol. 285, No. 13, pp. 9868-80

Graham, J. F., Kurian, D., Agarwal, S., Toovey, L., Hunt, L., Kirby, L., Pinheiro, T., J. T., Banner, S. J. & Gill, A. C. (2011). Na+/K+-ATPase is present in scrapie-associated fibrils, modulates PrP misfolding in vitro and links PrP function and dysfunction. PLOS One, Vol. 6, No. 11, pp. e26813

Graner, E., Mercadante, A. F., Zanata, S. M., Forlenza, O. V., Cabral, A. L., Veiga, S. S., Juliano, M. A., Roesler, R., Walz, R., Minetti, A., Izquierdo, I., Martins, V. R. & Brentani, R. R. (2000). Cellular prion protein binds laminin and mediates neuritogenesis. *Brain Res Mol Brain Res*, Vol. 76, No. 1, pp. 85-92

Gray, B. C., Siskova, Z., Perry, V. H. & O'Connor, V. (2009). Selective presynaptic degeneration in the synaptopathy associated with ME7-induced hippocampal pathology. *Neurobiol Dis*, Vol. 35, No. 1, pp. 63-74

Grosche, J., Matyash, V., Moller, T., Verkhratsky, A., Reichenbach, A. & Kettenmann, H. (1999). Microdomains for neuron-glia interaction: parallel fiber signaling to Bergmann glial cells. *Nat Neurosci*, Vol. 2, No. 2, pp. 139-143

Guenther, K., Deacon, R. M., Perry, V. H. & Rawlins, J. N. (2001). Early behavioural changes in scrapie-affected mice and the influence of dapsone. *Eur J Neurosci*, Vol. 14, No. 2, pp. 401-9

Haire, L. F., Whyte, S. M., Vasisht, N., Gill, A. C., Verma, C., Dodson, E. J., Dodson, G. G. & Bayley, P. M. (2004). The crystal structure of the globular domain of sheep prion protein. *J Mol Biol*, Vol. 336, No. 5, pp. 1175-83

Hegde, R. S., Mastrianni, J. A., Scott, M. R., DeFea, K. A., Tremblay, P., Torchia, M., DeArmond, S. J., Prusiner, S. B. & Lingappa, V. R. (1998). A transmembrane form of the prion protein in neurodegenerative disease. *Science*, Vol. 279, No. 5352, pp. 827-34

Herms, J. W., Tings, T., Dunker, S. & Kretzschmar, H. A. (2001). Prion protein affects Ca2+-activated K+ currents in cerebellar purkinje cells. *Neurobiol Dis*, Vol. 8, No. 2, pp. 324-30

Hooper, N. M. (2011). Glypican-1 facilitates prion conversion in lipid rafts. *J Neurochem*, Vol. 116, No. 5, pp. 721-5

Hope, J., Morton, L. J., Farquhar, C. F., Multhaup, G., Beyreuther, K. & Kimberlin, R. H. (1986). The major polypeptide of scrapie-associated fibrils (SAF) has the same size, charge distribution and N-terminal protein sequence as predicted for the normal brain protein (PrP). *Embo J*, Vol. 5, No. 10, pp. 2591-7

Horiuchi, M. & Caughey, B. (1999). Specific binding of normal prion protein to the scrapie form via a localized domain initiates its conversion to the protease-resistant state. *Embo J*, Vol. 18, No. 12, pp. 3193-203

Hornemann, S., Schorn, C. & Wuthrich, K. (2004). NMR structure of the bovine prion protein isolated from healthy calf brains. *EMBO Rep*, Vol. 5, No. 12, pp. 1159-64

Ikeda, S., Kobayashi, A. & Kitamoto, T. (2008). Thr but Asn of the N-glycosylation sites of PrP is indispensable for its misfolding. *Biochem Biophys Res Commun*, Vol. 369, No. 4, pp. 1195-8

Inouye, H., Bond, J., Baldwin, M. A., Ball, H. L., Prusiner, S. B. & Kirschner, D. A. (2000). Structural changes in a hydrophobic domain of the prion protein induced by hydration and by ala-->Val and pro-->Leu substitutions. *J Mol Biol*, Vol. 300, No. 5, pp. 1283-96

Jeffrey, M., Halliday, W. G., Bell, J., Johnston, A. R., MacLeod, N. K., Ingham, C., Sayers, A. R., Brown, D. A. & Fraser, J. R. (2000). Synapse loss associated with abnormal PrP precedes neuronal degeneration in the scrapie-infected murine hippocampus. *Neuropathol Appl Neurobiol*, Vol. 26, No. 1, pp. 41-54

Jeffrey, M., McGovern, G., Siso, S. & Gonzalez, L. (2011). Cellular and sub-cellular pathology of animal prion diseases: relationship between morphological changes, accumulation of abnormal prion protein and clinical disease. *Acta Neuropathologica*, Vol. 121, No. 1, pp. 113-134

Kayed, R., Sokolov, Y., Edmonds, B., McIntire, T. M., Milton, S. C., Hall, J. E. & Glabe, C. G. (2004). Permeabilization of lipid bilayers is a common conformation-dependent activity of soluble amyloid oligomers in protein misfolding diseases. *J Biol Chem*, Vol. 279, No. 45, pp. 46363-6

Kirby, L., Agarwal, S., Graham, J. F., Goldmann, W. & Gill, A. C. (2010). Inverse correlation of thermal lability and conversion efficiency for five prion protein polymorphic variants. *Biochemistry*, Vol. 49, No. 7, pp. 1448-59

Kirby, L., Birkett, C. R., Rudyk, H., Gilbert, I. H. & Hope, J. (2003). *In vitro* cell-free conversion of bacterial recombinant PrP to PrPres as a model for conversion. *J Gen Virol*, Vol. 84, No. 4, pp. 1013-20

Kirby, L., Goldmann, W., Houston, F., Gill, A. C. & Manson, J. C. (2006). A novel, resistance-linked ovine PrP variant and its equivalent mouse variant modulate the *in vitro* cell-free conversion of rPrP to PrP(res). *J Gen Virol*, Vol. 87, No. 12, pp. 3747-51

Knaus, K. J., Morillas, M., Swietnicki, W., Malone, M., Surewicz, W. K. & Yee, V. C. (2001). Crystal structure of the human prion protein reveals a mechanism for oligomerization. *Nat Struct Biol*, Vol. 8, No. 9, pp. 770-4

Kocisko, D. A., Come, J. H., Priola, S. A., Chesebro, B., Raymond, G. J., Lansbury, P. T. & Caughey, B. (1994). Cell-free formation of protease-resistant prion protein. *Nature*, Vol. 370, No. 6489, pp. 471-4

Kocisko, D. A., Priola, S. A., Raymond, G. J., Chesebro, B., Lansbury, P. T., Jr. & Caughey, B. (1995). Species specificity in the cell-free conversion of prion protein to protease-resistant forms: a model for the scrapie species barrier. *Proc Natl Acad Sci U S A*, Vol. 92, No. 9, pp. 3923-7

Kreft, M., Potokar, M., Pangrsic, T., Stenovec, M. & Zorec, R. (2009). Properties of Regulated Exocytosis and Vesicle Trafficking in Astrocytes. *Glia*, Vol. 57, No. 13, pp. S32-S32

Lasmezas, C. I., Deslys, J. P., Robain, O., Jaegly, A., Beringue, V., Peyrin, J. M., Fournier, J. G., Hauw, J. J., Rossier, J. & Dormont, D. (1997). Transmission of the BSE agent to mice in the absence of detectable abnormal prion protein. *Science*, Vol. 275, No. 5298, pp. 402-5

Lee, S., Antony, L., Hartmann, R., Knaus, K. J., Surewicz, K., Surewicz, W. K. & Yee, V. C. (2010). Conformational diversity in prion protein variants influences intermolecular beta-sheet formation. *Embo J*, Vol. 29, No. 1, pp. 251-62

Legname, G., Baskakov, I. V., Nguyen, H. O., Riesner, D., Cohen, F. E., DeArmond, S. J. & Prusiner, S. B. (2004). Synthetic mammalian prions. *Science*, Vol. 305, No. 5684, pp. 673-6

Lehmann, S. & Harris, D. A. (1997). Blockade of glycosylation promotes acquisition of scrapie-like properties by the prion protein in cultured cells. *J Biol Chem*, Vol. 272, No. 34, pp. 21479-87

Li, A., Christensen, H. M., Stewart, L. R., Roth, K. A., Chiesa, R. & Harris, D. A. (2007). Neonatal lethality in transgenic mice expressing prion protein with a deletion of residues 105-125. *Embo J*, Vol. 26, No. 2, pp. 548-58

Lopes, M. H., Hajj, G. N., Muras, A. G., Mancini, G. L., Castro, R. M., Ribeiro, K. C., Brentani, R. R., Linden, R. & Martins, V. R. (2005). Interaction of cellular prion and stress-inducible protein 1 promotes neuritogenesis and neuroprotection by distinct signaling pathways. *J Neurosci*, Vol. 25, No. 49, pp. 11330-9

Lysek, D. A., Schorn, C., Nivon, L. G., Esteve-Moya, V., Christen, B., Calzolai, L., von Schroetter, C., Fiorito, F., Herrmann, T., Guntert, P. & Wuthrich, K. (2005). Prion protein NMR structures of cats, dogs, pigs, and sheep. *Proc Natl Acad Sci U S A*, Vol. 102, No. 3, pp. 640-5

Ma, J., Wollmann, R. & Lindquist, S. (2002). Neurotoxicity and neurodegeneration when PrP accumulates in the cytosol. *Science*, Vol. 298, No. 5599, pp. 1781-5

Maglio, L. E., Martins, V. R., Izquierdo, I. & Ramirez, O. A. (2006). Role of cellular prion protein on LTP expression in aged mice. *Brain Res*, Vol. 1097, No. 1, pp. 11-8

Makarava, N., Kovacs, G. G., Bocharova, O., Savtchenko, R., Alexeeva, I., Budka, H., Rohwer, R. G. & Baskakov, I. V. (2010). Recombinant prion protein induces a new transmissible prion disease in wild-type animals. *Acta Neuropathol*, Vol. 119, No. 2, pp. 177-87

Makarava, N., Lee, C. I., Ostapchenko, V. G. & Baskakov, I. V. (2007). Highly promiscuous nature of prion polymerization. *J Biol Chem*, Vol. 282, No. 50, pp. 36704-13

Mallucci, G., Dickinson, A., Linehan, J., Klohn, P. C., Brandner, S. & Collinge, J. (2003). Depleting neuronal PrP in prion infection prevents disease and reverses spongiosis. *Science*, Vol. 302, No. 5646, pp. 871-4

Manson, J. C., Barron, R. M., Thomson, V., Jamieson, E., Melton, D. W., Ironside, J. & Will, R. (2001). Changing a single amino acid in the N-terminus of murine PrP alters TSE incubation time across three species barriers. *Embo J*, Vol. 20, No. 18, pp. 5070-5078

Manson, J. C., Clarke, A. R., Hooper, M. L., Aitchison, L., Mcconnell, I. & Hope, J. (1994a). 129/Ola Mice Carrying a Null Mutation in Prp That Abolishes Messenger-Rna Production Are Developmentally Normal. *Mol Neurobiol*, Vol. 8, No. 2-3, pp. 121-127

Manson, J. C., Clarke, A. R., McBride, P. A., McConnell, I. & Hope, J. (1994b). PrP gene dosage determines the timing but not the final intensity or distribution of lesions in scrapie pathology. *Neurodegeneration*, Vol. 3, No. 4, pp. 331-40

Martins, I. C., Kuperstein, I., Wilkinson, H., Maes, E., Vanbrabant, M., Jonckheere, W., Van Gelder, P., Hartmann, D., D'Hooge, R., De Strooper, B., Schymkowitz, J. & Rousseau, F. (2008). Lipids revert inert Abeta amyloid fibrils to neurotoxic protofibrils that affect learning in mice. *Embo J*, Vol. 27, No. 1, pp. 224-33

Miele, G., Jeffrey, M., Turnbull, D., Manson, J. & Clinton, M. (2002). Ablation of cellular prion protein expression affects mitochondrial numbers and morphology. *Biochem Biophys Res Commun*, Vol. 291, No. 2, pp. 372-7

Moore, R. A., Timmes, A., Wilmarth, P. A. & Priola, S. A. (2010). Comparative profiling of highly enriched 22L and Chandler mouse scrapie prion protein preparations. *Proteomics*, Vol. 10, No. 15, pp. 2858-69

Muramoto, T., DeArmond, S. J., Scott, M., Telling, G. C., Cohen, F. E. & Prusiner, S. B. (1997). Heritable disorder resembling neuronal storage disease in mice expressing prion protein with deletion of an alpha-helix. *Nat Med*, Vol. 3, No. 7, pp. 750-5

Nadal, R. C., Davies, P., Brown, D. R. & Viles, J. H. (2009). Evaluation of copper2+ affinities for the prion protein. *Biochemistry*, Vol. 48, No. 38, pp. 8929-31

Neuendorf, E., Weber, A., Saalmueller, A., Schatzl, H., Reifenberg, K., Pfaff, E. & Groschup, M. H. (2004). Glycosylation deficiency at either one of the two glycan attachment sites of cellular prion protein preserves susceptibility to bovine spongiform encephalopathy and scrapie infections. *J Biol Chem*, Vol. 279, No. 51, pp. 53306-16

Nishina, K. A., Deleault, N. R., Mahal, S. P., Baskakov, I., Luhrs, T., Riek, R. & Supattapone, S. (2006). The stoichiometry of host PrP^{C} glycoforms modulates the efficiency of PrP^{Sc} formation *in vitro*. *Biochemistry*, Vol. 45, No. 47, pp. 14129-39

Novitskaya, V., Bocharova, O. V., Bronstein, I. & Baskakov, I. V. (2006). Amyloid fibrils of mammalian prion protein are highly toxic to cultured cells and primary neurons. *J Biol Chem*, Vol. 281, No. 19, pp. 13828-36

Paludi, D., Thellung, S., Chiovitti, K., Corsaro, A., Villa, V., Russo, C., Ianieri, A., Bertsch, U., Kretzschmar, H. A., Aceto, A. & Florio, T. (2007). Different structural stability and toxicity of PrP(ARR) and PrP(ARQ) sheep prion protein variants. *J Neurochem*, Vol. 103, No. 6, pp. 2291-300

Pauly, P. C. & Harris, D. A. (1998). Copper stimulates endocytosis of the prion protein. *J Biol Chem*, Vol. 273, No. 50, pp. 33107-10

Pekny, M., Li, L. Z., Lundkvist, A., Andersson, D., Wilhelmsson, U., Nagai, N., Pardo, A. C., Nodin, C., Stahlberg, A., Aprico, K., Larsson, K., Yabe, T., Moons, L., Fotheringham, A., Davies, I., Carmeliet, P., Schwartz, J. P., Pekna, M., Kubista, M., Blomstrand, F., Maragakis, N. & Nilsson, M. (2008). Protective role of reactive astrocytes in brain ischemia. *J Cereb Blood Flow Metab*, Vol. 28, No. 3, pp. 468-481

Perez, D. R., Damberger, F. F. & Wuthrich, K. (2010). Horse prion protein NMR structure and comparisons with related variants of the mouse prion protein. *J Mol Biol*, Vol. 400, No. 2, pp. 121-8

Perry, V. H., Cunningham, C. & Boche, D. (2002). Atypical inflammation in the central nervous system in prion disease. *Curr Opin Neurol*, Vol. 15, No. 3, pp. 349-354

Perry, V. H., Cunningham, C. & Holmes, C. (2007). Systemic infections and inflammation affect chronic neurodegeneration. *Nat Rev Immunol*, Vol. 7, No. 2, pp. 161-167

Perry, V. H., Newman, T. A. & Cunningham, C. (2003). The impact of systemic infection on the progression of neurodegenerative disease. *Nat Rev Neurosci*, Vol. 4, No. 2, pp. 103-112

Perry, V. H. & O'Connor, V. (2010). The role of microglia in synaptic stripping and synaptic degeneration: a revised perspective. *Asn Neuro*, Vol. 2, No. 5, pp. 281-291
Petrakis, S., Malinowska, A., Dadlez, M. & Sklaviadis, T. (2009). Identification of proteins co-purifying with scrapie infectivity. *J Proteomics*, Vol. 72, No. 4, pp. 690-4
Piccardo, P., Manson, J. C., King, D., Ghetti, B. & Barron, R. M. (2007). Accumulation of prion protein in the brain that is not associated with transmissible disease. *Proc Natl Acad Sci U S A*, Vol. 104, No. 11, pp. 4712-7
Piro, J. R., Harris, B. T., Nishina, K., Soto, C., Morales, R., Rees, J. R. & Supattapone, S. (2009). Prion protein glycosylation is not required for strain-specific neurotropism. *J Virol*, Vol. 83, No. 11, pp. 5321-8
Priola, S. A. & Lawson, V. A. (2001). Glycosylation influences cross-species formation of protease-resistant prion protein. *Embo J*, Vol. 20, No. 23, pp. 6692-9
Prusiner, S. B. (1998). Prions. *Proc Natl Acad Sci U S A*, Vol. 95, No. 23, pp. 13363-13383
Quist, A., Doudevski, I., Lin, H., Azimova, R., Ng, D., Frangione, B., Kagan, B., Ghiso, J. & Lal, R. (2005). Amyloid ion channels: a common structural link for protein-misfolding disease. *Proc Natl Acad Sci U S A*, Vol. 102, No. 30, pp. 10427-32
Raeber, A. J., Race, R. E., Brandner, S., Priola, S. A., Sailer, A., Bessen, R. A., Mucke, L., Manson, J., Aguzzi, A., Oldstone, M. B., Weissmann, C. & Chesebro, B. (1997). Astrocyte-specific expression of hamster prion protein (PrP) renders PrP knockout mice susceptible to hamster scrapie. *Embo J*, Vol. 16, No. 20, pp. 6057-65
Ransom, B., Behar, T. & Nedergaard, M. (2003). New roles for astrocytes (stars at last). *Tr Neurosci*, Vol. 26, No. 10, pp. 520-2
Resenberger, U. K., Harmeier, A., Woerner, A. C., Goodman, J. L., Muller, V., Krishnan, R., Vabulas, R. M., Kretzschmar, H. A., Lindquist, S., Hartl, F. U., Multhaup, G., Winklhofer, K. F. & Tatzelt, J. (2011a). The cellular prion protein mediates neurotoxic signalling of beta-sheet-rich conformers independent of prion replication. *Embo J*, Vol. 30, No. 10, pp. 2057-70
Resenberger, U. K., Winklhofer, K. F. & Tatzelt, J. (2011b). Neuroprotective and Neurotoxic Signaling by the Prion Protein. *Top Curr Chem*, Vol. Prion Proteins, No. 305, pp. 101-119
Rezaei, H. (2008). Prion protein oligomerization. *Curr Alzheimer Res*, Vol. 5, No. 6, pp. 572-8
Ritchie, M. A., Gill, A. C., Deery, M. J. & Lilley, K. (2002). Precursor ion scanning for detection and structural characterization of heterogeneous glycopeptide mixtures. *J Am Soc Mass Spectrom*, Vol. 13, No. 9, pp. 1065-77
Robinson, S. R. & Dreher, Z. (1989). Evidence for three morphological classes of astrocyte in the adult rabbit retina: functional and developmental implications. *Neuroscience Letters*, Vol. 106, No. 3, pp. 261-8
Rossetti, G., Cong, X., Caliandro, R., Legname, G. & Carloni, P. (2011). Common Structural Traits across Pathogenic Mutants of the Human Prion Protein and Their Implications for Familial Prion Diseases. *J Mol Biol*, Vol. 411, No. 3, pp. 700-712
Rudd, P. M., Endo, T., Colominas, C., Groth, D., Wheeler, S. F., Harvey, D. J., Wormald, M. R., Serban, H., Prusiner, S. B., Kobata, A. & Dwek, R. A. (1999). Glycosylation differences between the normal and pathogenic prion protein isoforms. *Proc Natl Acad Sci U S A*, Vol. 96, No. 23, pp. 13044-9
Rudd, P. M., Merry, A. H., Wormald, M. R. & Dwek, R. A. (2002). Glycosylation and prion protein. *Curr Opin Struct Biol*, Vol. 12, No. 5, pp. 578-86

Saa, P., Castilla, J. & Soto, C. (2006). Ultra-efficient replication of infectious prions by automated protein misfolding cyclic amplification. *J Biol Chem*, Vol. 281, No. 46, pp. 35245-52

Saborio, G. P., Permanne, B. & Soto, C. (2001). Sensitive detection of pathological prion protein by cyclic amplification of protein misfolding. *Nature*, Vol. 411, No. 6839, pp. 810-3

Salamat, M. K., Dron, M., Chapuis, J., Langevin, C. & Laude, H. (2011). Prion propagation in cells expressing PrP glycosylation mutants. *J Virol*, Vol. 85, No. 7, pp. 3077-85

Sanghera, N., Wall, M., Venien-Bryan, C. & Pinheiro, T. J. (2008). Globular and pre-fibrillar prion aggregates are toxic to neuronal cells and perturb their electrophysiology. *Biochim Biophys Acta*, Vol. 1784, No. 6, pp. 873-81

Shmerling, D., Hegyi, I., Fischer, M., Blattler, T., Brandner, S., Gotz, J., Rulicke, T., Flechsig, E., Cozzio, A., von Mering, C., Hangartner, C., Aguzzi, A. & Weissmann, C. (1998). Expression of amino-terminally truncated PrP in the mouse leading to ataxia and specific cerebellar lesions. *Cell*, Vol. 93, No. 2, pp. 203-14

Silveira, J. R., Raymond, G. J., Hughson, A. G., Race, R. E., Sim, V. L., Hayes, S. F. & Caughey, B. (2005). The most infectious prion protein particles. *Nature*, Vol. 437, No. 7056, pp. 257-61

Simoneau, S., Rezaei, H., Sales, N., Kaiser-Schulz, G., Lefebvre-Roque, M., Vidal, C., Fournier, J. G., Comte, J., Wopfner, F., Grosclaude, J., Schatzl, H. & Lasmezas, C. I. (2007). *In vitro* and in vivo neurotoxicity of prion protein oligomers. *PLoS Pathog*, Vol. 3, No. 8, pp. e125

Siskova, Z., Page, A., O'Connor, V. & Perry, V. H. (2009). Degenerating synaptic boutons in prion disease: microglia activation without synaptic stripping. *Am J Pathol*, Vol. 175, No. 4, pp. 1610-21

Slezak, M. & Pfrieger, F. W. (2003). New roles for astrocytes: regulation of CNS synaptogenesis. *Tr Neurosci*, Vol. 26, No. 10, pp. 531-5

Smirnovas, V., Baron, G. S., Offerdahl, D. K., Raymond, G. J., Caughey, B. & Surewicz, W. K. (2011). Structural organization of brain-derived mammalian prions examined by hydrogen-deuterium exchange. *Nat Struct Mol Biol*, Vol. 18, No. 4, pp. 504-6

Solito, E., McArthur, S., Cristante, E., Paterno, M., Christian, H., Roncaroli, F. & Gillies, G. E. (2010). Annexin A1: A Central Player in the Anti-Inflammatory and Neuroprotective Role of Microglia. *J Immunol*, Vol. 185, No. 10, pp. 6317-6328

Stimson, E., Hope, J., Chong, A. & Burlingame, A. L. (1999). Site-specific characterization of the N-linked glycans of murine prion protein by high-performance liquid chromatography/electrospray mass spectrometry and exoglycosidase digestions. *Biochemistry*, Vol. 38, No. 15, pp. 4885-95

Stohr, J., Elfrink, K., Weinmann, N., Wille, H., Willbold, D., Birkmann, E. & Riesner, D. (2011). *In vitro* conversion and seeded fibrillization of posttranslationally modified prion protein. *Biol Chem*, Vol. 392, No. 5, pp. 415-21

Tahiri-Alaoui, A., Gill, A. C., Disterer, P. & James, W. (2004). Methionine 129 variant of human prion protein oligomerizes more rapidly than the valine 129 variant: implications for disease susceptibility to Creutzfeldt-Jakob disease. *J Biol Chem*, Vol. 279, No. 30, pp. 31390-7

Tahiri-Alaoui, A., Sim, V. L., Caughey, B. & James, W. (2006). Molecular heterosis of prion protein beta-oligomers. A potential mechanism of human resistance to disease. *J Biol Chem*, Vol. 281, No. 45, pp. 34171-8

Tanaka, M., Collins, S. R., Toyama, B. H. & Weissman, J. S. (2006). The physical basis of how prion conformations determine strain phenotypes. *Nature*, Vol. 442, No. 7102, pp. 585-9

Taubner, L. M., Bienkiewicz, E. A., Copie, V. & Caughey, B. (2010). Structure of the flexible amino-terminal domain of prion protein bound to a sulfated glycan. *J Mol Biol*, Vol. 395, No. 3, pp. 475-90

Thackray, A. M., Yang, S., Wong, E., Fitzmaurice, T. J., Morgan-Warren, R. J. & Bujdoso, R. (2004). Conformational variation between allelic variants of cell-surface ovine prion protein. *Biochem J*, Vol. 381, No. 1, pp. 221-9

Tobler, I., Gaus, S. E., Deboer, T., Achermann, P., Fischer, M., Rulicke, T., Moser, M., Oesch, B., McBride, P. A. & Manson, J. C. (1996). Altered circadian activity rhythms and sleep in mice devoid of prion protein. *Nature*, Vol. 380, No. 6575, pp. 639-42

Tuzi, N. L., Cancellotti, E., Baybutt, H., Blackford, L., Bradford, B., Plinston, C., Coghill, A., Hart, P., Piccardo, P., Barron, R. M. & Manson, J. C. (2008). Host PrP glycosylation: a major factor determining the outcome of prion infection. *PLoS Biol*, Vol. 6, No. 4, pp. e100

Tuzi, N. L., Clarke, A. R., Bradford, B., Aitchison, L., Thomson, V. & Manson, J. C. (2004). Cre-loxP mediated control of PrP to study transmissible spongiform encephalopathy diseases. *Genesis*, Vol. 40, No. 1, pp. 1-6

van der Kamp, M. W. & Daggett, V. (2010). Pathogenic mutations in the hydrophobic core of the human prion protein can promote structural instability and misfolding. *J Mol Biol*, Vol. 404, No. 4, pp. 732-48

Vanik, D. L. & Surewicz, W. K. (2002). Disease-associated F198S mutation increases the propensity of the recombinant prion protein for conformational conversion to scrapie-like form. *J Biol Chem*, Vol. 277, No. 50, pp. 49065-70

Waggoner, D. J., Drisaldi, B., Bartnikas, T. B., Casareno, R. L., Prohaska, J. R., Gitlin, J. D. & Harris, D. A. (2000). Brain copper content and cuproenzyme activity do not vary with prion protein expression level. *J Biol Chem*, Vol. 275, No. 11, pp. 7455-8

Wang, F., Wang, X., Yuan, C. G. & Ma, J. (2010). Generating a prion with bacterially expressed recombinant prion protein. *Science*, Vol. 327, No. 5969, pp. 1132-5

Weber, P., Giese, A., Piening, N., Mitteregger, G., Thomzig, A., Beekes, M. & Kretzschmar, H. A. (2007). Generation of genuine prion infectivity by serial PMCA. *Vet Microbiol*, Vol. 123, No. 4, pp. 346-57

Weissmann, C. (1991). A 'unified theory' of prion propagation. *Nature*, Vol. 352, No. 6337, pp. 679-83

Whittal, R. M., Ball, H. L., Cohen, F. E., Burlingame, A. L., Prusiner, S. B. & Baldwin, M. A. (2000). Copper binding to octarepeat peptides of the prion protein monitored by mass spectrometry. *Protein Sci*, Vol. 9, No. 2, pp. 332-43

Wille, H., Michelitsch, M. D., Guenebaut, V., Supattapone, S., Serban, A., Cohen, F. E., Agard, D. A. & Prusiner, S. B. (2002). Structural studies of the scrapie prion protein by electron crystallography. *Proc Natl Acad Sci U S A*, Vol. 99, No. 6, pp. 3563-8

Wong, B. S., Venien-Bryan, C., Williamson, R. A., Burton, D. R., Gambetti, P., Sy, M. S., Brown, D. R. & Jones, I. M. (2000a). Copper refolding of prion protein. *Biochem Biophys Res Commun*, Vol. 276, No. 3, pp. 1217-24

Wong, N. K., Renouf, D. V., Lehmann, S. & Hounsell, E. F. (2000b). Glycosylation of prions and its effects on protein conformation relevant to amino acid mutations. *J Mol Graph Model*, Vol. 18, No. 2, pp. 126-34, 163-5

Wuthrich, K. & Riek, R. (2001). Three-dimensional structures of prion proteins. *Adv Protein Chem*, Vol. 57, No. pp. 55-82

Yin, S., Pham, N., Yu, S., Li, C., Wong, P., Chang, B., Kang, S. C., Biasini, E., Tien, P., Harris, D. A. & Sy, M. S. (2007). Human prion proteins with pathogenic mutations share common conformational changes resulting in enhanced binding to glycosaminoglycans. *Proc Natl Acad Sci U S A*, Vol. 104, No. 18, pp. 7546-51

Zhang, C., Jackson, A. P., Zhang, Z. R., Han, Y., Yu, S., He, R. Q. & Perrett, S. (2010). Amyloid-like aggregates of the yeast prion protein ure2 enter vertebrate cells by specific endocytotic pathways and induce apoptosis. *PLoS One*, Vol. 5, No. 9, pp e12529.

5

Molecular Pathogenesis of Prion Diseases

Giuseppe Legname[1] and Gianluigi Zanusso[2]
[1]*Scuola Internazionale Superiore di Studi Avanzati,*
[2]*Università degli Studi di Verona,*
Italy

1. Introduction

Prion diseases or transmissible spongiform encephalopathies (TSEs) are rare, fatal and incurable neurodegenerative disorders of humans and animals (Prusiner, 1998).

In humans, prion diseases occur with unique aetiology as sporadic, genetic or infectious disorders. Sporadic cases of prion diseases, which account for the majority of casualties (up to 85% of all cases), are of unknown origin; the genetic forms are less frequent (up to 15%), while the infectious cases are extremely rare with an incidence of less than 1% (Prusiner, 2001). Creutzfeldt-Jakob disease (CJD), Gerstmann-Sträussler-Scheinker (GSS) syndrome, Fatal Familial Insomnia (FFI) are examples of human prion diseases. In animals the disease is mostly infectious and the mode of transmission is horizontal. Prion diseases include scrapie in sheep and goats, bovine spongiform encephalopathy (BSE) in cattle, and chronic wasting disease of deer, elk, and moose (Williams, 2005).

The agents responsible for prion diseases are infectious proteins named prions. The term 'prion' was coined when Stanley B. Prusiner introduced the concept of *proteinaceous infectious particles* (Prusiner, 1982). Since the introduction of this once heretical notion, mounting evidence has strengthened its validity.

In the next sections of this chapter we present and discuss the peculiar complexity of the molecular pathogenesis of prion diseases in humans and animals.

2. Prion protein and prions

2.1 The prion protein

The prion protein (PrP) is one of the most and best-studied models for misfolding diseases. The cellular form of PrP (PrP^C) is a glysosyl-phosphatidylinositol (GPI) anchored polypeptide present on the outer leaflet of the cellular membrane of most cell types in mammals. In humans, the *PRNP* gene, located in the short arm of chromosome 20 (Liao et al., 1986), features two exons. The second exon contains the entire open reading frame (ORF), which encodes for the protein. The PrP^C is composed of 253 amino acids in humans, including 22 amino acids of endoplasmic reticulum signal sequence at the N-terminus and 23 amino acids as GPI anchoring signal at the C-terminus (Stahl et al., 1990). The N-terminal region of PrP^C encompasses five characteristic amino acid octarepeats that coordinate copper and, to a lesser extent, other metal ions. The mature 208-residues protein possesses a single disulphide bridge between Cys179 and Cys214, and two sites for Asn-linked glycosylation within the carboxy-terminal region at position Asn181 and Asn197.

The protein is the first system where a polypeptide has been shown to exist in at least two significantly different conformations, associated with radically different functions.

The physiological function of PrP^C has not been established with certainty yet; nevertheless its evolutionarily conserved sequence suggests that it might play an important role in neuronal development and physiology. Indeed one recent finding indicates a possible involvement of this protein in neuronal differentiation and polarization (Kanaani et al., 2005). On account of additional evidence, it could also contribute to myelin formation and maintenance (Benvegnu et al., 2011a).

A strategy often employed to identify protein function is the development of transgenic mouse lines with a disabled gene. Many lines of knockout (KO) mice have been developed for PrP (Weissmann and Flechsig, 2003). In these models, typically either the entire ORF of exon 3 of *Prnp* (in mice), or the ORF as well as flanking sequences are deleted (Weissmann and Flechsig, 2003). The *Prnp* KO mice ($Prnp^{0/0}$) appear to develop and reproduce normally (Bueler et al., 1992), but their further evaluation found several abnormalities. The mice appear clinically asymptomatic yet they develop peripheral nerve demyelination, have increased susceptibility to ischemic brain injury, altered sleep and circadian rhythm, altered hippocampal neuropathology and physiology, including deficits in hippocampal-dependent spatial learning and hippocampal synaptic plasticity (Tobler et al., 1997, Nishida et al., 1999, Spudich et al., 2005, Criado et al., 2005). Mice with $Prnp^{0/0}$ are also more susceptible to oxidative stress, and PrP^C appears to play a neuroprotective role in cellular response to hypoxic-ischemic injury (Weise et al., 2006). Some $Prnp^{0/0}$ mouse lines in which the deletion extends beyond the ORF, although developing normally, acquire ataxia and Purkinje cell loss later in life (Moore et al., 1999).

Recent findings show development regional differences of the expression of PrP in mouse central nervous system (CNS), with specific white matter structures showing the earliest and highest expression of PrP^C. Indeed, all these regions are part of the thalamo-limbic neurocircuitry, hence suggesting a potential role of PrP^C in the development and functioning of this specific brain system (Benvegnu et al., 2010).

Furthermore, the transcriptome during development for the CNS of mice lacking a functional *Prnp* gene has recently been compared with that of wild-type animals (Benvegnu et al., 2011b). To assess the influence of PrP^C on gene expression profile in the mouse brain, a microarray analysis was undertaken using RNA isolated from the hippocampus at two different developmental stages: newborn (4.5-day-old) and adult (3-month-old) mice, both from wild-type and *Prnp* KO animals. Based on the comparison of these datasets, *commonly* co-regulated genes and *uniquely* de-regulated genes during postnatal development were identified. The absence of PrP^C affected several biological pathways, the most representative ones being cell signaling, cell-cell communication and transduction processes, calcium homeostasis, nervous system development, and synaptic transmission and cell adhesion. However, there was only a moderate alteration of the gene expression profile in our animal models. PrP^C deficiency did not lead to a dramatic alteration of gene expression profile, and produced moderately altered gene expression levels from young to adult animals. Hence, these results further support silencing endogenous PrP^C as therapeutic approach to prion diseases (Benvegnu et al., 2011b).

Concerning PrP^C cellular function, experiments have recently shown that PrP^C regulates the cleavage of neuregulin-1 proteins (NRG1). Neuregulins provide key axonal signals, which regulate processes, including glial cells proliferation, survival and myelination. Interestingly, $Prnp^{0/0}$ mice have recently been reported to have a late-onset demyelinating disease in the peripheral nervous system (PNS), but not in the CNS (Bremer et al., 2010). The comparison of wild-type and $Prnp^{0/0}$ mice showed that the NRG1 processing is developmentally regulated in the PNS and influenced by PrP^C in old but not in young animals. In addition, it has been found that neuregulin-3 processing – another neuregulin family member – is altered in the PNS of $Prnp^{0/0}$ mice. These differences in neuregulin proteins processing are not paralleled in the CNS, thus suggesting a different cellular function for PrP^C between the CNS and the PNS (Benvegnu et al., 2011a).

2.2 Prions and the biology of the conversion mechanism

Prion diseases are caused by changes in the conformation of the endogenous PrP^C, which turns into an alternatively folded, disease-causing form called the prion, or PrP^{Sc}. The normal PrP^C contains three α-helixes and two short β-sheet structures in its globular domain, whereas PrP^{Sc} contains fewer α-helical and mostly β-sheet structures (Prusiner, 1998). PrP^C and PrP^{Sc} possess the same primary polypeptide sequence, but different secondary and tertiary structures. PrP^{Sc} is produced by the conversion of existing PrP^C into PrP^{Sc}.

The process leading to PrP^{Sc} production from PrP^C is not completely understood. It is believed that this occurs when PrP^C comes into contact with PrP^{Sc} and is thus induced to take on the shape of PrP^{Sc} (Prusiner, 1998). The fact that mice devoid of PrP^C are resistant to infection, as they are unable to replicate prions, provides strong evidence that PrP^C is necessary for prion disease (Bueler et al., 1993). Although it is clear that PrP^C is necessary for prion disease, it is still debated whether other proteins or molecules are involved in the conformational change *in vivo* (Telling et al., 1995, Deleault et al., 2003). The conversion of monomeric PrP^C into insoluble, protease-resistant PrP^{Sc} is a process that seems to occur in structures denominated caveolae-like domains (CLDs) (Gorodinsky and Harris, 1995), and the resulting PrP^{Sc} subsequently traffics to other membranous compartments such as endosomes and lysosomes (Marijanovic et al., 2009). The membranes of CLDs seem to be composed of cholesterol-rich rafts and presumably provide the cellular environment for the formation of PrP^{Sc}. Two conversion and replication models have been proposed: (i) a nucleation-polymerization reaction, and (ii) a template-assisted conversion process. In the first model, the rate-limiting step is the formation of a critical amount of PrP^{Sc} to form a *seed* for the polymerization of PrP^{Sc}. In the template-assisted model, PrP^C must first undergo conversion toward a transition state that presumably corresponds to a partially destabilized structure (Aguzzi and Calella, 2009). The structural transition could be mediated by an auxiliary molecule, which facilitates the conversion to a nascent prion (Telling et al., 1995, Deleault et al., 2003). In disease-affected brain homogenates, limited proteolysis completely hydrolyzes PrP^C and produces a protease-resistant PrP^{Sc} molecule of about 140 amino acids, designated PrP27–30. In the presence of detergent, PrP27–30 polymerizes into amyloid (McKinley et al., 1991). Prion amyloids, or rods, formed by limited proteolysis and detergent extraction, are indistinguishable from the filaments that aggregate to form PrP amyloid plaques in the CNS, exhibiting similar ultrastructural morphology and tinctorial characteristics after staining with Congo red dye (Prusiner et al., 1983). So far, little is known about the structure of prions. Several models have been proposed, attempting to satisfy all available biophysical, biochemical and immunochemical data on infectious prions (Govaerts et al., 2004). The discovery that recombinant PrP, expressed in *Escherichia coli*, is infectious to mice when polymerized into amyloid fibrils has opened new avenues for research in the prion field (Legname et al., 2004). Characterization of these synthetic prions revealed novel distinctiveness associated with neuropathological changes in mouse models of prion disease (Legname et al., 2005). The conformational changes acquired by the synthetic prions confer increasing stability to PrP^{Sc}, as measured by the amount of chaotropic agents necessary to completely unfold PrP^{Sc}. Moreover, a linear correlation is established when the measure of stability of any particular isolate is expressed as a function of mouse survival times to the disease (Legname et al., 2006).

One of the strongest arguments for the existence of prions is the link between inherited prion diseases and mutations in the *PRNP* gene. Currently, almost 60 pathogenic mutations and several polymorphisms have been identified in the *PRNP* gene (Kovacs et al., 2002). They include missense point mutations, mostly located in the globular part, insertion or deletion mutations involving the N-terminal domain, and non-sense mutations resulting in the premature termination of PrP synthesis. Twelve polymorphisms are silent, while four of them alter the amino acid sequence. The most important one that markedly influences the disease is the M/V polymorphism at codon 129 (Collinge, 2001). The M/V polymorphism at position 129 is common; the homozygous M/M and V/V and the heterozygous M/V subjects account for 43%, 8% and 49%, respectively, in the Caucasian population (Zimmermann et al., 1999). This polymorphism is a key determinant of genetic susceptibility to acquired and sporadic prion diseases, the large majority of which occur in homozygous individuals (Collinge et al., 1991, Palmer et al., 1991, Windl et al., 1996). The *PRNP* heterozygotes appear to be protected from sporadic CJD (sCJD) compared to the *PRNP* homozygotes (Kobayashi et al., 2009, Baker et al., 1991, Hsiao et al., 1992). The M/V polymorphism at position 129 affects the disease phenotype when it is located on the mutant allele: D178N-129V causes familial CJD (fCJD), while D178N-129M is responsible for familial FFI. The M/V polymorphism located on the normal allele affects the age onset and duration of the disease. Patients carrying either M or V 129 codon have been observed in all inherited prion diseases. The altered conformation observed in human PrP mutants might lead to a different affinity for extracellular matrix components and cellular membranes and, consequently, to an aberrant localization of PrP in different cellular compartments, favoring formation of altered pathogenic topologies (Hegde et al., 1999). Independent evidence derived from cell culture studies, expressing some of the disease-linked mutants, showed that these mutations may affect folding and maturation of PrP^{C} in the secretory pathway of neuronal cells (Ashok and Hegde, 2009).

How mutations and polymorphisms can structurally modulate the diseases is not clear. In fact, until recently there was no evidence of a pathological point mutation causing substantial structural differences in PrP folding.

To shed new light on the role of pathological point mutations on PrP structure, a high-resolution 3D structure of the truncated recombinant human PrP containing the pathological

Q212P mutation has recently been determined and examined (Ilc et al., 2010). This mutation is responsible for a GSS syndrome characterized by mild amyloid PrP deposition in patients (Piccardo et al., 1998, Young et al., 1998). The high-resolution NMR structure of Q212P mutant revealed unique conformational features compared to the known structures of either human or other mammalian PrP^{C} (Christen et al., 2009, Christen et al., 2008, Gossert et al., 2005, Lopez Garcia et al., 2000, Riek et al., 1996).

The most remarkable differences involved the C-terminal end of the protein and the β_2–α_2 loop region. The Q212P mutant is the first known example of PrP structure where the α_3 helix between E200 and Y226 is broken into two helices. This breakage brings about dramatic changes in the hydrophobic interactions between the α_3 helix and the β_2–α_2 loop region. In the wild-type protein, long-range interactions between Y225 and M166 define the position of the β_2–α_2 loop and thus the tertiary structure of the protein. In this protein type, the solvent-exposed surface of the β_2–α_2 loop and the α_3 helix region is smaller, and Y169 is buried inside the hydrophobic cluster (Ilc et al., 2010).

When these structural findings are compared with the already resolved NMR structures of human PrP, carrying respectively the CJD-related E200K (Zhang et al., 2000) and the artificial R220K mutation, the α_3 helix appears well ordered up to the point mutation (Calzolai et al., 2000). After this mutation, the α_3 helix shows increased flexibility and significantly less order. At the same time, the R220K mutation does not alter the hydrophobic interactions between the aromatic residues of the β_2–α_2 loop and the α_3 helix.

Special interest in prion biology is therefore focused on the epitope formed by the β_2–α_2 loop and the α_3 helix, as this surface has been implicated in interactions with a hypothetical facilitator of prion conversion involved in the development of TSEs (Kaneko et al., 1997, Telling et al., 1995). Therefore, the plasticity of the loop may modulate the susceptibility to prion disease of a given species. While in PrP^{C} from most mammalian species this loop is flexible, it is well defined in PrP^{C} of elk (Gossert et al., 2005), bank vole (*Clethrionomys glareolus*) (Christen et al., 2008), tammar wallaby (Christen et al., 2009) and, as found out very recently, horse (Perez et al., 2010) and rabbit (Wen et al., 2010). Interestingly, elk and bank vole are highly susceptible to TSEs, whereas there have been no cases of prion diseases either in marsupials, horses or rabbits. The structure-function relationship suggested by these works may provide the molecular basis for understanding the generation of PrP^{Sc} in inherited prion diseases. In fact, the characterization of high-resolution structures of PrP pathological mutants and their comparison with the wild-type overall folding, highlights important regions in these proteins that could be involved in early events of PrP misfolding. This may also provide a molecular explanation for prion formation in the sporadic forms of prion disease.

3. Molecular pathogenesis of prion diseases

3.1 PrP^{Sc} conformers in human and animal prion disorders

Human and animal TSEs exist as different prion strains characterized by distinct biological properties. A prion strain is defined using several criteria, such as incubation time and lesion profile after transmission, as well as by physico-chemical characteristics of pathological PrP^{Sc} conformers (Bruce et al., 1994, Aguzzi et al., 2008).

Several studies demonstrated that prion strains can be distinguished based on different biochemical properties of PrP^{Sc}, encompassing conformation, glycoform profile, degrees of protease-resistance under different denaturing conditions, thus allowing a molecular strain typing classification of PrP^{Sc} (Wadsworth and Collinge, 2011). Treatment of PrP^{Sc} with proteinase K (PK) generates a large PK-resistant C-terminal core fragment termed PrP27-30 which is considered the pathogenic and infectious core of PrP^{Sc}. Full-length PrP^{Sc} and PrP27-30 are associated to the naturally occurring infectious agent causing prion diseases and are thought to be the primary cause of the histological changes in brains of subjects with prion diseases.

In human and animal prion disorders, the remarkable heterogeneity of disease phenotypes is influenced by the combination of either PrP^{Sc} type or relevant *PRNP* polymorphisms (Gambetti et al., 2011).

3.2 The biochemical phenotype of PrP^{Sc} in human and animal TSEs

In human prion disorders, several different types of PrP^{Sc} have been recognized. PrP^{Sc} types are distinguished based on the electrophoretic migration and the glycosylation profile of PrP27-30. This is composed of a major triplet of bands which represent the differently glycosylated isoforms of PrP^{Sc}.

Additional minor C-terminally truncated fragments (CTFs) resistant to proteases have been reported and they contribute to define the *biochemical strains* of PrP^{Sc}. The combination of PrP27-30 and CTFs is representative of specific patterns and correlates to distinct disease phenotypes (Zou et al., 2003, Zanusso et al., 2004).

In sCJD, three distinct PrP^{Sc} types have been described: type 1, type 2A and type U (Fig. 1A). Type 1 and type 2 PrP^{Sc} are distinguished based on the different electrophoretic mobility of the unglycosylated form of approximately 21kDa in type 1, and 19kDa in type 2, respectively (Parchi et al., 1999, Gambetti et al., 2003). In contrast, type U PrP^{Sc} shares apparent gel mobility with type 1, though it lacks the diglycosylated isoforms (Zanusso et al., 2007).

In variant CJD (vCJD), an unglycosylated band migrating at 19kDa and a highly glycosylated-dominant profile characterize PrP^{Sc}; wheresas type 2A PrP^{Sc} in sCJD is distinguished by the highly glycosylated-dominant profile. Accordingly, the current nomenclature defines type 2A-PrP^{Sc} associated to sCJD, and type 2B-PrP^{Sc} associated to vCJD, thus identifying BSE agent in humans (Collinge et al. 1996). In familial forms of CJD (E200K-129V) and FFI forms, a type 2B-like pattern is observed (Fig. 1A). The exception to the conventional definition of PrP^{Sc} typing is observed in GSS mutations. In GSS, PrP27-30 is absent and pathological PrP is composed of intermediate fragments (IFs) of ~11kDa and ~8kDa spanning residues ~90-150 and ~60-150 (Tagliavini et al., 1991, Tagliavini et al., 1994, Piccardo et al., 1998). According to their sequence, these IFs lack PrP post-translational modifications, including GPI-anchor.

However, in GSS P102L mutation, a hybrid phenotype of PrP^{Sc} is observed. In P102L, PrP^{Sc} is characterized by the presence of the 8kDa intermediate fragment (PrP8), as in other GSS, but also of PrP27-30 (Parchi et al., 1998) (Fig. 1A).

Although prion diseases are defined based on the presence of a disease-associated protease-resistant PrP that has been proven to retain infectivity, Gambetti *et al.* shifted this dogmatic definition. They reported on a series of individuals with dementia and spongiform encephalopathy but with a PrP resistant to minimal amount of PK, thus designating this novel form of prion disease as *variably protease-sensitive prionopathy* (or VPSPr) (Gambetti et al., 2008). Interestingly, in these cases the biochemical pattern of PrP is variable, as it contains both C-terminal fragments and intermediate fragments with molecular masses ranging from 20kDa to 7kDa (Zou et al., 2010) (Fig. 1A).

Over the last few years, the PrP^{Sc} biochemical types described in animal prion disorders have consistently increased, following the systematic testing of over 30-month-old cattle, carried out by several European countries in 2001. The diagnostic test relied on the detection of protease-resistant PrP by Western blot in the animals' brain tissue. This preventive measure allowed to detect all BSE-affected cattle, but also to recognize two additional BSE-associated PrP^{Sc} types, distinguished from classical BSE (C-BSE) for the different electrophoretic migration and pattern of PrP glycosylation. According to the higher and lower electrophoretic migration of the unglycosylated fragment of PrP^{Sc} compared to C-BSE, these "atypical" BSE forms were named H-type and L-type BSE, respectively (Biacabe et al., 2004, Casalone et al., 2004) (Fig. 1B).

The wide scale screening testing for prions on small ruminants resulted in similar findings, since additional PrP^{Sc} types were also found in scrapie. In particular, beside the classical scrapie strain, other atypical forms — originally named Nor 98 — have been reported; these are characterized by small intermediate truncated fragments of PrP associated to PrP27-30 (Benestad et al., 2003, Benestad et al., 2008) (Fig. 1C).

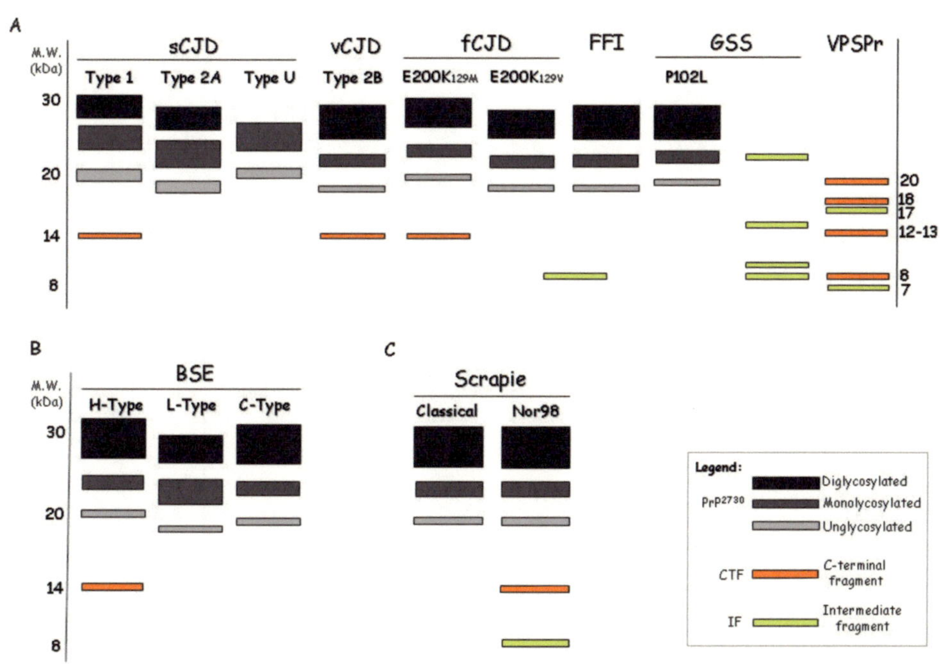

Fig. 1. PrP^{Sc} fragment patterns in human and animal prion disorders. Gel pattern of PrP^{Sc} in human forms (A), in BSE affected cattle (B), and in scrapie in sheep (C). Strains of TSE are defined in part by biochemical properties of PrP^{Sc} (glycosylation and size), pattern of PrP^{Sc} deposition in brain, and average age of disease onset.

3.3 Correlation between biochemical phenotypes of PrP^{Sc}, disease-phenotypes and prion strain biological properties

Several studies indicate that distinct PrP^{Sc} patterns represent the molecular signature of prion and have relevant biological implications including neuropathological phenotype and transmissibility. For instance, the occurrence of spongiform changes or amyloid deposits are strictly dependent on PrP^{Sc} species in brain tissue (Table 1).

	sCJD, fCJD, iCJD	vCJD	FFI	GSS		VPSPr
				Classic	P102L	
Clinical Phenotype	Subacute dementing illness with visual, cerebellar and/or extrapyramidal signs, myoclonus	Psychiatric features, painful distal sensations, cerebellar signs	Sleep disruption, dysautonomia, motor abnormalities	Slow progressive dementia and ataxia, pyramidal and extrapyramidal signs	As sCJD or classic GSS	Cognitive decline, mood or behavioural changes
Disease Duration	Weeks, months, less than two years	Months or years	15 months (6-42)	5-6 years	36 months (3-72)	20 months (10-60)
Pathological Phenotype	SD, astrogliosis, neuronal loss, amyloid plaques	SD, astrogliosis, neuronal loss, florid amyloid plaques	SD, astrogliosis, neuronal loss, mainly thalamic	Widespread amyloid deposits, neuronal loss, astrogliosis, NFTs	SD, astrogliosis or as classic GSS	SD, minimal astrogliosis
Pattern of PrP Deposition	Synaptic/punctate, and/or amyloid plaques	Synaptic/ punctate, florid plaques	Fine punctuate staining	Multi-centric amyloid plaques	As sCJD or in classic GSS	Intense staining, plaque- and dot-like
PrP^{Sc} Biochemical Phenotype	Type 1 Type 2A CTF12-14	Type 2B CTF12-14	Type 2B-like CTF12-14	PrP8 and 11kDa IFs	PrP27-30 and PrP8	CTFs IFs
Transmissible	Yes	Yes	Yes	No	Yes/No	Pending

Legend: iCJD: iatrogenic CJD; SD: spongiform degeneration; NFTs: neurofibrillary tangles; CTFs: C-terminal fragments; IFs: intermediate fragments; PsPr: protease-sensitive PrP;

Table 1. Disease characteristics of human prion disorders

However, this assumption is not fulfilled in GSS, since subjects carrying mutations, which segregate with GSS, except P102L, show a different disease phenotype, lacking PrP27-30 (Ghetti et al., 2003). As expected, spongiform changes are not observed and the intermediate fragments promote a PrP amyloidogenesis process widespread to all brain tissue.

Experimental studies *in vitro* showed the high propensity of these peptides to form amyloid aggregates (Salmona et al., 2003). Further, GSS does not propagate as a spongiform encephalopathy. In other words, unlike other prion diseases, GSS shares the disease characteristics of several other non-transmissible neurodegenerative disorders (Fig. 2).

A first link between PrP pattern and pathological phenotype involves PrP27-30 and the detection of spongiform degeneration. In general all prion disorders associated with PrP27-30, either in humans or in animals, are characterized by spongiform degeneration and astrogliosis. Further, the presence of PrP27-30 is related to transmissibility in susceptible recipients (Fig. 2).

In contrast, in P102L mutation spongiform changes and diffuse multicentre amyloid plaques are observed, sharing disease characteristics of both CJD and GSS. These findings correlate to the presence of both PrP27-30 and PrP8 (Wadsworth et al., 2006), and only P102L cases with PrP27-30 transmitted the disease, whereas others did not. In particular, a spongiform encephalopathy was observed only in transgenic mice challenged with P102L human cases showing spongiform degeneration and PrP27-30 (Piccardo et al., 2007).

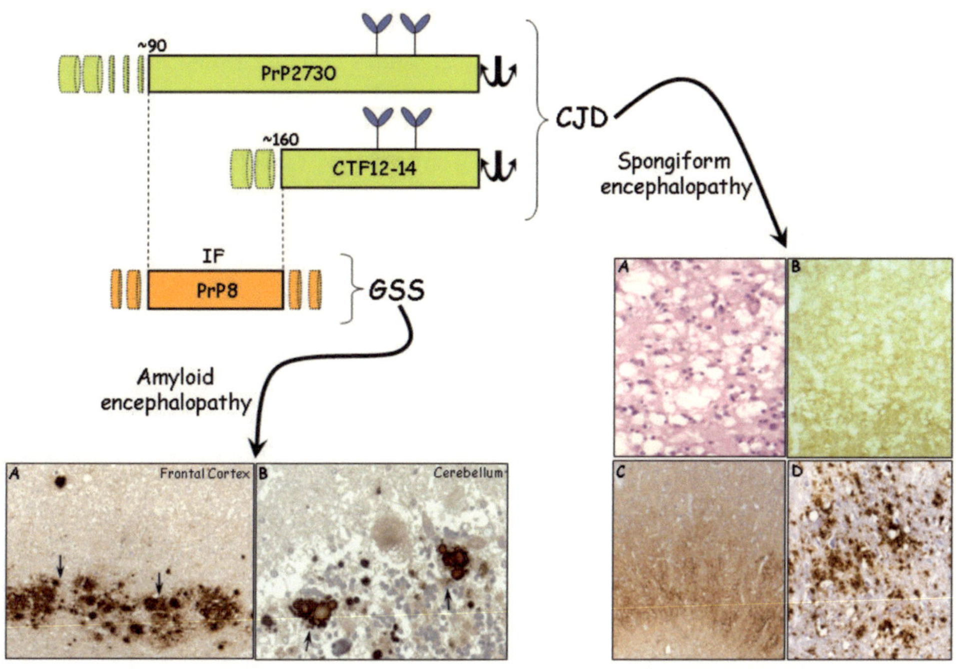

Fig. 2. Correlative analysis between PrP^{Sc} fragments and pathological phenotype.

In sCJD, the biochemical phenotype of PrP^{Sc} comprises both PrP27-30 and CTFs, resulting in a spongiform encephalopathy and different patterns of PrP deposition.

Conversely, in GSS, where PrP deposits consist of an intermediate fragment (PrP8), which lacks post-translational modifications including GPI anchor, the pathological phenotype is characterized by PrP amyloid multicentric plaques (arrows).

VPSPr-affected subjects have a weakly PK-resistant PrP and neuropathologically they show the distinct feature of a spongiform encephalopathy. As mentioned above, both PrP C-terminal fragments — indicating that most of them are GPI-anchored — consist mainly of those fragments forming the PrP pattern. Since IFs do not generate spongiform changes, these findings indicate that GPI-anchored PrP molecules might be associated with spongiform degeneration. As known from transgenic GPI anchorless mice, GPI anchorless PrP is able to replicate inducing an amyloidotic disease but not a spongiform encephalopathy (Chesebro et al., 2005).

3.4 The biological properties of prion strains are enciphered in the biochemical pattern of PrP^{Sc}: A lesson from two-dimensional analysis

In sCJD, a sextet of subtypes was recognized, characterized by disease phenotypic heterogeneity, which results from the combination of two PrP^{Sc} types and the polymorphism M/V at codon 129 (Parchi et al., 1999).

A decade ago we performed a 2D analysis — which separates proteins by molecular weight and isoelectric point — aimed at introducing a technique to better define the biochemical phenotype of PrP^{Sc}, beyond the conventional patterns obtained by SDS-PAGE (Zanusso et al., 2002). In particular, we argued whether additional PrP conformers might be observed within a given PrP27-30 band. In all sCJD cases associated with type 1 PrP^{Sc}, regardless of the polymorphism at codon 129, the 2D pattern of PrP27-30 and C-terminal fragments (CTFs) is identical (Fig. 3A). Conversely, we showed that type 2 PrP^{Sc} separated as two distinct patterns, one in MM2 cortical (MM2C) and the other in MV2 and VV2, which correlated with distinct pathological phenotypes. In particular, MM2 is characterized by a severe SD in the cerebral cortex with a relative spare of the cerebellum and a coarse pattern of PrP deposition, while in MV2 and VV2 the distribution of lesions is more diffuse, mostly concentrated in the cerebellum, with abundant amyloid plaques (Zanusso et al., 2004) (Fig. 3B and 3C).

PrP27-30 core fragment is depicted in black. The different spots composing PrP27-30 represent the N-terminally truncated fragments. The 16-17-kDa and the 12-14 kDa truncated fragments are seen in sCJD with type 1, and correlate to a synaptic PrP staining seen in the frontal cortex and cerebellum. MM2C and MV2/VV2 subtypes show distinct PrP 27-30 patterns and CTFs. In MM2C, CTFs are composed of 12-14 kDa species, while in MV2/VV2 these consist of 16-17kDa fragments. These biochemical patterns correlate to distinct pathological phenotypes.

These results were subsequently confirmed by transmission studies. In transgenic mice targeting and expressing different forms of *PRNP* (MM, MV, VV), MM1 and MV1 isolates showed similar biological properties, while the strain associated with an MV2 patient could not be distinguished from the VV2 strain, and MM2 isolate transmitted poorly (Bishop et al., 2010). In the bank vole, MM1 and MV1 CJD also behaved as similar agents, and differed from MM2 CJD. MV2 and VV2 did not transmit (Nonno et al., 2006).

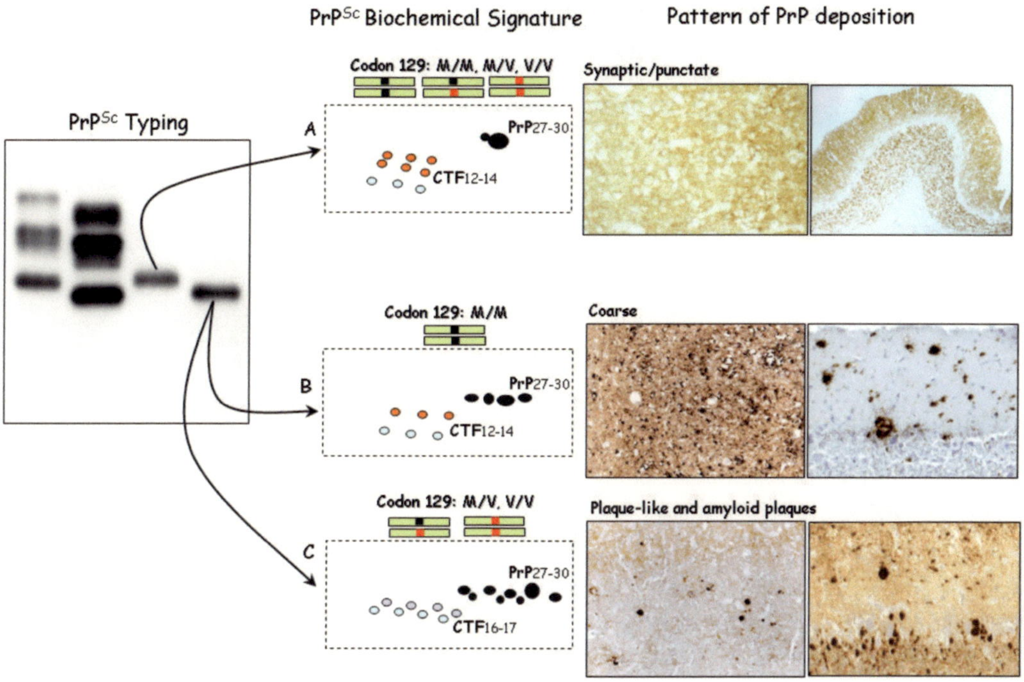

Fig. 3. Schematic diagram of PK-resistant C-terminal PrP core fragments in sCJD subtypes.

3.4.1 The biochemical link between animal and human prion forms is enciphered in PrP^{Sc}

We firstly proposed a parallel between sCJD in humans and BSE in cattle, by showing that MV2 sCJD subtype shared molecular similarities with cattle affected with bovine amyloidotic spongiform encephalopathy (BASE) including the pathological phenotype (Casalone et al., 2004, Brown et al., 2006). As in humans, two presumably sporadic forms of BSE are observed in cattle in addition to typical/classical BSE. Moreover, the apparent molecular weight of the unglycosylated band of bovine amyloidotic spongiform encephalopathy is identical to that of type 2A, while H-type BSE corresponds to type 1 PrP^{Sc} (Fig. 4). Of course, the link between C-BSE and vCJD had been largely demonstrated.

Wemheuer et al. proposed a correlation between classical and atypical/Nor98 scrapie in sheep and sCJD, showing that the two scrapie types share a number of striking similarities with human PrP^{Sc} types in sCJD (Wemheuer et al., 2009) (Fig. 4).

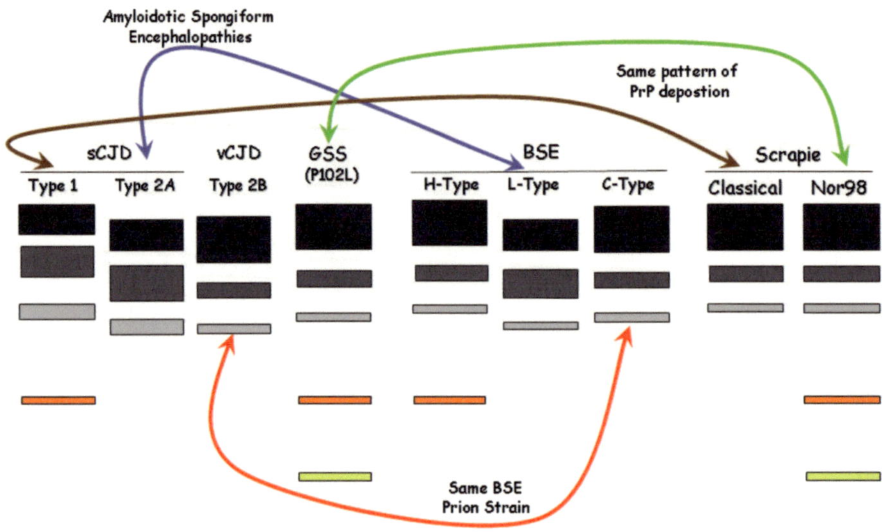

Fig. 4. Correlative analysis of PrP^{Sc} biochemical phenotype in different BSE, CJD and scrapie isolates. Arrows link human and animal forms.

4. Conclusion

The existence of different PrP^{Sc} types might be a common denominator of prion diseases in humans and animals and it might suggest the existence of different conformers within a given prion disorders. Further, although the biochemical approach is important for large-scale studies, it should be clear that for strain recognition and comparative analysis purposes, PrP^{Sc} biochemical similarity is only apparent evidence, and it does not reflect the biological properties of a given strain. These are revealed only after transmission.

In addition, the demonstration that synthetic prion strains can be made in the laboratory has ushered in a large set of experimental investigations that may help deciphering the structural determinants linked to different PrP^{Sc} types.

5. Acknowledgment

Giuseppe Legname has received funding from the European Community's Seventh Framework Programme (FP7/2007-2013) under grant agreement n° 222887 - the PRIORITY project - and from the *Ministero dell'Istruzione, dell'Università e della Ricerca* under the program PRIN 2008 *"Meccanismi Neurodegenerativi nelle Malattie da Prioni: Studi Conformazionali, Fisiopatologia della Proteina Prionica e Possibili Approcci Farmacologici"*.

6. References

Aguzzi, A. & Calella, A. M. 2009. Prions: protein aggregation and infectious diseases. *Physiol Rev*, 89, 1105-52.

Aguzzi, A., Sigurdson, C. & Heikenwaelder, M. 2008. Molecular mechanisms of prion pathogenesis. *Annu Rev Pathol*, 3, 11-40.

Ashok, A. & Hegde, R. S. 2009. Selective processing and metabolism of disease-causing mutant prion proteins. *PLoS Pathog,* 5, e1000479.

Baker, H. E., Poulter, M., Crow, T. J., Frith, C. D., Lofthouse, R. & Ridley, R. M. 1991. Aminoacid polymorphism in human prion protein and age at death in inherited prion disease. *Lancet,* 337, 1286.

Benestad, S. L., Arsac, J. N., Goldmann, W. & Noremark, M. 2008. Atypical/Nor98 scrapie: properties of the agent, genetics, and epidemiology. *Vet Res,* 39, 19.

Benestad, S. L., Sarradin, P., Thu, B., Schonheit, J., Tranulis, M. A. & Bratberg, B. 2003. Cases of scrapie with unusual features in Norway and designation of a new type, Nor98. *Vet Rec,* 153, 202-8.

Benvegnu, S., Gasperini, L. & Legname, G. 2011a. Aged PrP null mice show defective processing of neuregulins in the peripheral nervous system. *Mol Cell Neurosci,* 47, 28-35.

Benvegnu, S., Poggiolini, I. & Legname, G. 2010. Neurodevelopmental expression and localization of the cellular prion protein in the central nervous system of the mouse. *J Comp Neurol,* 518, 1879-91.

Benvegnu, S., Roncaglia, P., Agostini, F., Casalone, C., Corona, C., Gustincich, S. & Legname, G. 2011b. Developmental influence of the cellular prion protein on the gene expression profile in mouse hippocampus. *Physiol Genomics,* 43, 711-25.

Biacabe, A. G., Laplanche, J. L., Ryder, S. & Baron, T. 2004. Distinct molecular phenotypes in bovine prion diseases. *EMBO Rep,* 5, 110-5.

Bishop, M. T., Will, R. G. & Manson, J. C. 2010. Defining sporadic Creutzfeldt-Jakob disease strains and their transmission properties. *Proc Natl Acad Sci U S A,* 107, 12005-10.

Bremer, J., Baumann, F., Tiberi, C., Wessig, C., Fischer, H., Schwarz, P., Steele, A. D., Toyka, K. V., Nave, K. A., Weis, J. & Aguzzi, A. 2010. Axonal prion protein is required for peripheral myelin maintenance. *Nat Neurosci,* 13, 310-8.

Brown, P., Mcshane, L. M., Zanusso, G. & Detwile, L. 2006. On the question of sporadic or atypical bovine spongiform encephalopathy and Creutzfeldt-Jakob disease. *Emerg Infect Dis,* 12, 1816-21.

Bruce, M., Chree, A., Mcconnell, I., Foster, J., Pearson, G. & Fraser, H. 1994. Transmission of bovine spongiform encephalopathy and scrapie to mice: strain variation and the species barrier. *Philos Trans R Soc Lond B Biol Sci,* 343, 405-11.

Bueler, H., Aguzzi, A., Sailer, A., Greiner, R. A., Autenried, P., Aguet, M. & Weissmann, C. 1993. Mice devoid of PrP are resistant to scrapie. *Cell,* 73, 1339-47.

Bueler, H., Fischer, M., Lang, Y., Bluethmann, H., Lipp, H. P., Dearmond, S. J., Prusiner, S. B., Aguet, M. & Weissmann, C. 1992. Normal development and behaviour of mice lacking the neuronal cell-surface PrP protein. *Nature,* 356, 577-82.

Calzolai, L., Lysek, D. A., Guntert, P., Von Schroetter, C., Riek, R., Zahn, R. & Wuthrich, K. 2000. NMR structures of three single-residue variants of the human prion protein. *Proc Natl Acad Sci U S A,* 97, 8340-5.

Casalone, C., Zanusso, G., Acutis, P., Ferrari, S., Capucci, L., Tagliavini, F., Monaco, S. & Caramelli, M. 2004. Identification of a second bovine amyloidotic spongiform encephalopathy: molecular similarities with sporadic Creutzfeldt-Jakob disease. *Proc Natl Acad Sci U S A,* 101, 3065-70.

Chesebro, B., Trifilo, M., Race, R., Meade-White, K., Teng, C., Lacasse, R., Raymond, L., Favara, C., Baron, G., Priola, S., Caughey, B., Masliah, E. & Oldstone, M. 2005. Anchorless prion protein results in infectious amyloid disease without clinical scrapie. *Science,* 308, 1435-9.

Christen, B., Hornemann, S., Damberger, F. F. & Wuthrich, K. 2009. Prion protein NMR structure from tammar wallaby (Macropus eugenii) shows that the beta2-alpha2 loop is modulated by long-range sequence effects. *J Mol Biol,* 389, 833-45.

Christen, B., Perez, D. R., Hornemann, S. & Wuthrich, K. 2008. NMR structure of the bank vole prion protein at 20 degrees C contains a structured loop of residues 165-171. *J Mol Biol,* 383, 306-12.

Collinge, J. 2001. Prion diseases of humans and animals: their causes and molecular basis. *Annu Rev Neurosci,* 24, 519-50.

Collinge J, Sidle KC, Meads J, Ironside J, Hill AF. 1996. Molecular analysis of prion strain variation and the aetiology of 'new variant' CJD. *Nature.* 383:685-90.

Collinge, J., Palmer, M. S. & Dryden, A. J. 1991. Genetic predisposition to iatrogenic Creutzfeldt-Jakob disease. *Lancet,* 337, 1441-2.

Criado, J. R., Sanchez-Alavez, M., Conti, B., Giacchino, J. L., Wills, D. N., Henriksen, S. J., Race, R., Manson, J. C., Chesebro, B. & Oldstone, M. B. 2005. Mice Devoid Of Prion Protein have cognitive deficits that are rescued by reconstitution of PrP in neurons. *Neurobiol Dis,* 19, 255-65.

Deleault, N. R., Lucassen, R. W. & Supattapone, S. 2003. RNA molecules stimulate prion protein conversion. *Nature,* 425, 717-20.

Gambetti, P., Cali, I., Notari, S., Kong, Q., Zou, W. Q. & Surewicz, W. K. 2011. Molecular biology and pathology of prion strains in sporadic human prion diseases. *Acta Neuropathol,* 121, 79-90.

Gambetti, P., Dong, Z., Yuan, J., Xiao, X., Zheng, M., Alshekhlee, A., Castellani, R., Cohen, M., Barria, M. A., Gonzalez-Romero, D., Belay, E. D., Schonberger, L. B., Marder, K., Harris, C., Burke, J. R., Montine, T., Wisniewski, T., Dickson, D. W., Soto, C., Hulette, C. M., Mastrianni, J. A., Kong, Q. & Zou, W. Q. 2008. A novel human disease with abnormal prion protein sensitive to protease. *Ann Neurol,* 63, 697-708.

Gambetti, P., Kong, Q., Zou, W., Parchi, P. & Chen, S. G. 2003. Sporadic and familial CJD: classification and characterisation. *Br Med Bull,* 66, 213-39.

Ghetti, B., Tagliavini, F., Takao, M., Bugiani, O. & Piccardo, P. 2003. Hereditary prion protein amyloidoses. *Clin Lab Med,* 23, 65-85, viii.

Gorodinsky, A. & Harris, D. A. 1995. Glycolipid-anchored proteins in neuroblastoma cells form detergent-resistant complexes without caveolin. *J Cell Biol,* 129, 619-27.

Gossert, A. D., Bonjour, S., Lysek, D. A., Fiorito, F. & Wuthrich, K. 2005. Prion protein NMR structures of elk and of mouse/elk hybrids. *Proc Natl Acad Sci U S A,* 102, 646-50.

Govaerts, C., Wille, H., Prusiner, S. B. & Cohen, F. E. 2004. Evidence for assembly of prions with left-handed beta-helices into trimers. *Proc Natl Acad Sci U S A,* 101, 8342-7.

Hegde, R. S., Tremblay, P., Groth, D., Dearmond, S. J., Prusiner, S. B. & Lingappa, V. R. 1999. Transmissible and genetic prion diseases share a common pathway of neurodegeneration. *Nature,* 402, 822-6.

Hsiao, K., Dlouhy, S. R., Farlow, M. R., Cass, C., Da Costa, M., Conneally, P. M., Hodes, M. E., Ghetti, B. & Prusiner, S. B. 1992. Mutant prion proteins in Gerstmann-Straussler-Scheinker disease with neurofibrillary tangles. *Nat Genet,* 1, 68-71.

Ilc, G., Giachin, G., Jaremko, M., Jaremko, L., Benetti, F., Plavec, J., Zhukov, I. & Legname, G. 2010. NMR structure of the human prion protein with the pathological Q212P mutation reveals unique structural features. *PLoS ONE,* 5, e11715.

Kanaani, J., Prusiner, S. B., Diacovo, J., Baekkeskov, S. & Legname, G. 2005. Recombinant prion protein induces rapid polarization and development of synapses in embryonic rat hippocampal neurons in vitro. *J Neurochem,* 95, 1373-86.

Kaneko, K., Zulianello, L., Scott, M., Cooper, C. M., Wallace, A. C., James, T. L., Cohen, F. E. & Prusiner, S. B. 1997. Evidence for protein X binding to a discontinuous epitope on the cellular prion protein during scrapie prion propagation. *Proc Natl Acad Sci U S A,* 94, 10069-74.

Kobayashi, A., Hizume, M., Teruya, K., Mohri, S. & Kitamoto, T. 2009. Heterozygous inhibition in prion infection: the stone fence model. *Prion,* 3, 27-30.

Kovacs, G. G., Trabattoni, G., Hainfellner, J. A., Ironside, J. W., Knight, R. S. & Budka, H. 2002. Mutations of the prion protein gene phenotypic spectrum. *J Neurol,* 249, 1567-82.

Legname, G., Baskakov, I. V., Nguyen, H. O., Riesner, D., Cohen, F. E., Dearmond, S. J. & Prusiner, S. B. 2004. Synthetic Mammalian Prions. *Science,* 305, 673-6.

Legname, G., Nguyen, H. O., Baskakov, I. V., Cohen, F. E., Dearmond, S. J. & Prusiner, S. B. 2005. Strain-specified characteristics of mouse synthetic prions. *Proc Natl Acad Sci U S A,* 102, 2168-73.

Legname, G., Nguyen, H. O., Peretz, D., Cohen, F. E., Dearmond, S. J. & Prusiner, S. B. 2006. Continuum of prion protein structures enciphers a multitude of prion isolate-specified phenotypes. *Proc Natl Acad Sci U S A,* 103, 19105-10.

Liao, Y. C., Lebo, R. V., Clawson, G. A. & Smuckler, E. A. 1986. Human prion protein cDNA: molecular cloning, chromosomal mapping, and biological implications. *Science,* 233, 364-7.

Lopez Garcia, F., Zahn, R., Riek, R. & Wuthrich, K. 2000. NMR structure of the bovine prion protein. *Proc Natl Acad Sci U S A,* 97, 8334-9.

Marijanovic, Z., Caputo, A., Campana, V. & Zurzolo, C. 2009. Identification of an intracellular site of prion conversion. *PLoS Pathog,* 5, e1000426.

Mckinley, M. P., Meyer, R. K., Kenaga, L., Rahbar, F., Cotter, R., Serban, A. & Prusiner, S. B. 1991. Scrapie prion rod formation in vitro requires both detergent extraction and limited proteolysis. *J Virol,* 65, 1340-51.

Moore, R. C., Lee, I. Y., Silverman, G. L., Harrison, P. M., Strome, R., Heinrich, C., Karunaratne, A., Pasternak, S. H., Chishti, M. A., Liang, Y., Mastrangelo, P., Wang, K., Smit, A. F., Katamine, S., Carlson, G. A., Cohen, F. E., Prusiner, S. B., Melton, D. W., Tremblay, P., Hood, L. E. & Westaway, D. 1999. Ataxia in prion protein (PrP)-deficient mice is associated with upregulation of the novel PrP-like protein doppel. *J Mol Biol,* 292, 797-817.

Nishida, N., Tremblay, P., Sugimoto, T., Shigematsu, K., Shirabe, S., Petromilli, C., Erpel, S. P., Nakaoke, R., Atarashi, R., Houtani, T., Torchia, M., Sakaguchi, S., Dearmond, S. J., Prusiner, S. B. & Katamine, S. 1999. A mouse prion protein transgene rescues mice deficient for the prion protein gene from purkinje cell degeneration and demyelination. *Lab Invest,* 79, 689-97.

Nonno, R., Di Bari, M. A., Cardone, F., Vaccari, G., Fazzi, P., Dell'omo, G., Cartoni, C., Ingrosso, L., Boyle, A., Galeno, R., Sbriccoli, M., Lipp, H. P., Bruce, M., Pocchiari, M. & Agrimi, U. 2006. Efficient transmission and characterization of Creutzfeldt-Jakob disease strains in bank voles. *PLoS Pathog,* 2, e12.

Palmer, M. S., Dryden, A. J., Hughes, J. T. & Collinge, J. 1991. Homozygous prion protein genotype predisposes to sporadic Creutzfeldt-Jakob disease. *Nature,* 352, 340-2.

Parchi, P., Chen, S. G., Brown, P., Zou, W., Capellari, S., Budka, H., Hainfellner, J., Reyes, P. F., Golden, G. T., Hauw, J. J., Gajdusek, D. C. & Gambetti, P. 1998. Different patterns of truncated prion protein fragments correlate with distinct phenotypes in P102L Gerstmann-Straussler-Scheinker disease. *Proc Natl Acad Sci U S A,* 95, 8322-7.

Parchi, P., Giese, A., Capellari, S., Brown, P., Schulz-Schaeffer, W., Windl, O., Zerr, I., Budka, H., Kopp, N., Piccardo, P., Poser, S., Rojiani, A., Streichemberger, N., Julien, J., Vital, C., Ghetti, B., Gambetti, P. & Kretzschmar, H. 1999. Classification of sporadic Creutzfeldt-Jakob disease based on molecular and phenotypic analysis of 300 subjects. *Ann Neurol,* 46, 224-33.

Perez, D. R., Damberger, F. F. & Wuthrich, K. 2010. Horse prion protein NMR structure and comparisons with related variants of the mouse prion protein. *J Mol Biol,* 400, 121-8.

Piccardo, P., Dlouhy, S. R., Lievens, P. M., Young, K., Bird, T. D., Nochlin, D., Dickson, D. W., Vinters, H. V., Zimmerman, T. R., Mackenzie, I. R., Kish, S. J., Ang, L. C., De Carli, C., Pocchiari, M., Brown, P., Gibbs, C. J., Jr., Gajdusek, D. C., Bugiani, O., Ironside, J., Tagliavini, F. & GhettI, B. 1998. Phenotypic variability of Gerstmann-Straussler-Scheinker disease is associated with prion protein heterogeneity. *J Neuropathol Exp Neurol,* 57, 979-88.

Piccardo, P., Manson, J. C., King, D., Ghetti, B. & Barron, R. M. 2007. Accumulation of prion protein in the brain that is not associated with transmissible disease. *Proc Natl Acad Sci U S A,* 104, 4712-7.

Prusiner, S. B. 1982. Novel proteinaceous infectious particles cause scrapie. *Science,* 216, 136-44.

Prusiner, S. B. 1998. Prions. *Proc Natl Acad Sci U S A,* 95, 13363-83.

Prusiner, S. B. 2001. Shattuck lecture--neurodegenerative diseases and prions. *N Engl J Med,* 344, 1516-26.

Prusiner, S. B., Mckinley, M. P., Bowman, K. A., Bolton, D. C., Bendheim, P. E., Groth, D. F. & Glenner, G. G. 1983. Scrapie prions aggregate to form amyloid-like birefringent rods. *Cell,* 35, 349-58.

Riek, R., Hornemann, S., Wider, G., Billeter, M., Glockshuber, R. & Wuthrich, K. 1996. NMR structure of the mouse prion protein domain PrP(121-321). *Nature,* 382, 180-2.

Salmona, M., Morbin, M., Massignan, T., Colombo, L., Mazzoleni, G., Capobianco, R., Diomede, L., Thaler, F., Mollica, L., Musco, G., Kourie, J. J., Bugiani, O., Sharma, D., Inouye, H., Kirschner, D. A., Forloni, G. & Tagliavini, F. 2003. Structural properties of Gerstmann-Straussler-Scheinker disease amyloid protein. *J Biol Chem,* 278, 48146-53.

Spudich, A., Frigg, R., Kilic, E., Kilic, U., Oesch, B., Raeber, A., Bassetti, C. L. & Hermann, D. M. 2005. Aggravation of ischemic brain injury by prion protein deficiency: role of ERK-1/-2 and STAT-1. *Neurobiol Dis,* 20, 442-9.

Stahl, N., Borchelt, D. R. & Prusiner, S. B. 1990. Differential release of cellular and scrapie prion proteins from cellular membranes by phosphatidylinositol-specific phospholipase C. *Biochemistry*, 29, 5405-12.

Tagliavini, F., Prelli, F., Ghiso, J., Bugiani, O., Serban, D., Prusiner, S. B., Farlow, M. R., Ghetti, B. & Frangione, B. 1991. Amyloid protein of Gerstmann-Straussler-Scheinker disease (Indiana kindred) is an 11 kd fragment of prion protein with an N-terminal glycine at codon 58. *EMBO J*, 10, 513-9.

Tagliavini, F., Prelli, F., Porro, M., Rossi, G., Giaccone, G., Farlow, M. R., Dlouhy, S. R., Ghetti, B., Bugiani, O. & Frangione, B. 1994. Amyloid fibrils in Gerstmann-Straussler-Scheinker disease (Indiana and Swedish kindreds) express only PrP peptides encoded by the mutant allele. *Cell*, 79, 695-703.

Telling, G. C., Scott, M., Mastrianni, J., Gabizon, R., Torchia, M., Cohen, F. E., Dearmond, S. J. & PruSINER, S. B. 1995. Prion propagation in mice expressing human and chimeric PrP transgenes implicates the interaction of cellular PrP with another protein. *Cell*, 83, 79-90.

Tobler, I., Deboer, T. & Fischer, M. 1997. Sleep and sleep regulation in normal and prion protein-deficient mice. *J Neurosci*, 17, 1869-79.

Wadsworth, J. D. & Collinge, J. 2011. Molecular pathology of human prion disease. *Acta Neuropathol*, 121, 69-77.

Wadsworth JD, Joiner S, Linehan JM, Cooper S, Powell C, Mallinson G, Buckell J, Gowland I, Asante EA, Budka H, Brandner S, Collinge J. 2006. Phenotypic heterogeneity in inherited prion disease (P102L) is associated with differential propagation of protease-resistant wild-type and mutant prion protein. *Brain* 129:1557-69.

Weise, J., Sandau, R., Schwarting, S., Crome, O., Wrede, A., Schulz-Schaeffer, W., Zerr, I. & Bahr, M. 2006. Deletion of cellular prion protein results in reduced Akt activation, enhanced postischemic caspase-3 activation, and exacerbation of ischemic brain injury. *Stroke*, 37, 1296-300.

Weissmann, C. & FlechsiG, E. 2003. PrP knock-out and PrP transgenic mice in prion research. *Br Med Bull*, 66, 43-60.

Wemheuer, W. M., Benestad, S. L., Wrede, A., Schulze-Sturm, U., Wemheuer, W. E., Hahmann, U., Gawinecka, J., Schutz, E., Zerr, I., Brenig, B., Bratberg, B., Andreoletti, O. & Schulz-Schaeffer, W. J. 2009. Similarities between forms of sheep scrapie and Creutzfeldt-Jakob disease are encoded by distinct prion types. *Am J Pathol*, 175, 2566-73.

Wen, Y., Li, J., Yao, W., Xiong, M., Hong, J., Peng, Y., Xiao, G. & Lin, D. 2010. Unique structural characteristics of the rabbit prion protein. *J Biol Chem*, 285, 31682-93.

Williams, E. S. 2005. Chronic wasting disease. *Vet Pathol*, 42, 530-49.

Windl, O., Dempster, M., Estibeiro, J. P., Lathe, R., De Silva, R., Esmonde, T., Will, R., Springbett, A., Campbell, T. A., Sidle, K. C., Palmer, M. S. & Collinge, J. 1996. Genetic basis of Creutzfeldt-Jakob disease in the United Kingdom: a systematic analysis of predisposing mutations and allelic variation in the PRNP gene. *Hum Genet*, 98, 259-64.

Young, K., Piccardo, P., Kish, S. J., Ang, L. C., Dlouhy, S. & Ghetti, B. 1998. Gerstmann-Sträussler-Scheinker disease (GSS) with a mutation at prion protein (PrP) residue 212. *Journal of Neuropathology & Experimental Neurology*, 57, 518.

Zanusso, G., Farinazzo, A., Prelli, F., Fiorini, M., Gelati, M., Ferrari, S., Righetti, P. G., Rizzuto, N., Frangione, B. & Monaco, S. 2004. Identification of distinct N-terminal truncated forms of prion protein in different Creutzfeldt-Jakob disease subtypes. *J Biol Chem,* 279, 38936-42.

Zanusso, G., Polo, A., Farinazzo, A., Nonno, R., Cardone, F., Di Bari, M., Ferrari, S., Principe, S., Gelati, M., Fasoli, E., Fiorini, M., Prelli, F., Frangione, B., Tridente, G., Bentivoglio, M., Giorgi, A., Schinina, M. E., Maras, B., Agrimi, U., Rizzuto, N., Pocchiari, M. & Monaco, S. 2007. Novel prion protein conformation and glycotype in Creutzfeldt-Jakob disease. *Arch Neurol,* 64, 595-9.

Zanusso, G., Righetti, P. G., Ferrari, S., Terrin, L., Farinazzo, A., Cardone, F., Pocchiari, M., Rizzuto, N. & Monaco, S. 2002. Two-dimensional mapping of three phenotype-associated isoforms of the prion protein in sporadic Creutzfeldt-Jakob disease. *Electrophoresis,* 23, 347-55.

Zhang, Y., Swietnicki, W., Zagorski, M. G., Surewicz, W. K. & Sonnichsen, F. D. 2000. Solution structure of the E200K variant of human prion protein. Implications for the mechanism of pathogenesis in familial prion diseases. *J Biol Chem,* 275, 33650-4.

Zimmermann, K., Turecek, P. L. & Schwarz, H. P. 1999. Genotyping of the prion protein gene at codon 129. *Acta Neuropathol,* 97, 355-8.

Zou, W. Q., Capellari, S., Parchi, P., Sy, M. S., Gambetti, P. & Chen, S. G. 2003. Identification of novel proteinase K-resistant C-terminal fragments of PrP in Creutzfeldt-Jakob disease. *J Biol Chem,* 278, 40429-36.

Zou, W. Q., Puoti, G., Xiao, X., Yuan, J., Qing, L., Cali, I., Shimoji, M., Langeveld, J. P., Castellani, R., Notari, S., Crain, B., Schmidt, R. E., Geschwind, M., Dearmond, S. J., Cairns, N. J., Dickson, D., Honig, L., Torres, J. M., Mastrianni, J., Capellari, S., Giaccone, G., Belay, E. D., Schonberger, L. B., Cohen, M., Perry, G., Kong, Q., Parchi, P., Tagliavini, F. & Gambetti, P. 2010. Variably protease-sensitive prionopathy: a new sporadic disease of the prion protein. *Ann Neurol,* 68, 162-72.

6

Acute Encephalopathies and Psychiatry

Karim Sedky[1], Racha Nazir[1] and Steven Lippmann[2]
[1]Penn State College of Medicine, Hershey, PA
[2]University of Louisville School of Medicine, Louisville, KY
USA

1. Introduction

An encephalopathic delirium occurs due to a disturbance of brain function leading to a change in mental status. Fluctuating consciousness, hallucinations, disorientation, and short-term memory deficits are common presentations. This syndrome is more frequent among elderly people and occurs in up to 30% of hospitalized patients[1]. There are many medical conditions that can cause a delirium, including organ failures and electrolyte imbalances, etc. Polypharmacy and/or toxicities increase the risk of developing a confusional state. When considering a delirium diagnosis, a thorough evaluation is mandatory. This includes history taking from patients and their family, a physical examination, and a neurological evaluation. Laboratory investigations include a basic metabolic panel, a complete blood count, liver function tests, a calcium assay, toxicology or plasma drug level screening, thyroid stimulating hormone, urine analysis, and in certain cases, a rapid plasma reagin (RPR) and/or human immunodeficiency viral levels (HIV), etc. A computerized tomography scan of the head or magnetic resonance imaging is obtained in most cases. Early, prompt management of delirium decreases morbidity and mortality.

Patients suffering from certain psychiatric conditions can be misdiagnosed as having an encephalopathy and vice versa. Psychosis is common in many psychiatric disorders and may include auditory hallucinations. Psychoses in confusional states will prompt the search for medical causes. Visual hallucinations are most typically observed in cases of a delirium due to a medical condition (e.g., electrolyte imbalance, brain tumor, toxicities, and/or seizures, etc). Tactile hallucinations, or formications, are a feeling that bugs are crawling under the skin and are common with drug use (e.g., cocaine) or alcohol withdrawal. Olfactory hallucinations are often noted in individuals suffering from seizures or brain disorders. Delirium diagnosis becomes especially challenging in people with history of a psychiatric disorder presenting with a new change in mental status. It is important for physicians to be aware of such disorders and to quickly recognize adverse-events caused by psychotropic medications and/or the occurrence of new onset medical disorders. Diagnosis is especially difficult in chronically ill patients, who are poor historians with inability to communicate coherently. This chapter reviews causes of delirium that are secondary to psychiatric drugs as well as reviewing psychiatric mimickers of delirium.

2. Encephalopathy secondary to psychiatric treatments

There are a vast variety of psychiatric medications available. These include antidepressant drug, anxiolytic agents, antipsychotic medications, and mood stabilizers (e.g., antiepileptic pharmacueticals and/or lithium). Through different mechanisms of action, these medications can result in causing an acute or chronic encephalopathy. Older versions of the psychopharmaceuticals are the most common offending agents. For example, tricyclic antidepressant drugs are more likely to cause anticholinergic induced delirium as compared to the selective serotonin reuptake inhibitors. Neuroleptic malignant syndrome occurs with higher frequency when utilizing older neuroleptic medications versus experience with the newer generation of antipsychotic agents.

2.1 Medications with anticholinergic effects

There are multiple medications that induce anticholinergic effects that include cognitive dysfunction, decreased concentration, confusion, and memory deficits[2] (see Table-1). Delirium occur especially in elderly persons secondary to anticholinergic side-effects caused by antipsychotic and antidepressant medications. A survey of elderly patients hospitalized with an acute medical illness revealed that a significant number were prescribed antipsychotic agents and experienced a delirium, as compared to those not receiving them (10% versus 0%)[3].

Many tricyclic and tetracyclic antidepressant medicines are high in anticholinergic potential. Amitriptyline, protriptyline, doxepin, imipramine, and trimipramine are the most notable. In one study, such antidepressant agents were responsible for causing an acute delirium in 13.6% of patients[4]. The second generation antidepressant medications usually have less anticholinergic side-effects[5].

Clozapine, chlorpromazine, and thioridazine are the antipsychotic agents that have the most anticholinergic potential for causing a delirium[6]. Olanzapine has a moderate affinity to this receptor[7]; other antipsychotic drugs are less likely to cause encephalopathy due to anticholinergia.

First generation antipsychotic agents and risperidone often can result in parkinsonian signs and symptoms that include resting tremors, shuffling gait, a flat affect, cog-wheel muscular rigidity, and bradykinesia. Benzotropine and trihexyphenidyl are frequently co-utilized to medicate this adversity, but particularly in elderly patients adding these medicines can induce a delirium.

2.2 Neuroleptic Malignant Syndrome (NMS)

Antipsychotic medications are prescribed to treat people with psychotic disorders and acute agitation. Haloperidol is frequently used in acute medical settings due to its low anticholinergic effects and wide availability in oral and parenteral forms. Delirium can signify the induction of neuroleptic malignant syndrome by antipsychotic drugs. Other medications with similar properties include metoclopramide and prochlorperazine. Dopamine receptor blockade is hypothesized as the pathology behind NMS, but other etiologies might include sympathetic or adrenal dysregulation. Sudden discontinuation of dopaminergic agonists like bromocriptine can also lead to a similar condition.

ANTIDEPRESSANT		**ANTIPSYCHOTIC**	
DRUGS		**DRUGS**	
SSRIs		**LOW POTENCY**	
fluoxetine, paroxetine,	-	**NEUROLEPTICS**	
fluvoxamine, sertraline,	except paroxetine	chlorpromazine	++++
citalopram, &	and fluvoxamine	thioridazine	++++
escitalopram	(+)	mesoridazine	++++
Bupropion		**HIGH POTENCY**	
	-	**NEUROLEPTICS**	
SNRIs		haloperidol	+
nefazdone, venlafaxine,		perphenazine	++
desvenlafaxine, &	-	fluphenazine	++
duloxetine		loxapine	++
		thiothixene	++
TCAs			
(tri- & tetracyclic			
antidepressants)		**2ND GENERATION**	
amitriptyline		**ANTIPSYCHOTIC**	
trimipramine		**DRUGS**	
doxepine	++++	clozapine	++++
clomipramine	+++	risperidone	+
imipramine	++/+++	paliperidone	+
desipramine	+++/++++	olanzapine	+
nortriptyline	++	quetiapine	+
	+	ziprasidone	++
MAOIs	+/++	aripiprazole	+
phenelzine			
tranylcypromine			
isocarboxazid	+		
	+		
	+		

SSRI: Selective Serotonin Reuptake Inhibitor; SNRI: Selective Norepinephrine Reuptake Inhibitor; TCA: Tri- and Tetracyclic Antidepressant; MAOI: Monoamine Oxidase Inhibitor.

Table 1. Anticholinergic Effects of Psychotropic Medications

Neuroleptic malignant syndrome occurs in up to 0.02% of individuals medicated with antipsychotic agents[8]. It was previously thought to be of a higher incidence; however, early detection, cautious neuroleptic dosing, and the introduction of second generation antipsychotic medicines might have contributed to this decrease in frequency. NMS is more common in people with dehydration, agitation, iron deficiency, and in rapid antipsychotic medication increases or high dosage applications. Risk may increase also when antipsychotic medicines are co-prescribed with lithium and in patients with a history of NMS. The onset can be within a week of medication initiation[8].

Autonomic dysfunction is a prominent part of the presentation. Confusion and muscle stiffness are noted. Laboratory findings include elevated transaminases, aldolase, lactic acid dehydrogenase, leucocytosis, and/or metabolic acidosis. High creatinin phosphokinase induced by rhabdomyolysis might result in kidney failure.

Differentiate this syndrome from central nervous system infections which are associated with headaches, fever and localizing signs. Heatstroke can also present with hyperthermia, tachycardia, and confusion; yet, it is differentiated by findings of dry skin and hypotonia. Serotonin syndrome is related to taking serotonergic agents and evidences muscle tremors rather than stiffness. Malignant hyperthermia is a reaction to anesthetic agents. In the workup always rule out psychiatric cases of malignant catatonia.

NMS varies from a life-threatening situation to a self-limited condition, with 63% of cases taken off of the drug recovering within several days[8]. Parenteral depot medication exposure greatly prolongs the course. Fatalities are observed in up to 10% of patients. Immediate discontinuation of the antipsychotic drug is essential.

2.3 Sedative-hypnotic agents

Benzodiazepines and barbiturates can precipitate delirium. Up to 13.9% of patients presenting with acute encephalopathy due to medication, were caused by benzodiazepine intake[6]. In elderly individuals and/or those with liver disease, medication levels can quickly become toxic causing an encephalopathy, even at normal medication dosages. The longer acting benzodiazepines might have a higher risk of causing delirium as compared to shorter acting variants (relative ratio was 5.4 versus 2.6)[9]. Higher dosages are also more likely to cause an encephalopathy than lower ones (relative ratio was 3.3 versus 2.6).

Benzodiazepines are usually indicated as a short-term treatment for anxiety, insomnia, and alcohol withdrawal. Yet, very often these medicines are utilized over the long-term. After prolonged duration use or abuse, sudden dosage taper or discontinuation can lead to severe withdrawal symptoms including convulsions and an encephalopathy. Deaths from benzodiazepine withdrawal occur. Thus, seizure precautions and prompt replacement of the sedative medication is emergently required at dosages that stop seizures and suppress hyperadrenergic withdrawal signs[10].

Barbiturates are no longer commonly utilized; they are mainly prescribed to treat seizure disorders or alcohol withdrawal delirium, especially since some of them have a long half-life and are inexpensive. Sedative toxicity with psychosis has been reported particularly during medication overdoses. Withdrawal delirium (i.e., delirium tremens) can occur after sudden decreases or discontinuation of barbiturates. Isolated visual hallucinations, without overt toxicity or withdrawal, are reported in adults and children[11].

2.4 Serotonin syndrome

Serotonin syndrome occurs due to hyperstimulation of the 5-HT_{1A} receptors[12]. Etiologies include taking serotonin precursors or agonists (e.g., buspirone and trazodone), neurotransmitter releasers (e.g., amphetamines), reduced serotonin-reuptake from selective serotonin reuptake inhibitor (SSRI) drugs and related agents, or diminishing serotonin metabolism by taking monoamine oxidase inhibitors (MAOIs). Co-prescribing serotonergic medicines, as in MAOIs with SSRIs or sumatriptan and related drugs, must be avoided. Drug interaction through inhibitors of cytochrome P450 can lead to inhibition of hepatic degradation of the SSRIs, leading to a high blood levels and toxicity risk[13].

Serotonin syndrome is an uncommon side-effect of antidepressant drugs, but it is more likely once utilizing medications with a long half-life (e.g., flouxetine). This adversity usually occurs within the first few days of medication initiation[13]. Three different levels of the disorder are described[13]: 1. a mild form with tremors, myoclonus, diaphoresis, and restlessness; 2. a syndrome of impaired consciousness or coma, neurological features of myoclonus, tremors or rigidity, autonomic hyperactivity, or breathing difficulties; and 3. a dangerous, toxic condition with coma, seizures, and fever. Deaths occur in the more severe versions, with brain edema and a coagulopathy. Laboratory findings include elevation of the creatinin kinase, transaminases, and leukocytosis.

2.5 Lithium

Lithium is a salt frequently used to treat bipolar disorders or as an augmenting agent for those who suffer from depression. It is effective for controlling manic symptoms at blood levels of 0.6 to 1.2 μg/ml and for maintenance therapy at 0.3 to 0.6 μg/dl. Lithium toxicity is common in dehydrated individuals (see Table-2). Nephrogenic diabetes insipidus occurs in 10% of treated patients and causes dehydration, possibly precipitating toxicity and an encephalopathy. For people over 65 years-of-age, with impaired renal function and polypharmacy, the risk for this adversity increases by two-fold[14,15]. When co-prescribed with diuretics (e.g., hydrochlorthiazide), non-steriodal anti-inflammatory drugs (e.g., ibuprofen), and/or angiotensin converting enzyme inhibitors (e.g., captopril), lithium excretion is reduced leading to potential toxicity if dose adjustment is not made[15].

Toxic symptoms are generally correlated to serum blood lithium levels. Mild cases occur when concentrations are between 1.5 to 2μg/ml, presenting with gastrointestinal upset, mild tremors, and weakness. With moderate toxicity, concentrations range from 2 to 2.5μg/ml and complaints include tinnitus, muscle twitches, dysarthria, and hyperreflexia manifest. At higher blood levels, severe toxicity includes delirium, seizures, coma, and even death; in these cases, blood concentrations are less well correlated to clinical status. Neurotoxicity with permanent sequellae follows high level intoxication[15]. Thus, significant toxicity mandates hydration and immediate discontinuation of lithium; hemodialysis maybe required.

[1]	Dehydration
	a. Increased perspiration
	b. Nephrogenic diabetes insipidus
[2]	Impaired renal function-nephritis or renal tubular nephrosis
[3]	Medications
	a. Loop diuretics e.g., hydrochlorothiazide
	b. Angiotensin converting enzyme inhibitor e.g., captopril
	c. Non-steroidal anti-inflammatory drugs e.g., ibuprofen

Table 2. Causes of Lithium Toxicity

There is controversy about the safety of combing lithium with antipsychotic medications; several sporadic cases of encephalopathy have been reported with such combinations[16]. This might be explained by lithium enhancing dopamine receptor blockade[17]. Otherwise, co-prescribing leads to a higher concentration of intracellular lithium, in a dose-dependent nature[16]. One retrospective study documented low encephalopathy rates[18]. Nevertheless, such combinations remain frequently utilized, effective, and safe.

2.6 Medication causing hepatotoxicity

Many psychopharmaceuticals can cause liver damage (see Table-3). Acute hepatic failure is an idiosyncratic reaction to medications and can lead to encephalopathy within weeks of first symptom development. Chronic hepatotoxicity and fibrosis usually occurs with long-term treatment; delirium occurs later in the disease process.

ANTIDEPRESSANT DRUGS		**ANTIPSYCHOTIC DRUGS**	
SSRIs		**FIRST GENERATION AGENTS**	
Fluoxetine	+	Phenothiazine (Chlorpromazine)	++
Paroxetine	+	Butyrophenones (Haloperidol)	++
Sertraline	+	**SECOND GENERATION AGENTS**	
Citalopram	+/-	Clozapine	+++
Escitalopram	?	Risperidone	++
Bupropion	+	Paliperidone	?
SNRIs		Olanzapine	++
Nefazdone	++++	Quetiapine	+
Venlafaxine	++	Ziprasidone	-
Desvenlafaxine	+	Aripiprazol	-
Duloxetine	++	**MOOD STABILIZERS**	
OTHERS		Carbamazepine	+++
Trazdone	?	Oxcarbazepine	++
Mirtazapine	?	Divalproex	+++
TRI- & TETRACYCLICS		Lamotrigine	++
Cloimpramine, Imipramine, Amitriptyline, etc	++/+++	Topiramate	?
MAOIs		Gabapentine	?
Phenelzine, Tranylcypromine	++	Lithium	?
		OTHERS	
		Pemoline	++++
		Atomoxetine	++
		Tacrine	++++

SSRI: Selective Serotonin Reuptake Inhibitor; SNRI: Selective Norepinephrine Reuptake Inhibitor; MAOI: Monoamine Oxidase Inhibitor.

Table 3. Psychiatric Medications and Hepatotoxicity

A prominent example was the selective serotonin-norepinephrine reuptake inhibitor, nefazdone, and it has been withdrawn from the market due to this problem. Other drugs can also result in hepatotoxicity; pemoline and tacrine are major offending agents and are rarely utilized now due to this adverse-event. Antiepileptic/mood stabilizer medicines, too, sometimes can induce liver dysfunction[19]. Carbamazepine and valproate products, like divalproex, may cause hepatic inflammation and an encephalopathy. Hyperammonemia might develop even in the absence of other abnormal liver function tests[20].

2.7 Electrolyte abnormalities

Several psychotropic medications may lead to hyponatremia, including antidepressant and antiepileptic/mood stabilizer drugs. Carbamazepine is a well-established offender. Although the mechanism is unknown, stimulation of the 5-HT_2 and 5-HT_{1c} might lead to increased release of antidiuretic hormone (ADH) and water retention at renal tubules[21]. Inhibition of norepinephrine reuptake can also lead to increased ADH through α_1-adrenergic receptor stimulation[21].

People with serum sodium concentrations at 125-130 mEq/l would present with gastrointestinal complaints of nausea and vomiting and the neurological symptoms of fatigue, headaches, and muscle cramps. Delirium ensues with levels below 125mEq/l[22]. At concentrations lower than 120 mEq/l, convulsions, respiratory failure, and death are reported[21]. However, some individuals with chronic hyponatremia might be asymptomatic even at more severely low sodium levels. Laboratory evidence includes lower than normal serum osmolality and increased urine sodium or osmolality[21].

Hyponatremia can occur just weeks after medication initiation[21]. Selective serotonin reuptake inhibitors may have a greater potential for causing this side-effect compared to other antidepressant drugs (ranging from 0.5-32%)[21,22]. Patients older than age 65 carry a six-fold increased risk. Female gender, high medication doses, low baseline sodium levels, being underweight, co-treatment with diuretic agents, and smoking tobacco are other risk factors (nicotine stimulates vasopressin causing enhancement of water reabsorption from renal tubules)[22].

2.8 Leucopenia, neutropenia and/or agranulocytosis

It is important to note that psychotropic medications have been attributed to leucopenia and in rare cases neutropenia[23]. This can predispose people to infections, septicemia, delirium, and death. Clozapine is the antipsychotic drug most associated with bone marrow suppression and use requires special registry for patients and their physicians. A complete blood cell count with white cell differentials is indicated weekly following drug initiation in the first few weeks; the frequency then can be decreased to every other week. Since agranulocytosis develops usually in the first 18 months of this pharmacotherapy, frequency of blood counts can be decreased to monthly intervals after six months of stability. Nevertheless, bone marrow suppression has been reported years after uncomplicated therpy[24]. Immediate medication discontinuation is mandated in all cases of agranulocytosis.

Antiepileptic drugs also have a risk of causing bone marrow suppression. This is especially true with carbamazepine and valproate products. Other medications only rarely cause this side-effect. In contrast, lithium may induce leucocytosis.

2.9 Electroconvulsive Therapy (ECT)

Electroconvulsive therapy is frequently used to treat patient suffering from depression. Delirium can result from the pre-treatment anesthesia or due to the ECT itself. An ECT-induced delirium occurs in up to 12% of individuals, usually resolving spontaneously within an hour[25]. Assurance and benzodiazepines are used to treat any associated agitation. Older age, comorbid neurological disorders, and rapid discontinuation of benzodiazepines after long-term treatment during an ECT series increases the incidence of delirium. Since continued seizures leading to status epilepticus should be ruled out, many physicians continue electroencephalographic monitoring in the post-convulsive period to detect such ictus. A higher incidence of confusion might follow co-prescribing lithium or dopaminergic agents during ECT.

3. Psychiatric disorders mimicking encephalopathy

3.1 Schizophrenia and schizoaffective disorder

Schizophrenia occurs in up to 1% of the population and usually presents first in the late teens and early twenties. According to the Diagnostic and Statistical Manual for Mental Disorders-fourth edition-revised (DSM-IV-R) criteria, to fit this diagnosis, the individual has to have at least two major symptoms for at least six months[26]: delusions which are false fixed beliefs, hallucinations which are misperception of stimuli by the five senses in the absence of stimulation, disorganization of speech, behavior, and/or thought disorder, catatonia or negative symptoms. The negative symptom profile includes apathy, slow movements, ambivalence, and a blunted affect. Catatonia includes motor hyperactivity or excitability, negativism, mutism, waxy flexibility of limbs, and echolalia or echopraxia[27].

Only one presenting symptom might be enough to diagnose this disorder if there are at least two voices talking to each other in the patient's mind, "commentary voices", and/or if the delusion is bizarre. This is particularly so when premorbid social dysfunction has long proceeded the acute psychotic episode, with compromised interpersonal relationships, oddities in behaviors, and low school performance.

There are five sub-types of schizophrenia. This includes a catatonic type; a disorganized version with disorganization of speech, behavior, or thought process; a paranoid type with delusions; an undifferentiated form which has a mixture of symptoms; and a residual one which is less specific but more chronic. Patients presenting with catatonia or disorganization are the ones most easily misdiagnosed.

History taking, with collateral information from the families helps to differentiate schizophrenia from an encephalopathy. A long history of mental illness and its onset during teenage years are usually prominent in schizophrenia; this psychiatric illness has little variation within the day, is characterized by psychotic relapse, and generally evidences intact cognition. Delirium waxes and wanes over time and evidences confusion, poor memory, and disorientation. Preserved cognition is the best clue to ruling out a delirium. Visual hallucinations occur during delirium, while auditory hallucinations more common to schizophrenia. Schizoaffective disorder is a psychosis with a mood disorder component.

3.2 Depressive disorder and bipolar spectrum

Major depressive disorder affects up to 20% of the population, with a higher prevalence among females. Symptoms include feeling sad or irritable, decrease in energy and interest, change in appetite and weight, sleep problems, guilt, anhedonia, and thoughts of suicide. Four to five symptoms are required for at least a duration of two weeks. This syndrome can be associated with psychoses, disorganization, and/or catatonia. Delusions are usually related to one theme and can include nihilistic themes (e.g., the world is coming to an end) and Cotard syndrome (i.e., feeling one is dead and internal organs are decaying). Thorough history gathering and clinical evaluation usually aids in diagnosis. Antidepressant medication alone may not be adequate in psychotic cases, when the addition of an antipsychotic drug is indicated. Since this syndrome is frequently associated with suicidality, medication overdoses should be considered, especially when confusion or a change of mental status is observed. In cases presenting with tricyclic or tetracyclic antidepressant overdose, cardiac monitoring is mandated. Frequent blood work is required for patients on polypharmacy or clozapine. Liver function monitoring is essential in persons medicated with antiepileptic/mood stabilizer drugs.

Bipolar Disorders occur at a rate of 1% in the general population. This cyclic ailment alternates between depression and mania/hypomania, which is characterized by elated or irritable mood, decreased need for sleep, grandiosity, pressured speech, risk taking behaviors, impulsivity, flight of ideas or racing thoughts, and/or distractibility. Three or four symptoms are needed to confirm this diagnosis. Psychoses can also be observed. "Delirious mania" has been described in individuals presenting initially with grandiosity, excitement, and psychosis. They are disorganized and can become delirious. Such cases have been described frequently in younger populations with catatonia evident[28]. This can be challenging to differentiate from delirium alone, especially in elderly cases. History taking, physical examination, and laboratory investigations are important to reach a sound diagnosis. This illness is characterized by acute onset, history of an affective disorder, mania, and response to bipolar treatment. Overt delirium cases evidence cognitive abnormalities, such as disorientation, and require a medical evaluation to rule out toxicities, electrolyte abnormalities, or organ failures, etc.

3.3 Dementia

This disorder is more common in elderly patients and increases in frequency as the individual ages. It can be multifactorial and includes Alzheimer disease, Lewy body dementia, vascular causes, vitamin deficiency, or even infectious offenders (e.g., syphilis). Individuals or relatives usually complain of gradual memory deterioration, aphasia (impairment in language or speech), apraxia (inability to perform complex movements in presence of normal motor function), and problems with executive function. Dementia has a more constant memory deficit pattern, without a waxing and weaning course. Aside from Lewy body dementia, in which visual hallucinations are common, hallucinations usually occur late in the disease or when comorbid delirium exists. Treatable etiologies such as vitamin deficiency, infectious etiologies, and vascular disease should be detected and promptly managed to prevent irreversible disease progression.

3.4 Alcohol and substance-induced delirium

The American Psychiatric Association manual, the DSM-IV-R, has standardized psychiatric disorders that include delirium due to drugs or alcohol. Encephalopathies can occur in individuals consuming alcohol during two stages: 1. alcohol intoxication with delirium and 2. alcohol withdrawal delirium. There is also an alcohol-induced, persisting amnestic disorder with residual dementia that presents initially in a delirium (with Wernicke's Korsakoff syndrome). Amphetamine, cannabis, cocaine, hallucinogen, inhalant, opioid, and phencyclidine (PCP) drugs can be related to a delirium. Other substances are associated with disorientation and are categorized under a substance-induced delirium group [e.g., gamma hydroxybutyrate (GHB)].

3.4.1 Alcohol withdrawal / delirium tremens

Alcohol is a very frequently abused substance. A single 12-ounce drink of beer, 4-ounces of wines, or a 1-1.5 ounces of 80-proof of spirits raises the blood alcohol level by 15-20mg/dl, in a 150-pound normal male[29]. It takes 30-90 minutes to reach a peak concentration and in healthy people, a further hour to be metabolized[29]. Detoxification is dependent on alcohol dehydrogenase metabolizing alcohol to acetaldehyde, and aldehyde dehydrogenase converting acetaldehyde into acetic acid. Alcohol intoxication can occur more readily, even with less ethanol consumption, in persons lacking these enzymes, as in some Asian populations. Symptoms of ethanol intoxication are correlated to blood alcohol levels. Alcohol dependency involves a need to increase the amount of alcohol to achieve a past same effect and unsuccessful efforts to diminish use despite the knowledge of its deleterious effects. Social and occupational dysfunction is common.

3.4.1.1 Alcohol intoxication

Toxicity occurs within hours of drinking. At levels of 0.05 mg/dl, disinhibition and disturbed judgment becomes evident in non-addicted persons. Motor function disruption is apparent at concentrations above 0.1%. Confusion and encephalopathy occurs near 0.3%, while coma is often observered at concentrations above 0.4%. Death is most commonly secondary to respiratory inhibition[29]. Signs of intoxication include slurring of speech, motor clumsiness, nystagmus, impaired cognition with delirium, and respiratory depression[26]. In such circumstances, it may be necessary to rule out intracranial hemorrhage, by obtaining a brain imaging scan of the head.

3.4.1.2 Alcohol withdrawal

In ethanol addicted individuals, a withdrawal syndrome can occur within half a day from the last drink or lower alcohol ingestion depending on the amount consumed, other substances used, patient's tolerance, hepatic status, and enzymatic activity. Withdrawal is associated with autonomic hyperactivity of vital signs, tremors, sweating, anxiety, decreased sleep, and/or perceptual disturbance (visual or tactile hallucinations). Grand-mal seizures can develop in up to 3% of this population[29].

Delirium Tremens (DTs) is a life threatening degree of withdrawal. It develops, within days to two weeks in addicted individuals after abrupt abstinence or reduced ethanol consumption. The DTs is characterized by severe withdrawal symptoms, seizures, fever, and a delirium[27].

Thiamine deficiency while metabolizing glucose without vitamin B1 can lead to a **Wernicke Korsakoff syndrome**. Wernickes is an acute, sometimes reversible condition, secondary to thiamine deficiency leading to bleeding in the mammillary bodies and related areas. It is characterized by delirium, ataxia, and ophthalmoplegia. Korsakoff is a related disorder presenting with confusion and confabulation. Both can result in a residual dementia.

3.4.2 Encephalopathy related to substance use

3.4.2.1 Cannabis

The effects of marijuana usually lasts for up to three hours; yet, its metabolite, tetrahydrocannabinol, can accumulate in adipose tissue, lasting for a much longer duration. This natural substance may cause a delirium[30]. Chronic use can lead to respiratory epithelial damage, increased risk of infections, autonomic hyperactivity, cognitive deficits, and teratogenicity [31]. Synthetic marijuana is sometimes more common and cheaper than natural cannabis. It may be preferred by those who are monitored for drug abuse intake since it is not detected by regular urine drug screens.

3.4.2.2 Stimulants

Cocaine: Several fatal cocaine-induced agitated encephalopathy cases have been reported[32]. Cocaine-associated delirium usually presents with hyperthermia, bizarre behavior, and delirium. It may herald cardiovascular collapse and death.

3.4.2.3 Hallucinogens

Ecstasy (3,4 methylenedioxymethamphetamine) or MDMA: Several post-ecstasy ingestion reports of delirium have been described in the literature [33]. This drug is thought to combine the effects of lysergic acid diethylamide (LSD) and amphetamines, leading to higher serotonin and dopamine levels. Intake of this substance leads initially to elevation in mood and increased sociability; while in individuals naïve to the drug, it can lead to anorexia, sweating, and elevated vital signs. Psychosis, confusion, and disorganization are sometimes documented[34]. This is mediated by hyperthermic effects of the drug, resulting in electrolyte imbalance with neurotoxicity that can precipitate seizures.

Gamma-hydroxybutyrate (GHB): This substance is a naturally occurring analog of gamma-aminobutyric acid (GABA). There are two other precursor drugs that are inactive unless metabolized into GHB within the body. Cross tolerance between ethanol and these substances do exist[35].

Intoxication with these short-acting agents can leads to euphoria, disinhibition, respiratory depression, and significant central nervous system depression. Combativeness is observed during such intoxications. Hypotension and/or bradycardia are documented. The toxicity usually resolves within a few hours due to the short half-life of the drug[35]. With medical intervention, fatalities are uncommon.

Withdrawal has been reported after drug discontinuation in individuals abusing GHB for long periods. High doses of benzodiazepines are required to treat withdrawal tremors, seizures, hallucinations, delusions, autonomic hyperactivity, and delirium[36]. Deaths are reported[10]. Diagnosis is difficult since GHB is non-detectable by routine drug screening and even with special urine testing it is usually no longer detected 12 hours after ingestion[10].

3.4.2.4 Opiates

This group of medication has been linked to hypoactive delirium[37]. Sedation, sleep disturbances, slowed mentation, and inattention are frequent signs. The mechanism is probably multifactorial; yet, anticholinergic effects of these agents might be prominent. Methadone has unpredictable pharmacokinetics and varies from one person to another. Naltrexone, a long-acting opioid antagonist, has frequently been used for rapid detoxification from opiates and blunts the pleasurable effects of opiates. In rare instances, naltrexone leads to delirium[38]. Disorientation, psychosis, and poor attention or concentration are documented and followed by evidence for withdrawal that includes mydriasis, diarrhea, lacrimation, muscle aches, abdominal discomfort, piloerection, and yawning.

Dextromethorphan is a frequently used antitussive drug that is a dextrorotatory isomer of codeine. When degraded by the liver, it forms a phencyclidine (PCP)-like substance, dextrorphan[39]. This over-the-counter preparation is frequently abused, and in high dosage can lead to a delirium with euphoria, autonomic hyperactivity, psychosis, agitation, and violent behavior. Ataxia, dysarthria, and seizures have also been reported. Elderly people are more prone to these ill effects, even at conventional doses[40].

3.4.2.5 Others

Nicotine Withdrawal: Sudden discontinuation of smoking tobacco leads to bradycardia, agitation, and irritability. On very rare occasions, a delirium or psychosis is documented after discontinuation of nicotine[41,42].

Ketamine: This agent is related to phencyclidine and is utilized as an anesthetic due to its analgesic and amnestic effects. Due to its tendency to cause psychoses with illusions, depersonalization, and even delirium, it is not commonly prescribed, but remains in a research status. Such encephalopathies are thought to be more frequent among females using rapid and/or high drug dosage[43].

4. Capacity and competency of the patient to make a decision

In a medical setting it is challenging when an ill patient decides not to proceed with an investigation, procedure, and/or treatment. Yet, imposing a decision on someone is only legitimate in certain situations. Forced interventions against an individual's stated wishes can only be done if the patient is legally declared not competent or found not to be clinically of decisional capacity.

Competency can only be determined in a judicial setting by a court order. The judge permanently appoints a medical guardian to make all future medical decisions. Arranging this may take several days to weeks, rending it unpractical in emergencies.

A medical team might consult with a psychiatrist for a bedside evaluation to determine whether a patient has the **"decisional capacity"** to make their own medical decisions. The capacity to make a decision must be specific to a particular procedure or plan at a specific time. Unless the individual is overtly delirious or unable to understand their situation, a thorough evaluation is necessary. Decisional capacity can vary between being present or absent quickly over time or vacillate back and forth. The psychiatrist must collaborate with the treating physician to understand the necessity of a procedure and consequences if it is not done in order to communicate this to the patient during the assessment.

There are several issues that must be documented as to reasons why a person is determined to be non-decisional at specific time[44]. They must understand information about their disease, its prognosis, and the suggested procedure. These individuals must understand their own decision and the reasoning behind it. Patients should comprehend alternatives and be able to choose between them. It is helpful to ask all evaluated persons to repeat back their understandings. To be decisional, the patient must demonstrate acceptance of the pathology diagnosed, the advantages and disadvantages of the proposed intervention, and the pros and cons of refusing the medical recommendations. A limited understanding may render people as non-decisional. For example, someone in a coma is never decisional. The individuals involved should be able to clearly communicate their wishes. Communication usually is in the form of speaking or writing, and it must always reflect good understanding of the clinical circumstances. If the patient's wishes are inconsistent or unclear, this infers a lack of decisional capacity.

All decisional patients are able to coherently clarify their decision and reasoning. Once found to be non-decisional, relatives or medical surrogates are called upon for making medical decisions. In overt emergencies, physicians may become the surrogate when family or guardians are not available; documented collaboration with colleagues and a hospital medical ethics committee consultation is helpful and provides some legal protection. In non-emergent cases, seek permission from a court to obtain guardianship for the non-decisional patient when surrogate decision makers are not available.

5. References

[1] Lonergan E, Luxenberg J, Areosa SA. Benzodiazepines for delirium. Cochrane Database Syst Rev 2009; (4):CD006379.

[2] Bosshart H. Withdrawal-induced delirium associated with a benzodiazepine switch: a case report. *J Med Case Reports* 2011; 5:207-11.

[3] Flacker JM, Cummings V, Mach JR Jr, Bettin K, Kiely DK, Wei J. The association of serum anticholinergic activity with delirium in elderly medical patients. *AM J Geri Psych* 1998; 6:31-41.

[4] Hufschmidt A, Shabarin V, Zimmer T. Drug-induced confusional states: the usual suspects? *Acta Neurol Scand* 2009; 120(6):436-8.

[5] Schatzberg AF, Cole JO, DeBattista C. Manual of Clinical Psychopharmacology; seventh edition. American Psychiatric Publishing Co, Washington, DC 2010.

[6] Baweja R, Sedky K, Lippmann S. Clozapine associated delirium. *East J Med* 2010; 15: 71-2.

[7] Lieberman JA. Managing anticholinergic side effects. *Prim Care Companion J Clin Psychiatry* 2004; 6(suppl 2):20-3.

[8] Strawn JR, Keck PE, Caroff SN. Neuroleptic Malignant Syndrome. *Am J Psych* 2007; 164(6):870-6.

[9] Marcantonio ER, Juarez G, Goldman L, Mangione CM, Ludwig LE, Lind L, Katz N, Cook EF, Orav EJ, Lee TH. The relationship of postoperative delirium with psychoactive medications. *J Am Med Assoc* 1994; 272:1518–22.

[10] Wojtowicz JM, Yarema MC, Wax PM. Withdrawal from gamma-hydroxybutyrate, 1,4-butanediol and gamma-butyrolactone: a case report and systematic review. *CJEM* 2008; 10(1):69-74.

[11] Marin LL, Garcia-Penas JJ, Herguedas JL, Gutierrez-Solana LG, Ruiz-Falco M, Rodriguez AD, Extremera VC. Phenytoin-induced visual disturbances mimicking delirium tremens in a child. *Eur J Pediatr Neurol* 2010; 14(5):460-3.

[12] Birmes P, Coppin D, Schmitt L, Lauque D. Serotonin syndrome: A brief review. *Can Med Assoc J* 2003; 168(11):1439-42.

[13] Radomski JW, Dursun SM, Reveley MA, Kutcher SP. An exploratory approach to the serotonin syndrome: An update of clinical phenomenology and revised diagnostic criteria. *Med Hypotheses* 2000; 55(3):218-24.

[14] Timmer RT, Sands JM. Lithium Intoxication. *J Am Soc Nephrol* 1999; 10:666-74.

[15] Oakley PW, Whyte IM, Carter GL. Lithium toxicity: An iatrogenic problem in susceptible individuals. *Aust N Z J Psych* 2001; 35(6):833-40.

[16] Boora K, Xu J, Hyatt J. Encephalopathy with combined lithium-risperidone administration. *Act Psychiatr Scand* 2008; 117:394-6.

[17] Sternberg DE, Bowers MB Jr, Heninger GR, Charney DS. Lithium prevents adaptation of brain dopamine systems to haloperidol in schizophrenic patients. *Psychiatry Res* 1983; 10:79-86.

[18] Baastrup P, Hollnagel P, Sorensen R, Schou M. Adverse reactions in treatment with lithium carbonate and haloperidol. *JAMA* 1976; 236:2645-6.

[19] Bjornsson E. Hepatotoxicity associated with antiepileptic drugs. *Acta Neurol Scand* 2008; 118:281-90.

[20] Carr RB, Shrewsbury K. Hyperammonia due to valproic acid in the psychiatric setting. *Am J Psych* 2007; 164:1020-7.

[21] Jacob S, Spinler SA. Hyponatremia associated with selective serotonin-reuptake inhibitors in older adults. *Ann Pharmacotherapy* 2006; 40:1618-22.

[22] Movig KL, Leufkens HG, Lenderink AW, van den Akker VG, Hodiamont PP, Goldschmidt HM, Egberts AC. Association between antidepressant drug use and hyponatraemia: a case-control study. *Br J Clin Pharmacol* 2002; 53(4):363–9.

[23] Sedky K, Lippmann S. Psychotropic medications and leukopenia. *Curr Drug Targets* 2006; 7(9):1191-4.

[24] Sedky K, Shaughnessy R, Hughes T, Lippmann S. Clozapine-induced agranulocytosis after 11 years of treatment. *Am J Psych* 2005; 162:814.
[25] Fink M. Post-ECT delirium. *Convulsive Therapy* 1993; 9(4):326-30.
[26] Diagnostic and Statistical Manual of Mental Disorders-IV-revised. American Psychiatric Association, Washington, DC, 2000.
[27] Fornaro M. Catatonia: A narrative review. *Cent Nerv Syst Agents Med Chem* 2011; 11(1): 73-9.
[28] Weintraub D, Lippmann S. Delirium mania in the elderly. *Int J Ger Psych* 2001; 16:374-7.
[29] Synopsis of psychiatry, 10th edition, 2007. Sadock BJ and Sadock VA. Lippincott Williams and Wilkins, Philadelphia, PA. Chapter 12; Substance-related disorders.
[30] Andre C, Jaber-Filho JA, Bent RM, Damasceno LM, Aquino-Neto FR. Delirium following ingestion of marijuana present in chocolate cookies. *CNS Spectr* 2006; 11(4):262-4.
[31] Hubbard JR, Franco SE, Onaivi ES. Marijuana: medical implications. *Am Fam Physician* 1999; 60(9):2583-8.
[32] Wetli CV, Mash D, Karch SB. Cocaine-associated agitated delirium and the neuroleptic malignant syndrome. *Am J Emerg Med* 1996; 14:425-8.
[33] Alciati A, Scaramelli B, Fusi A, Butteri E, Cattaneo ML, Mellado C. Three cases of delirium after "Ecstasy" ingestion. *J Psychoactive Drugs* 1999; 31(2):167-70.
[34] Gowing LR, Henry-Edwards SM, Irvine RJ, Ali RL. The health effects of ecstasy: a literature review. *Drug Alcohol Review* 2002; 21:53-63.
[35] Mason PE, Kerns II WP. Gamma hydroxybutyric acid (GHB) intoxication. *Acad Emerg Med* 2002; 9:730-9.
[36] Van Noorden MS, Van Dongen LC, Zitman FG, Vergouwen T. Gamma-hydroxybutyrate withdrawal syndrome: dangerous but not well-known. *Gen Hosp Psych* 2009; 31:394-6.
[37] Slatkin N, Rhiner M. Treatment of opiod-induced delirium with acetylcholinesterase inhibitors: a case report. *J Pain Symptom Management* 2004; 27(3):268-73.
[38] Das PP, Grover S, Kumar S. Naltrexone-precipitated delirium. *German J Psych* 2005; 8:101-3.
[39] Tobias JD. Dexmedetomidine to control agitation and delirium from toxic ingestions in adolescents. *J Pediatr Pharmacol* 2010; 15(1):43-8.
[40] Lotrich FE, Rosen J, Pollock BG. Detromethorphan-induced delirium and possible methadone interaction. *Am J Geriat Pharmacotherapy* 2005; 3(1):17-20.
[41] Gallagher R. Nicotine withdrawal as an etiologic factor in delirium. *J Pain Symptom Management* 1998; 16(2):76-7.
[42] Lucidarme O, Seguin A, Daubin C, Ramakers M, Terzi N, Beck P, Charbonneau P, Cheyron D. Nicotine withdrawal and agitation in ventilated critically ill patients. *Critical Care* 2010; 14(2):R58.
[43] Nguyen HT, Tran MCJ, Patel A. Pediatric emergence delirium with ketamine: a current and comprehensive literature review. http://www.pedsanesthesia.org/meetings/2007winter/pdfs/P88.pdf. Last accessed July 21, 2011.

[44] Appelbaum PS. Assessment of patients' competence to consent to treatment. *N Eng J Med* 2007; 357(18):1834-40.

7

Current Advances in Cerebral Malaria Associated Encephalopathy

Mingli Liu, Shanchun Guo, Monica Battle and Jonathan K. Stiles
Microbiology, Biochemistry & Immunology,
Morehouse School of Medicine,
Atlanta, GA
USA

1. Introduction

Malaria (*Plasmodium falciparum*) infects 200 to 300 million people globally and kills 900,000 (mostly children) every year. Severe malaria-related pathogeneses impacts a broad spectrum of host system and multiple organs (Zhu, Wu et al. 2009). Up to 20% of fatal cases are due to cerebral malaria (CM) and other severe forms of malaria such as severe malaria anemia (SMA). The precise mechanisms responsible for fatal CM-induced brain damage are unclear. To date, two main hypotheses have been proposed for human cerebral malaria. The first is the mechanical hypothesis, which proposes that infected or parasitized red blood cells (iRBC, or pRBC) bind to endothelial cells (EC), thus obstructing blood flow in micro capillaries leading to low tissue perfusion, compromised oxygenation and tissue damage. The second is the immunopathological hypothesis which proposes that hyper-inflammatory responses responsible for eliminating *P. falciparum* parasite cause edema, dysfunction in blood brain barrier (BBB), and organ failure and death.

Current anti-malaria drugs, such as quinine and artemisinin derivatives can effectively clear the parasites in blood, however a significant segment of severe malaria patients including CM patients still die or develop severe sequelae regardless of treatment (Taoufiq, Gay et al. 2008; Balachandar and Katyal 2010). Therefore important questions remain to be answered concerning the mechanism/(s) governing CM pathogenesis and appropriate therapies. The existing anti-malaria therapies are not sufficient partly due to drug resistance and various side effects, but beyond that these treatments mainly focus on the clearance of parasite, a direct antiplasmodial strategy, and are unable to prevent secondary changes such as encephalopathy resulting from parasite derived factors. The molecular mechanisms involved in malaria pathogenesis are highly complex and multifactorial. Recent studies have demonstrated that many pathological changes result from malaria-induced secondary effects involving various signaling molecules of the host (Armah, Wilson et al. 2007; Pamplona, Ferreira et al. 2007; Pamplona, Hanscheid et al. 2009). A better understanding of malaria host-parasite interactions will facilitate the development of novel strategies for intervention.

2. Pathological abnormalities associated with CM

2.1 Histopathologic hallmarks of the CM

The histopathologic hallmark of CM is sequestration of infected red blood cells in the microcirculation of the brain and retina (White 2011). A study performed in South Asia to quantitatively analyze the microvascular sequestration of *P. falciparum* in human brain demonstrated that sequestration occurs in all patients with *falciparum* malaria and is a consistent characteristic of severe malaria (Silamut, Phu et al. 1999). Fibrin thrombi and perivascular ring hemorrhages are also frequently found intravascular and extravascular. Diffuse petechial hemorrhages are seen in the cerebrum and cerebellum (Patankar, Karnad et al. 2002). Red blood cells (RBCs) around capillaries with hemorrhages are usually non-infected, because parasitized RBCs (pRBCs) are adherent to the endothelial cells in the vessel walls and are unable to freely bleed into the parenchyma (sequestration theory) (White 2011). Patches of necrosis are present around vessels with thrombi, with or without hemorrhages. Inflammation in the parenchyma of the brain or retina is not significant. Anti-malaria therapy could effectively eliminate parasites from the brains, but such interventions cannot always reverse malaria-induced primary or secondary pathological processes in severely diseased individuals. Circulating pRBCs will sequester as they mature (schizonts and trophozoites) (Silamut, Phu et al. 1999; Rogerson, Grau et al. 2004), but it is unclear what determines adherence to sites where severe pathology is common in the brain compared to sites where consequences appear minor such as in gastrointestinal tract and skin (Rogerson, Grau et al. 2004). Histopathological studies from animal models have also indicated that experimental cerebral malaria (ECM) is associated with microvascular plugging (sequestration of pRBCs, leukocytes and platelets), blood brain barrier (BBB) compromise, parenchymal petechial hemorrhages and edema (Medana, Chaudhri et al. 2001; Penet, Viola et al. 2005). Histology is the least expensive morphological technique, which enables examination of large areas of tissue, but all the lesions described above are not specific for malaria.

2.2 Retinal changes associated with CM

A postmortem study from Taylor et al (Taylor, Fu et al. 2004) raised an important question of how to accurately diagnose cerebral malaria. They found that one quarter of patients clinically diagnosed as cerebral malaria had an alternative cause of death, with no histopathologic findings typical of cerebral malaria. The retinal and cerebral circulations share a common embryologic origin, therefore changes identified by ophthalmoscopy at the fundus could be very helpful to accurately diagnose cerebral malaria (White, Lewallen et al. 2009; Beare, Lewallen et al. 2011). To this end, a case-control study was conducted during 1996 to 2008 in Malawi to analyze the differences in clinical and/or pathological alterations between children dying from CM and those dying of other deadly infectious diseases (White 2011). This project [supported by the National Institutes of Health (NIH) and named the Blantyre Malaria Project (BMP)] emphasized the application of the fundus as a tool to help diagnosis and prognosis for CM. All of the CM patients were asked to receive a full examination of eyes. At the end of 2008, 90 autopsies were performed among 352 deceased individuals. The patients' eyes were also removed for pathological analysis and clinicopathological correlation. Through this project, a clinicopathologic correlation of retinal hemorrhages with brain bleeding was substantially established, and they established the diagnostic criteria for malaria retinopathy based on their findings of retinal hemorrhages as well as three other pathological changes (White 2011), papilledema, an unusual discoloration of the retinal vessels, and a patchy whitening of the retina surrounding the fovea and in the periphery (White 2011). Today, malarial retinopathy is widely accepted as a diagnostic and prognostic factor in human cerebral malaria (White, Lewallen et al. 2009; Combes, El-Assaad et al. 2010). It has been strongly recommended that retina examination become a routine technique to assess a comatose child or adult when CM is a possible diagnosis (Beare, Lewallen et al. 2011). However, a key limitation of the retinal assessment is the subjective nature of ophthalomoscopy and its dependence on the expertise of the examining physician.

2.3 Magnetic resonance imaging

The first *in vivo* magnetic resonance on experimental CM was performed by Penet et al in 2005 (Penet, Viola et al. 2005). Magnetic resonance imaging (MRI) and magnetic resonance spectroscopy (MRS) are noninvasive and quantitative techniques which can identify not only structural but also functional and metabolic changes in experimental CM. They have confirmed characteristics of severe brain edema, parechymal tissue damage, cerebral hemorrhages, BBB disruption (Penet, Viola et al. 2005), and reduced cerebral blood flow in ECM (Penet, Viola et al. 2005). The hemorrhages mostly occurred in the corpus callosum. Crushing of the cerebellum and the pituitary gland, distortion of the brain stem and cerebellum are also frequently observed. These noninvasive and quantitative techniques will be as promising as surrogate tools used to monitor the progression of malaria and the efficacy of anti-malaria treatments (Penet, Viola et al. 2005; Vyas, Gupta et al. 2010; Rasalkar, Paunipagar et al. 2011). The BMP project (see 2.2) is conducting a magnetic resonance imaging scan to assess association between the brains of living individuals and prognosis of CM (White 2011). However, MRI systems are very expensive, emphasize the need to consider strategies that most severe malaria patients who are from underdeveloped African countries could afford.

3. Functional abnormalities commonly associated with CM

Cognitive impairment. CM in children is not only related to high mortality but also long-term neurocognitive sequelae (Casals-Pascual, Idro et al. 2008). Children with CM developed new neurological deficits such as gross motor, sensory, and language problems significantly more than corresponding controls (Birbeck, Molyneux et al. 2010). Many children with severe malaria suffer from intracranial hypertension caused by brain endothelial injury, apoptosis, and BBB dysfunction (Idro, Marsh et al. 2010). Intracranial hypertension compromises brain perfusion, nutrient and oxygen delivery leading to global ischemic injury, herniation, brainstem compression, and death (Walker, Salako et al. 1992; Newton, Crawley et al. 1997). Many children with severe malaria are discharged with spastic quadriplegia and severe learning disability (Newton, Crawley et al. 1997). Even if the gross neurological function can be almost completely recovered, hypoxia due to under-perfusion in multiple small areas still leaves many children with cognitive deficiencies (Idro, Marsh et al. 2010). In several retrospective and prospective studies, cognitive dysfunction in children with CM have been found to occur more frequently, and persist far longer than physical and neurologic deficits (Dugbartey, Spellacy et al. 1998; Holding, Stevenson et al. 1999; Carter,

Mung'ala-Odera et al. 2005; Carter, Lees et al. 2006; Boivin, Bangirana et al. 2007; John, Bangirana et al. 2008). 11.8% of surviving children had deficits particularly in vocabulary, receptive and expressive speech, word finding and phonology, concomitant with concurrent impairment in nonverbal functioning, memory or attention (Carter, Lees et al. 2006). The duration of seizures and extended comas are related to persistent cognitive deficits (Boivin, Bangirana et al. 2007).

Coma. Marsh et al (Marsh, English et al. 1996; Idro, Marsh et al. 2010) divided CM into four distinct groups based on the severity of neurological dysfunction (Marsh, English et al. 1996; Idro, Marsh et al. 2010). They are summarized as follows: 1) prolonged postictal state, patients in this group usually become conscious within 6 hours with complete neurological recovery. 2) covert status epilepticus, patients in this group are at high risk of aspiration resulting from hypoxic and hypercarbic status caused by hyperventilation. The length of the seizure will determine the patients' neurocognitive outcome. 3) severe metabolic derangement, deaths of patients were reported to be highly related to hypoglycemia and acidosis. 4) primary neurological syndrome, coma which may be caused by intracranial sequestration may persist for one to two days, often accompanied by intracranial hypertension (Marsh, English et al. 1996; Idro, Marsh et al. 2010).

Epilepsy. The incidence of epilepsy occurs in around 10% of children months to years after exposure to hypoxia (Ngoungou and Preux 2008; Birbeck, Molyneux et al. 2010), and increases with time (Opoka, Bangirana et al. 2009). Epilepsy in malaria is believed to be caused by the focal hypoxic/ischemic neural injury or global ischemic injury (Newton, Peshu et al. 1994; Crawley, Smith et al. 1996; Potchen, Birbeck et al. 2010). The morbidity of epilepsy is positively associated with the timing of exposure to hypoxia (Ngoungou and Preux 2008; Opoka, Bangirana et al. 2009). However, behavior and neuropsychiatric disorders did not differ significantly (Birbeck, Molyneux et al. 2010).

Malaria prophylaxis using sulphadoxine-pyrimethamine combined with amodiaquine was reported to improve cognitive function and school performance in clinical trials when compared to placebo groups (Clarke, Jukes et al. 2008). Similar phenomenon was found in an animal study by Reis et al (Reis, Comim et al. 2010), who support the view that cognitive dysfunction is sustained after rescue treatment in PbA-infected CM-sensitive C57BL/6 mice, an animal model for CM. In addition, treatment of CM-sensitive C57BL/6 mice with additive antioxidants such as malondialdehyde, MDA and conjugated dienes along with chloroquine prevented the development of persistent cognitive damage. This indicates that cognition problems may be associated with deleterious reactive oxygen species released during infection.

4. Effects of cellular and humoral components in CM pathogenesis

4.1 Endothelial cells and parasitized red blood cells

Endothelial cells. One major feature of CM is the sequestration of pRBCs in brain microcirculation through adhesion between pRBCs and endothelial cells. The adhesion of *falciparum* parasitized erythrocytes to the human cerebral microvascular endothelium enables the parasites to avoid splenic clearance (D'Ombrain, Voss et al. 2007) providing the biological basis for the sequestration of pRBCs, and the major feature of CM. The surface receptors on endothelial cells are responsible for adhesion. The major surface receptors on endothelial cells are Intercellular Adhesion Molecule 1 (ICAM-1) and CD36 (Collins, Read et al. 1995; Tripathi, Sullivan et al. 2006; Tripathi, Sha et al. 2009). CD36 is an 88-kDa integral protein found on the surface of not only endothelial cells, but adipocytes, platelets, monocytes, and macrophages. ICAM-1 is a 90–115 kDa transmembrane glycoprotein expressed on a variety of cell types including endothelial cells (Ochola, Siddondo et al. 2011). Other endothelial surface antigens include PECAM-1, hyaluronic acid, chondroitin sulfate A (CSA), thrombospondin (TSP),αvβ3 and E-selectin, P-selectin, vascular cell adhesion molecule-1 (VCAM-1) (Schofield and Hackett 1993; Ho, Hickey et al. 2000; Craig and Scherf 2001; Yipp, Hickey et al. 2007). The sequestration of pRBCs in brain microcirculation in CM is due to the erythrocyte membrane protein 1 (pfEMP-1) expressed on *P.falciparum* parasitized RBCs adhere to endothelium through the endothelial surface receptors (Kang and McGavern 2010), mainly ICAM-1 and CD36. The interactions between pRBCs (not normal erythrocytes) and vascular endothelium through cellular adhesion molecules induce the deleterious endothelial cell responses (Combes, El-Assaad et al. 2010), including inflammation, endothelial activation, and apoptosis of microvascular endothelial cells resulting in the disruption of the blood-brain barrier (Idro, Marsh et al. 2010) in *P. falciparum* malaria. Apoptosis sequentially occurred in different cells. In murine models, apoptosis occurs in endothelial cells first, and is followed by neuronal and glia cells (Lackner, Burger et al. 2007). *P. falciparum*-pRBCs increase the expression of ICAM-1 and CD36 (Collins, Read et al. 1995; Tripathi, Sullivan et al. 2006; Tripathi, Sha et al. 2009) which strengthens sequestration, probably through NF-kappa B (Collins, Read et al. 1995; Tripathi, Sullivan et al. 2006; Tripathi, Sha et al. 2009) and MAP Kinase activation (Yipp, Robbins et al. 2003). In addition, pRBC adhesion to endothelium was found to up regulate several TNF-superfamily genes and apoptosis-related genes such as Bad, Bax, caspase-3, SARP2, DFF45/ICAD, IFN-g receptor2, Bcl-w, Bik, and iNOS (Pino, Vouldoukis et al. 2003). It is worthy to note that direct contact between pRBC and microvascular EC may not be required for triggering apoptosis, because soluble factors released from parasitized erythrocytes have apoptotic effects on HBVEC and neuroglia cells (Wilson, Huang et al. 2008). The heterogeneity of endothelium in various locations of the body, characterized by the difference in expression levels of CD36 or ICAM-1 would probably determine the type and severity of malaria. Most recent results indicated that increased binding to CD36 by parasites is associated with uncomplicated malaria, since little CD36 is expressed on brain microvasculature (Ochola, Siddondo et al. 2011); while binding to ICAM-1 by parasites is increased and is associated with cerebral malaria (Ochola, Siddondo et al. 2011). Chilongola et al argued Ochola's finding, and they suggested that CD36 deficiency may protect against *falciparum* malarial anemia (Chilongola, Balthazary et al. 2009). Further studies are required to clear out these arguments. Another big change in endothelial cells in CM is the damage of microvasuclar repair which is associated with low levels of circulating endothelial progenitor cells (CD34+/VEGF2+ and CD34+/CD133+) (Gyan, Goka et al. 2009). Together, activation of endothelial cells in brain vascular system by pRBC is one of the key events leading to encephalopathy.

Parasitized red blood cells. pfEMP-1, a variable antigen expressed by *P. falciparum* (D'Ombrain, Voss et al. 2007), is encoded by the var-gene family of *P. falciparum* (Ikenoue, Kawazu et al. 2002). As we described before, this knob protein plays a significant role in the pathophysiology of CM (Sharma 1997). pfEMP-1protein (Ikenoue, Kawazu et al. 2002) interacts with the endothelial cell through adhesion molecules in a receptor-ligand dependent manner (D'Ombrain, Voss et al. 2007). Ultrastructural studies found an attachment between pRBC knobs and endothelial cell microvillus protrusions (Tripathi, Sullivan et al. 2006). pfEMP-1 has been considered a good candidate antigen for vaccination and a molecular therapeutic target to reverse the cytoadherence process (Sharma 1997). In addition, PfEMP-1 suppresses the production of the cytokine interferon-gamma (IFNγ) produced by human peripheral blood mononuclear cells (γδT, NK, and αβT cells), which is a receptor (CD36)- independent (D'Ombrain, Voss et al. 2007). Down-regulation of the proinflammatory IFN-γ responses has some beneficial effects for parasite growth. Taken together, changes in RBCs phenotype by *falciparum* infections trigger activation of cerebral microvascular endothelial cells resulting in *falciparum* related encephalopathy.

4.2 Leukocytes

Monocyte sequestration has recently been acknowledged to play a role in human CM and murine ECM (Grau, Fajardo et al. 1987; Combes, El-Assaad et al. 2010). Fatal malaria caused by *P. falciparum* is associated with both neutrophil activation and subsequent endothelial damage. For example, apoptosis induced by secretory products of neutrophils plays a key role in endothelial cell damage (Hemmer, Lehr et al. 2005). An antioxidant such as ascorbic acid and a protease inhibitor such as ulinastatin have been used to dramatically decrease *falciparum*-activated neutrophil-associated endothelial apoptosis (Hemmer, Lehr et al. 2005). The role of CD4+, CD8+, NKT and σγT cells will be described elsewhere (see 4.5 Immunity to malaria).

4.3 Platelets

Endothelial cell activation plays an important role in the pathogenesis of cerebral malaria. Rosetting pRBCs bind to the endothelial cells and occlude microvessels in the brain (Cox and McConkey 2010). Therefore, it is not surprising that thrombocytopenia is a common feature in both murine ECM and human CM (Wassmer, Combes et al. 2003; Combes, El-Assaad et al. 2010). Thus, it is essential to understand the association between platelets, pRBCs, leukocytes and endothelial cells in CM. CM is characterized by the accumulation of circulating cells including platelets within brain microvessels (Faille, Combes et al. 2009). Sequestration and accumulation of platelets in various organs, especially in the brain may partly explain the decrease in platelet count in circulation (Wassmer, Combes et al. 2003; Combes, El-Assaad et al. 2010) in malaria disease.

There is increasing evidence that platelets contribute to the pathogenesis of cerebral malaria. Platelets modulate cytoadherence of pRBCs to brain endothelial cells *in vitro* (Faille, Combes et al. 2009). Animal studies indicate that blocking platelet function in mice is protective against severe malaria (Sun, Chang et al. 2003; van der Heyde, Gramaglia et al. 2005; Wassmer, Combes et al. 2006). Platelets and endothelial cells share common receptors, such as CD36, the complement receptor gC1qR/HABP/p32, and PECAM-1. CD36 and PECAM-1 are receptors for pRBCs (Treutiger, Heddini et al. 1997; Pain, Ferguson et al. 2001; Biswas, Hafiz et al. 2007). Interactions between PfEMP1 on *Plasmodium* and CD36 on platelets possibly lead to platelet activation. The platelet activation aggregates pRBCs and platelets resulting in occlusion of microcirculation and activation of the endothelial cells (Cox and McConkey 2010). gC1qR/HABP/p32 interacts with both pRBCs and platelets potentiating clumping of pRBCs (Biswas, Hafiz et al. 2007). The pathogenic role of platelets can be summarized as follows. First, *in vitro* cocultures from Wassmer et al (Wassmer, de Souza et al. 2006) showed that platelets or pRBC have a direct cytotoxic effect on TNF- or LT-alpha-activated human brain vascular endothelial cells (HBVEC); second, platelets potentiate the cytotoxicity of pRBC activated HBVEC cells. Both permeability and trans-endothelial electrical resistance (TEER) are strongly affected, and the apoptosis rate of HBVEC cells dramatically increase. Inhibition of platelet adherence to brain microvessels protects against severe *P. berghei* malaria (Sun, Chang et al. 2003; van der Heyde, Gramaglia et al. 2005); third, studies evaluating interactions of platelet-RBC-endothelium suggest that pathogenic effects of platelets are not caused by adherence to the endothelial cells but result from the regulation of cytokine production (van der Heyde, Gramaglia et al. 2005; Cox and McConkey 2010). It has also been reported that there are more than 300 biologically active proteins in platelet extracts (Coppinger, Cagney et al. 2004), which play a crucial role in activation of endothelial cells (Coppinger, Cagney et al. 2004). As such, platelets can increase leukocyte adhesion to endothelial cells via IL-1, fibrinogen, ICAM-2 and P-secletin (McEver 2001); fourth, micro-particles released from platelets can increase adhesion between endothelium and leukocytes and platelets via ICAM-1 (Barry and FitzGerald 1999; Combes, El-Assaad et al. 2010).

However, effects to target platelets as therapy for cerebral malaria have resulted in controversy. Some studies argue that platelets have a protective role in malaria (Polack, Delolme et al. 1997; Wassmer, Taylor et al. 2008), while others argue the opposite view. Such inconsistencies might be explained by the different roles platelets play. For example, platelet activation will produce thrombocytopenia, which may be an adaptive response to platelet-induced RBC clumping (Wassmer, Taylor et al. 2008).

4.4 Immunity to malaria

Immune responses are crucial factors in the pathophysiology of cerebral malaria, both in its initiation and progression. Parasite-triggered immune response and inflammation are considered to be a probable cause of death from CM associated encephalopathy. Innate immunity is generated by neutrophils, NK, NKT, dentritic cell (DCs) and σγT cells; while adaptive immunity is produced by CD4+, CD8+ T cells. B cells and NK cells are not requisite for CM pathology (Yanez, Manning et al. 1996), but NK cells are involved in CXCL10-induced CXCR3+T cells trafficking leading to cerebral diseases and fatalities (Hansen, Bernard et al. 2007). NKT cells are specialized cells coexpressing NK and T cell receptors. They produce high levels of IFN-γ and IL-4 after activation, and therefore influence Th1/Th2 immune responses. Thus, the polarization of Th1/Th2 immune responses will determine malarial fatalities (Hansen, Siomos et al. 2003). In a mouse model utilized by Seixas et al, DCs are activated in response to pRBCs internalization, and are important in shaping the adaptive immune response to severe malaria (Seixas, Moura Nunes et al. 2009).

ECM involving *P. berghei* ANKA is considered a T cell-mediated disease. Both CD4+ and CD8+ T cells are involved in ECM (Belnoue, Potter et al. 2008). Treatment with anti-CD4 or anti-CD8 antibodies protected against ECM (Hermsen, van de Wiel et al. 1997). Studies in malaria patients also indicate higher frequencies of peripheral blood CD4(+) Foxp3(+) CD25(+) regulatory T (Treg) cells which correlate with increased blood parasitemia (Haque,

Best et al. 2010). In contrast, CD4+ natural regulatory T cells [CD4(+) Foxp3(+) CD25(+), Treg] in animals prevent cerebral malaria via CTLA-4 (but not IL-10) when expanded *in vivo*. In addition to CD4+ T cells, studies from a murine CM model also confirmed that CXCL10/CXCR3 interactions in the pathogenesis of fatal CM is through the recruitment and activation of pathogenic CD8+ T cells (Belnoue, Potter et al. 2008; Van den Steen, Deroost et al. 2008). The reason why CXCR3-/- mice were resistant to CM is potentially due to a reduction in the number of CD8+ T cells (Miu, Mitchell et al. 2008). Consistent with this, adoptive transfer of CD8+ cells abrogated protection of CM in CXCR3-/- and CXCL10-/- mice against *P. berghei*-mediated ECM. CD8+ cytotoxic T cells are involved in the disruption of BBB by perforin-dependent process. Interestingly, only CD8+ cells which were located in microvessels, expressed perforin, induced granule exocytosis and cytolysis (Nitcheu, Bonduelle et al. 2003; Miu, Mitchell et al. 2008), and activated cytotoxicity in a Fas dependent pathway (Nitcheu, Bonduelle et al. 2003; Miu, Mitchell et al. 2008). ECM induction was not only dependent on CD8(+) T cell-derived perforin but also on granzyme B (GzmB) (Haque, Best et al. 2011). CD8+ T cell-mediated CM pathology is characterized as organ-specific; it only occurs in the brain not the liver (Haque, Best et al. 2011). McQuillan et al (McQuillan, Mitchell et al. 2011) indicated that protection against CM was associated with a reduction in the accumulation and activation of CD8+ T cells in the cerebral microcirculation, along with reduction in malaria parasite burden in the same area (McQuillan, Mitchell et al. 2011). A breakthrough in malaria immunity research is that classical anti-plasmodial drugs act on the immune system in addition to their anti-plasmodial activities. Quinine treatment reduced local cytokines and chemokines and coincided with protection against the disease (McQuillan, Mitchell et al. 2011). Artemisinin and its derivatives have been shown to reduce CD4+ and CD8+ T cell inflammatory responses (Veerasubramanian, Gosi et al. 2006; Wang, Tang et al. 2007; Wang, Qiu et al. 2007; Xu, He et al. 2007). Yanez et al indicated that γδ T cells, in addition to CD4+ and CD8+ T cells, have an essential role to play in the pathogenesis of CM (Yanez, Batchelder et al. 1999).

4.5 Astrocytes, microglia, blood brain barrier

Studies from a rodent model and human postmortem tissue suggest that the activation of astrocytes and microglial cells occurs during pathogenesis of CM (Medana, Hunt et al. 1997; Medana, Day et al. 2002; Medana and Turner 2006; Szklarczyk, Stins et al. 2007). Accumulation of macrophages and proliferation of microglial cells in the brain play important roles in CM. They increase the adherence of pRBCs to the cerebral microvasculature by secretion of proinflammatory mediators, disruption of BBB, and recruitment of inflammatory cells to the local area, resulting in the brain pathophysiological changes in these patients. An elegant study on the retina by Medana et al (Medana, Chan-Ling et al. 1996; Medana, Chan-Ling et al. 2000) emphasized the importance of the immune system in the activation of glial cells and consequently in the formation of CM. Because the retina and the brain share similarities in development and function, they used retinal astrocytes and microglial cells to study the function of astrocytes and microglia in the pathogenesis of ECM (Medana, Chan-Ling et al. 1996; Medana, Chan-Ling et al. 2000). Activation of astrocytes and microglia were both observed during fatal murine cerebral malaria using the retinal whole-mount technique (Medana, Chan-Ling et al. 1996; Medana, Chan-Ling et al. 2000). They found that the disruption of blood retinal barrier (BRB)/BBB by parasites initiated morphological and distributional changes in astrocytes and microglia. However these mild changes and redistribution were not sufficient for the development of cerebral pathology. The loss of astrocyte ensheathment of vessel segments and the reactive microglia changes resulting in severe cerebral pathology will require immune system activation triggered by the malaria parasites (Medana, Chan-Ling et al. 1996; Medana, Chan-Ling et al. 2000).

Activated astrocytes and microglial cells are capable of secreting a wide range of cytokines/chemokines, expressing MHC class II and co-stimulatory molecules (Dong and Benveniste 2001; Combes, El-Assaad et al. 2010). Thus they contribute to inflammatory responses within the brain parenchyma in CM (Deininger, Kremsner et al. 2002). Microglia and astrocytes produce TNF-alpha during the course of the disease (Medana, Hunt et al. 1997), which plays a key role in the pathogenesis of fatal CM (Lucas, Lou et al. 1997). Astrocytes express TNF receptor 1 (TNFR1), TNF receptor 2 (TNFR2), IL-1 receptor 1, IFN α/β receptor, IFN-γ receptor, and macrophage colony-stimulating factor (M-CSF) receptor (Tada, Diserens et al. 1994). TNF-α induces astrocytes to generate and secret colony stimulating factors M-CSF, granulocyte colony-stimulating factor (G-CSF) and granulocyte macrophage colony-stimulating factor (GM-CSF), IL-6 and TNF-α itself (Benveniste 1992). TNF-α and IL-1 induce astrocytes to produce pro-inflammatory cytokines and nitric oxide (Aloisi, Borsellino et al. 1995). Nevertheless, *in vivo*, astrocytes limit the immune response within the central nervous systems (CNS) and initiate repair processes (Eddleston and Mucke 1993; Mucke and Eddleston 1993). Microglia, when stimulated by LPS and IFN-γ (Giulian, Baker et al. 1986; Frei, Siepl et al. 1987), produce and release IL-1 (Giulian and Lachman 1985; Giulian, Baker et al. 1986; Giulian, Young et al. 1988), IL-6 and TNF-α (Frei, Malipiero et al. 1989; Medana, Hunt et al. 1997). IL-1 is mitogenic to astroglia (Giulian, Baker et al. 1986). In malaria, any factors (such as CD8+T cells) inducing damage to the microvascular endothelium can result in the leakage of cytokines, malaria antigens and other potentially harmful molecules across the BBB into the brain parenchyma. All of these, in turn, result in the activation of microglia and the activation and apoptosis of astrocytes (Hunt, Golenser et al. 2006) to exacerbate the CM syndrome.

The degree of immune activation and degeneration of glial cells reflect the extent of neurological complications in murine ECM (Medana, Chaudhri et al. 2001). Astrocyte disruption will cause acute or chronic damage to brain function. Damage to astrocytes, a major source of kynurenic acid may result in reduced production of the neuroprotectant molecule kynurenic acid (Medana, Hien et al. 2002; Medana, Day et al. 2003; Hunt, Golenser et al. 2006), causing a decrease in its ratio relative to the neuroexcitotoxic molecule quinolinic acid, which might contribute to some of the neurological symptoms of ECM and CM (Medana, Hien et al. 2002; Medana, Day et al. 2003; Hunt, Golenser et al. 2006). Redistribution, changes in gene expression, and the death of astrocytes have all been reported in human CM and ECM (Medana, Idro et al. 2007). Astrocyte ensheathment of vessels was associated with a big increase in BBB permeability that occurs at the time of neurological complications in the murine models of malaria. The loss of astrocyte processes was associated with the adherence of monocytes to the vascular endothelium, suggesting that toxic products produced by monocytes might play a role in astrocyte degeneration (Medana, Chaudhri et al. 2001). Microglia were found to be concentrated around capillaries in the grey matter. However microglia containing neutral lipid and iron pigment were found in large perivascular lesions in the white matter. In addition, microglia were associated with perivenular haemorrhages (Medana, Chaudhri et al. 2001). Activation of microglia might damage astrocytes via Fas/FasL interactions (Potter, Chan-Ling et al. 2006). These findings underline the important contribution within the CNS of glia and their secreted products, such as cytokines, in the development of human CM.

4.6 Microparticles (MP) and CM

Eukaryotic cells, after activation by a variety of stimuli, shed components of their plasma membranes into circulation. Such submicron particles may include cytoplasmic and nuclear (Roos, Gennero et al. 2010) elements and are known colloquially as microparticles (MPs) (Barry and FitzGerald 1999; Doeuvre, Plawinski et al. 2009). Monocytes, lymphocytes, endothelial cells, erythrocytes, granulocytes and platelets have been shown to vesiculate either *in vitro* or *in vivo* (Barry and FitzGerald 1999). MPs, exposing the phospholipid phosphatidyl serine (PS) on the external surface of the cell membrane (Schroit, Madsen et al. 1985), have been identified increasingly in a broad range of diseases (Roos, Gennero et al. 2010) where vascular dysfunction and inflammation are important pathophysiological mechanisms (Lynch and Ludlam 2007).

Human studies (Combes, Taylor et al. 2004) on MPs in CM were first conducted in Malawian patients demonstrated that increased release of circulating endothelial cell-derived MP- (EMPs) correlate with malaria severity. EMPs are increased in patients with severe CM complicated with coma (Barry and FitzGerald 1999; Doeuvre, Plawinski et al. 2009), but not with those with malaria complicated by anemia. The high concentrations of plasma TNF in patients with CM may enhance endothelial vesiculation both *in vivo* and *in vitro* (Combes, Simon et al. 1999). In a *P. berghei* (PbA) infected ECM mouse model, ABCA1, a gene determining the lipid transbilayer remodeling was found to be responsible for external exposure of PS to generate EMPs in malaria (Combes, Coltel et al. 2005).

Apart from endothelium, other cell types including erythrocytes, platelets and monocytes also release microparticles and contribute to the pathogenesis in patients with malaria. Red blood cell–derived microparticles (RMPs) were increased in patients with *P. falciparum, P. vivax,* and *P. malariae* compared with healthy controls (Nantakomol, Dondorp et al. 2011). RMPs were highest in severe *falciparum* malaria patients. RMPs released from either parasitized erythrocytes or uninfected red blood cells (URBCs) are pathogenic. pRBCs released 10 times more RMPs than did URBCs. Overall, the majority of RMPs were derived from URBCs (Nantakomol, Dondorp et al. 2011). *In vitro,* RMPs production increased as the parasites matured. Some biological molecules can trigger RMPs release. For example, hemin-mediated oxidative stress was associated with the production of RMPs (Nantakomol, Dondorp et al. 2011). Hemin induced RMP formation in URBCs was inhibited by N-acetylcysteine. In PbA infected C57 BL/6 mice (Couper, Barnes et al. 2010), malaria parasite-derived plasma MPs which are derived primarily from pRBCs, induced severe inflammation through potent macrophage activation as indicated by CD40 up-regulation and TNF production. Consistent with this, *in vitro* experiments confirmed that these MPs produced higher levels of macrophage activation than intact infected red blood cells. MPs driven macrophage activation was dependent on MyD88 and TLR-4 signaling (Couper, Barnes et al. 2010).

Platelets vesiculate particles following activation by complement proteins C5b-9 (Sims, Faioni et al. 1988). It was demonstrated that platelet-derived MPs (PMPs) may modulate adhesive interactions between endothelial cells and monocytes resulting in human atherosclerosis and inflammation (Sims, Faioni et al. 1988). In 2009, Grau's group (Faille, Combes et al. 2009) showed that PMPs derived from activated platelets are able to bind to *falciparum*-infected RBCs (pRBCs), thereby transferring platelet antigens to the PRBCs surface. PMPs uptake by HBVECs induce changes in the endothelial phenotype, dramatically increasing pRBCs cytoadherence to HBVECs and playing a role in the pathogenesis of *P.falciparum* (Faille, Combes et al. 2009). PMPs adherence is specific to pRBCs, and require the expression of the pfEMP variant on pRBCs. Not surprisingly, this binding to pRBCs decreases either after digestion of pRBCs surface proteins by trypsin or neutralization of PMPs with a mAb to platelet-endothelial cell adhesion molecule-1 (CD31) and glycoprotein IV (CD36) (Faille, Combes et al. 2009).

In a recent human study conducted in Douala, Cameroon (Pankoui Mfonkeu, Gouado et al. 2010) indicated that not only plateletic, erythrocytic and endothelial but also leukocytic MPs levels were elevated in CM patients with neurological dysfunctions but return to normal levels after recovery of patients. This vesiculation in the vascular compartment is a characteristic of CM but not of SMA. Platelet MPs were the most abundant and their levels significantly correlated with the depth of unconsiousness and thrombocytopenia. Their findings raise the importance of MP as a biomarker of cerebral involvement and the importance of the intervention to block MPs production as a new therapeutic strategy in CM (Pankoui Mfonkeu, Gouado et al. 2010). Whether MPs can be detected and identified in CSF or other body compartments (saliva) as a predictor of cerebral tissue damage is unclear.

Various techniques including flow cytometry (FC), enzyme-linked immunosorbent assay (ELISA), and functional assays have been used to detect circulating MPs (Azevedo, Pedro et al. 2007; Lynch and Ludlam 2007). 1) FC is the most common method to quantify MPs. The advantages of FC are simplicity and the wealth of data generated from study samples. However, the small size of MPs and the lack of uniformity in methodology complicate measurement of outcomes. As MPs contain surface and cytoplasmic contents of the parent cells (particles which reflect their cell of origin and its state of activation) and contain phosphatidylserine, antibodies against specific cell surface markers and annexin V can be used for detection. FC can be used to quantify and identify MPs of different cellular origin (Doeuvre, Plawinski et al. 2009; Campos, Franklin et al. 2010; Roos, Gennero et al. 2010). 2) Since FC is too expensive and not feasible in most clinical centers, an ELISA for PMPs has recently been developed as a viable alternative for the clinical measurement of PMPs levels (Shirafuji, Hamaguchi et al. 2008; Nomura, Shouzu et al. 2009). ELISA can be performed after freezing the sample, allowing samples to be batched for assays, and thus reducing expenses. The PMPs ELISA kit used two monoclonal antibodies against glycoprotein CD42b and CD42a (Shirafuji, Hamaguchi et al. 2008; Nomura, Shouzu et al. 2009). One unit/milliliter of PMPs was defined as 24,000 platelets/ml of solubilized platelets in this ELISA system.

Recently, new methods have been introduced to assay for MPs. SYTO 13 is a more sensitive quantitative assay for MPs (Ullal, Pisetsky et al. 2010). The emergence of SYTO13 dyes for detection of MPs is attributed to limitation of FC with either light scatter or surface marker staining due to the small size of MPs (0.05 to 1.5µm). The SYTO 13 assay is based on the principle that MPs contain DNA and RNA, thus allowing SYTO13 to bind both DNA and

RNA within particles. STYO 13 enhanced the ability of the detection for particles 1.5–2.9 times more than did light scatter in FC (Ullal, Pisetsky et al. 2010). Circulating nucleic acids (CNAs) have been increasingly recognized as powerful diagnostic and prognostic tools for various inflammatory diseases (Ullal, Pisetsky et al. 2010). For example, CNAs level as measured by amplification of the human telomerase reverse transcriptase (hTERT) gene, or the dsDNA quantification were significantly increased in plasma from *P. vivax* patients compared with healthy controls (Ullal, Pisetsky et al. 2010). No such report is available for malaria encephalopathy.

5. Molecular pathogenesis of CM

5.1 Crosstalk and signaling pathways in CM

5.1.1 Cytokines and chemokines

Cytokines and chemokines exert both protective and harmful effects during CM pathogenesis. Antigen-like components released from malaria induce both pro and anti-inflammatory cytokines and chemokines. The balance between these biological mediators is crucial for parasite control and for the contribution to the pathogenesis of severe malaria and CM encephalopathy (Idro, Marsh et al. 2010).

5.1.1.1 Th1 and Th2 cytokines

The harmful, dysregulated immune response resulting in CM or ECM is mainly due to the imbalance between Th1 and Th2 types with overproduction of some cytokines, such as IFNγ combined with underproduction of others such as IL-10.

Th1 cytokines include IFN-γ and lymphotoxin (TNF-beta). CD4+ Th cells are subdivided into two different types, known as type 1 Th (Th1) and type 2 Th (Th2). Th1 cells produce cytokines, such as IL-2, IFN-γ (at a later stage also by CD8+ cytotoxic T cells), tumor necrosis factor (TNF-alpha) and TNF-beta, which cause the activation of macrophages and the process of opsonization and cytotoxicity (Romagnani 1997). In contrast, Th2 cells are considered to play a regulatory and protective role, since cytokines produced by these cells [e.g., IL-10, transforming growth factor-β (TGF-β), IL-4 and IL-13] inhibit the production of Th1 cytokines and activation of macrophages (Romagnani 1997; Hunt and Grau 2003). A recent study in Ghanaian and Indian patients demonstrated an association between fatal CM and increased serum and cerebrospinal fluid (CSF) levels of proinflammatory and proapoptotic factors including CXCL10, IL-1ra, sTNFR1, sTNFR2, sFas and decreased serum and CSF levels of neuroprotective angiogenic growth factors (PDGFb) (Armah, Wilson et al. 2007). In children with CM, cytokine TNF-α level in CSF is associated with subsequent neurological and cognitive morbidity (John, Panoskaltsis-Mortari et al. 2008).

Th2 cytokines include IL-4, IL-10 and TGF-beta. IL-10 not only plays an important role in cerebral malaria pathogenesis (Yanez, Manning et al. 1996; John, Panoskaltsis-Mortari et al. 2008), but also is associated with asymptomatic malaria in pregnant women (Wilson, Bythwood et al. 2010). TGFβ isoforms were shown to accumulate in the brain of CM patients. Members of the TGFβ cytokine family have been associated with the control of malaria infection and parasite growth (Omer and Riley 1998; Hunt and Grau 2003; Chaiyaroj, Rutta et al. 2004); TGFβ1 levels were significantly reduced in peripheral plasma of children with CM (Omer and Riley 1998; Hunt and Grau 2003; Chaiyaroj, Rutta et al.

2004). However, a mechanism for CM was found through TGFβ1 released from activated platelets, by which TGFβ1 induces TNF-mediated apoptosis in human brain endothelium (Wassmer, de Souza et al. 2006).

Other host serological factors contain CXCL10, interleukine (IL-1), IL-6, IL-8, MCP-1, RANTES. In 2003, CXCL10 was first reported to be a host-protective factor in ECM (Hunt and Grau 2003). CXCL10 expression was expressed early in either cerebral malaria-susceptible or -resistant strains of mice to *P. berghei* ANKA infection (Chen and Sendo 2001; Hanum, Hayano et al. 2003). More recently, a pioneering study conducted both in India and Ghana, identified CXCL10 as a serum and CSF biomarker associated with increased risk of fatal *P. falciparum*-mediated CM in humans (Armah, Wilson et al. 2007; Jain, Armah et al. 2008; Wilson, Huang et al. 2008). Subsequently, studies from a murine CM model also confirmed the importance of CXCL10/CXCR3 interactions in the pathogenesis of fatal CM through the recruitment and activation of pathogenic CD8+ T cells (Belnoue, Potter et al. 2008; Van den Steen, Deroost et al. 2008). CXCL10-/- and CXCR3-/- mice are partially resistant to *P. berghei*-mediated CM. Furthermore, the study also revealed that CXCR3-/- mice were resistant to CM as a result of a reduction in the number of CD8+ T cells (Miu, Mitchell et al. 2008). Adoptive transfer of CD8+ cells abrogated protection of CM in CXCR3-/- mice while CXCL10-/- mice were partially resistant to *P. berghei*-mediated CM. A proposed cellular pathways of CXCL10-mediated severe malaria is presented in Figure 1 [(Adapted with permission from Cytokine and Growth Review (Liu, Guo et al. 2011)]. Endothelial cells, astrocytes and microglia are a prominent source of CXCL10 and CXCL9. 1) Through T cells sequestration (Belnoue, Kayibanda et al. 2002; Nitcheu, Bonduelle et al. 2003; Campanella, Tager et al. 2008; Miu, Mitchell et al. 2008). CXCL10 could attract activated T cells and mediate Th1-type response, characterized by the sequestration of monocytes and T cells (mainly CD8+) in cerebral microvessels. Granule exocytosis and Fas/Fas ligand activation pathways are two distinct mechanisms involved in the death of brain endothelial cells by CD8+ lymphocytes. 2) Through NK cell sequestration (Hansen, Siomos et al. 2003; Hansen, Bernard et al. 2007), NK cells mediate direct cytotoxic activity or reconstitution capacity of T cells to migrate in response to CXCL10 to the CNS. 3) Through up-regulation of ICAM-1 on brain microvascular endothelial cells (Bauer, Van Der Heyde et al. 2002). LTα and IFN-γ are required for PbA-induced endothelial ICAM-1 up-regulation and PbA-induced increased cytoadherence of sequestered of pRBC to the endothelium of cerebral vessels. This results in hypoxia, hemorrhage and pathology, and represents another potential mechanism of CM pathogenesis.

CXCL10 is elevated in association with chills, rigors, anemia (Jain, Singh et al. 2009) and pre-chloroquine/primaquine chemotherapy and disappears after chemotherapy against malaria. Interestingly, HIV infection increases susceptibility to malaria when CXCL10 levels are elevated (Chaisavaneeyakorn, Moore et al. 2002) while filariasis produces resistance to malaria by down-regulating CXCL10 (Metenou, Dembele et al. 2009). Recent studies suggest that altered levels of CXCL4 and CXCL10 play a prominent role in the pathogenesis of fatal CM and may be used as functional or surrogate biomarkers for predicting CM severity (Wilson, Jain et al. 2011). This remarkable link between increased CXCL10 and the severity of parasitic diseases suggest further studies needed to be conducted on the mechanisms involved. (Campanella, Tager et al. 2008). Our recent *in vitro* cell culture studies (Liu & Stiles, manuscript in review) revealed that Heme regulates CXCL10 at the transcriptional level [See 5.1.3.1 Heme/ Heme oxygenase-1 (HO-1)].

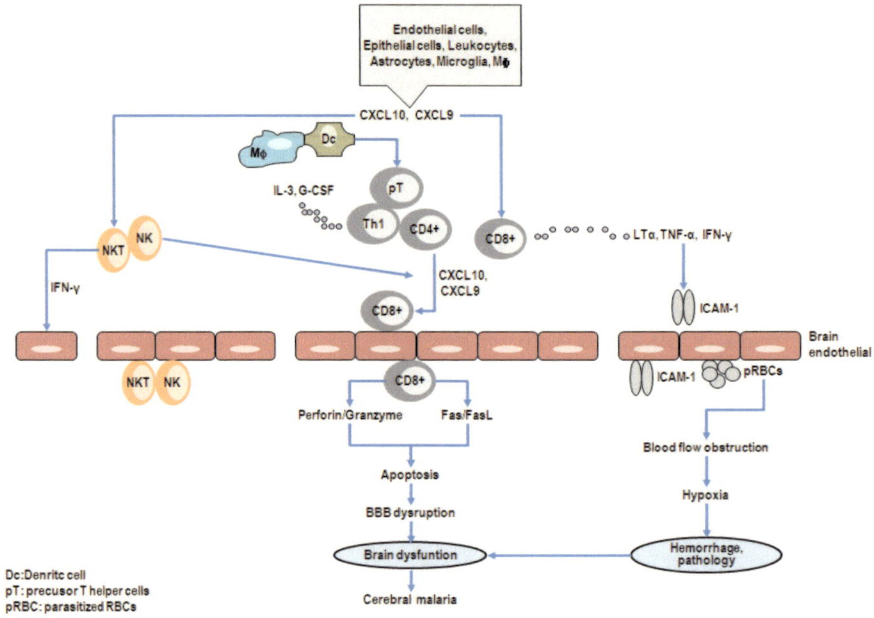

Fig. 1. Proposed cellular pathways in CXCL10-mediated severe malaria.

IL-1 and IL-6 are key pathogenic factors in malaria (John, Panoskaltsis-Mortari et al. 2008). Significantly elevated levels of IL-1, G-CSF and monocyte chemoattractant protein-1 (MCP-1) but not IL-8 have been reported in children who died of CM than children without the disease (UM) (John, Park et al. 2008). However, a study on the global transcriptome of HBVEC after exposure to *P.falciparum*-infected RBCs showed that proinflammatory molecule IL-8 together with CCL20, CXCL11, CXCL2 and IL-6 were increased more than 100-fold consistent with the critical role of the endothelium in promoting leukocyte infiltration (Tripathi, Sha et al. 2009). Low levels of the chemokine RANTES are independently associated with mortality (John, Opika-Opoka et al. 2006). In summary, the role of cytokines/chemokines and corresponding receptor interactions appear to be highly associated with severity of CM encephalopathy.

5.1.1.2 Angiopoiesis and CM (angiogenic/angiostatic factors)

Vascular endothelial growth factor (VEGF) and Angiopoietin-1 (Ang-1)/ Ang-2. Severe and cerebral malaria are associated with endothelial activation (Conroy, Lafferty et al. 2009). The role of VEGF in CM encephalopathy remains to be clarified. Increased production of VEGF is able to trigger vascular leakage in the circulation of mice, and promote injury in ECM (Epiphanio, Campos et al.) although it can induce antiapoptotic proteins like Bcl2 in endothelial cells (Ferrara 2004). In our study performed in Indian angiogenic and anti-apoptotic factors, VEGF was found to be negatively correlated with mortality associated with CM (Jain, Armah et al. 2008), and to be protective against fatal CM (Jain, Armah et al. 2008). ANG-1 and ANG-2 are major regulators of endothelial activation and integrity (Conroy, Lafferty et al. 2009). CM patients have significantly lower ANG-1 levels, significantly higher ANG-2 levels and ANG-2/ANG-1 ratio than non-malaria or malaria patients without cerebral involvement (Conroy, Lafferty et al. 2009). ANG-2 has dual functions depending on the activity of endogenous VEGF-A. Lobov et al (Lobov, Brooks et al. 2002) stated that VEGF acts through the conversion of ANG-2 stimulation from anti- to pro-angiogenic to regulate vascularity (Lobov, Brooks et al. 2002). ANG-2 *in vivo* increases capillary diameter, remodels the basal lamina, promotes proliferation and migration of endothelial cells, and stimulates sprouting of blood vessels when VEGF-A is activated; whereas, ANG-2 promotes endothelial apoptosis and vessel regression if the VEGF activity is inhibited. Plasma levels of ANG-1 and -2 predict cerebral malaria outcome in Central India (Jain, Lucchi et al, 2011). Malar J. 2011 Dec 23;10(1):383.

5.1.1.3 Erythropoietin and CM

Erythropoietin (Epo) regulates the production of new erythrocytes in blood trough binding to its receptor (EpoR) which is expressed on the cell surface of bone marrow erythroid precursors (Casals-Pascual, Idro et al. 2009). During this process, tissue hypoxia activates *Epo* gene expression (Casals-Pascual, Idro et al. 2009). Epo has recently been recognized as a tissue-protective cytokine (Brines, Grasso et al. 2004). The tissue-protective effects of Epo are mediated by EpoR located on neurons, astrocytes, microglia and endothelial cells (Masuda, Nagao et al. 1993; Masuda, Okano et al. 1994; Bernaudin, Nedelec et al. 2002; Sargin, El-Kordi et al. 2011). In other words, the non-hematopoietic function of Epo occurs in organs outside the bone marrow such as brain, retina, spinal cord, peripheral nerves, heart, kidney, and skin (Ghezzi and Brines 2004; Maiese, Li et al. 2005; Arcasoy 2008; Casals-Pascual, Idro et al. 2009). In this case, hypoxia does not have a key role in the regulation of EpoR, whereby Epo, pro-inlammatory cytokines IL-1 and TNF regulate EpoR (Nagai, Nakagawa et al. 2001; Brines and Cerami 2005; Siren, Fasshauer et al. 2009). The distinct functions of Epo are thought to be mediated via different receptors (Brines, Patel et al. 2008; Casals-Pascual, Idro et al. 2009). EpoR homodimers induce the haematopoietic response, whereas tissue-protective actions are induced by a heterocomplex composed of the Epo receptor and other cytokine receptors such as CD131, the beta-common receptor (mediating signals from GM-CSF, IL-3 and IL-5) (Brines, Patel et al. 2008). The pleiotropic action of Epo through the heterodimeric EpoR causes anti-apoptotic, anti-inflammatory, anti-angiogenic and anti-oxidatory effects in a variety of neuropathological disorders (Brines, Grasso et al. 2004; Hasselblatt, Ehrenreich et al. 2006), which might be potentially beneficial in CM. In the *P. berghei*-infected mouse model, Epo activated neural stem cells (NSC) and caused proliferation of NSC and neuronal precursor cells in sub ventricular zone (Core, Hempel et al. 2011). Emerging evidence has shown beneficial effects of recombinant human erythropoietin (rHuEpo) in both experimental and human CM (Casals-Pascual, Idro et al. 2008; Casals-Pascual, Idro et al. 2009; Mishra and Wiese 2009). Experimental CM studies have shown that Epo increases survival, shortens coma recovery times (Bienvenu, Ferrandiz et al. 2008) and decreases the inflammatory response and neuronal apoptosis in the brain (Kaiser, Texier et al. 2006; Wiese, Hempel et al. 2008). Human studies in African children with CM have indicated that Epo prevents brain damage (Casals-Pascual, Idro et al. 2009) and protects against neurological sequelae (Casals-Pascual, Idro et al. 2008). Although a safety profile for short-term (7 days) administration of erythropoietin at high does (1,500U/kg/day during 3 days) combined to quinine have recently been assessed in Mali (Picot, Bienvenu et al. 2009), a multicenter study using Epo as an adjunctive therapy to improve survival during CM is necessary. In summary, the interactions between Epo and EpoR in organs outside bone marrow appear to contribute to the protection against fatal CM pathogenesis although the mechanism is not completely understood.

5.1.2 Signaling pathways in CM encephalopathy

Cytoadherence between pRBC and endothelial cells is increased by up regulation of endothelial molecules such as ICAM-1, CD36 (Combes, El-Assaad et al.) in severe malaria. The proinflammaotry NF-kappaB pathway (Tripathi, Sha et al. 2009; Labbe, Miu et al. 2010), Src family kinase (Yipp, Robbins et al. 2003; Gillrie, Krishnegowda et al. 2007) and Rho kinase (Taoufiq, Gay et al. 2008) play certain roles in modulating the host response to *P. falciparum*, especially in the interaction between sequestered pRBC and specific endothelium [Fig. 2, Adapted with permission from Cytokine and Growth Review (Liu, Guo et al. 2011)]. A better understanding of host-parasite interactions will facilitate the development of novel strategies for interventions.

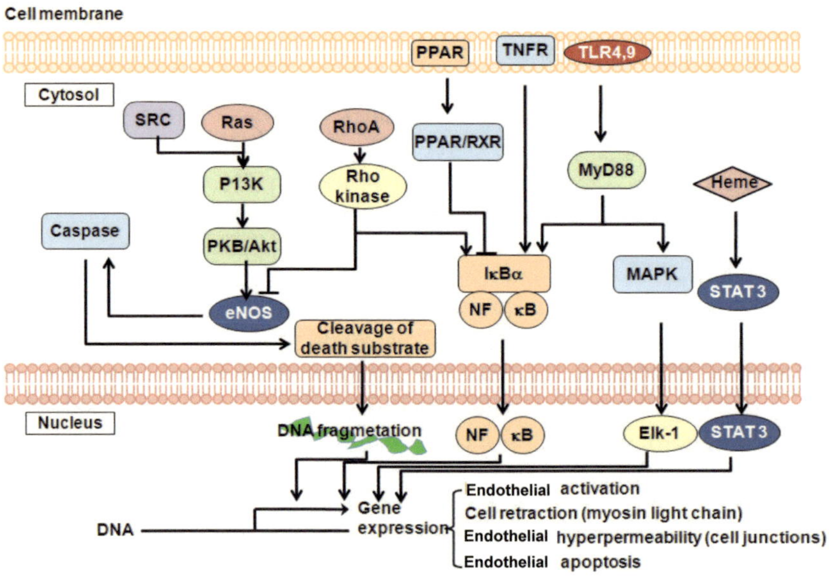

Fig. 2. Kinases and transcription factors in cerebral malaria.

5.1.2.1 Rho kinase signaling pathway

Some endothelial cell surface receptors have an intracellular domain coupled to G-protein and Rho signaling (Taoufiq, Gay et al. 2008). GDP/GTP exchanges and the activation of RhoA activate its downstream molecule Rho kinase. Activated Rho A/Rho kinase pathway leads to endothelial dysfunction by increasing cell retraction (through phosphorylation of myosin light chain) and endothelial hyperpermeability (through tight junction). Rho kinase also downregulates PI3K/Akt/eNOS cell growth pathway (Taoufiq, Gay et al. 2008). Rho kinase inhibitor (HA-1077), a drug already in clinical use, was reported to decrease both NF-kappaB activation and endothelial apoptosis (Taoufiq, Gay et al. 2008; Zang-Edou, Bisvigou et al. 2010), increase survival, and delay or prevent development of cerebral malaria (Waknine-Grinberg, McQuillan et al. 2010).

5.1.2.2 NF-κB signaling pathway

pRBCs exposure induced nuclear translocation of NF-κB in HBVEC, which is related to ICAM-1 expression. In this way, pRBCs may increase their sequestration, thereby exacerbating CM (Tripathi, Sullivan et al. 2006). A global gene profile study on HBVECs after interaction with pRBCs emphasized that the proinflammatory NF-κB pathway was central to the regulation of the *P.falciparum*-modulated endothelium transcriptorme (Tripathi, Sha et al. 2009).

5.1.2.3 Toll-like receptor (TLR) signaling pathway

MyD88 is a necessary adaptor molecule for intracellular signaling induced by most TLRs (Coban, Ishii et al. 2007). TLR4, TLR9 and MyD88 were described to play a role in pro-inflammatory responses to malaria infection following interaction of DC with the malaria parasite (Seixas, Moura Nunes et al. 2009). Both TLR4 and TLR9 besides MyD88 are required for complete DC activation, and consequently up regulation of co-stimulatory molecules, NF-κB nuclear tanslocation and production of cytokines (Seixas, Moura Nunes et al. 2009). Among the MyD88-dependent CM-related innate immunity signaling, TLR2 or TLR9 increases susceptibility to CM-related mortality, suggesting that these two TLRs play a critical role in the pathogenesis, and not in protective immunity (Coban, Ishii et al. 2007). TLR2 stimulation with *P. falciparum* glycosylphosphatidylinositol (*Pf*GPI) increases pRBCs uptake and clearance by macrophage as another example of the role of innate immunity responses to malaria (Erdman, Cosio et al. 2009).

5.1.2.4 Peroxisome proliferator activating receptor (PPAR)/PKC signaling pathway

PPAR-retinoid X receptor (PPARγ/RXR) activated phagocytosis of pRBCs and decreased malaria-induced TNF-α secretion by monocytes/macrophages (Serghides and Kain 2001). PPAR has been reported to inhibit the induction of inflammatory genes via PPARγ-dependent mechanisms, an effect mediated, at least partially, by inhibition of transcription factors NF-kB (Straus, Pascual et al. 2000). *Pf*GPI from *P. falciparum* has also been shown to be a potent inducer of inducible NO synthase system through the activation of NF-kB (Schofield, Novakovic et al. 1996).

5.1.2.5 Signal transducer and activator of transcription (STAT3) signaling pathway

STAT3 is a signaling cascade activated by pro-inflammatory stimuli and cellular stresses. This protein located in the cytoplasm is in its inactive form and is activated via phosphorylation (pSTAT3) by the Janus tyrosine kinases (JAKs). The active form of STAT3 quickly translocates to the nucleus. pSTAT3 is a potent negative modulator of the Th1-mediated inflammatory response, and also an activator of a variety of genes which are important for immune modulation (Yu and Jove 2004; El Kasmi, Holst et al. 2006). Chen's group has reported that lethal *Plasmodium yoelii (P.yoelii)* induced activation of STAT3 in the early phase of infection. The dominant pSTAT3 response may dampen the development of protective immunity, resulting in high parasitemia and death (Shi, Qin et al. 2008). Our data (Liu & Stiles, manuscript in review) showed that STAT3 is activated by PbA infection *in vivo* and Heme *in vitro*, while HO-1 regulates STAT3 signaling.

5.1.2.6 TNF/TNFR (LTαβ/LTβR) signaling pathway

TNF, the most extensively investigated cytokine in CM, up regulates ICAM-1 expression on the cerebral vascular endothelial cells and enhances the cytoadhesion of pRBCs (Idro, Marsh et al. 2010). Local synthesis is enhanced close to the sequestration sites. TNF has dual functions in malaria: it may be cytoprotective in the early phase, but its sustained high levels leads to complications (Hunt and Grau 2003; Idro, Marsh et al. 2010). Signaling through TNF receptors activate the classic NF-κB/RelA pathway resulting in the expression of a large number of genes involved in inflammatory responses, cell adhesion or cell growth (Togbe, de Sousa et al. 2008). Unfortunately, neither pentoxifylline, which reduces macrophage TNF synthesis, nor anti-TNF monoclonal antibody increased the survival of patients (Looareesuwan, Wilairatana et al. 1998; Wenisch, Looareesuwan et al. 1998; Idro, Marsh et al. 2010) although the coma period was shortened (Di Perri, Di Perri et al. 1995) or the levels of TNF/TNFR and IL-6 were decreased (Looareesuwan, Wilairatana et al. 1998; Wenisch, Looareesuwan et al. 1998).

5.1.2.7 MAP kinase/ Src family kinase pathway

MAPKs and downstream activation of the ERK and p38 pathways (not shown in Fig.2 for clarity) triggered by *Pf*GPIs regulate TNF-α and IL-12 production, two of the major inflammatory cytokines produced by macrophages stimulated with *Pf*GPIs (Zhu, Wu et al. 2009). Src-family kinase signaling was found to modulate the adhesion of *P. falciparum* on human microvasculature (Yipp, Robbins et al. 2003; Gillrie, Krishnegowda et al. 2007). A novel mechanism for the regulation of pRBCs adhesion on human microvascular endothelial cells is through CD36, Src-family kinase, and ectoalkaline phosphatase (Yipp, Robbins et al. 2003).

5.1.2.8 Apoptosis-related genes

See 4.1 Endothelial progenitor cells and endothelial cell markers

5.1.3 Other signaling pathways

5.1.3.1 Heme/Heme oxygenase-1 (HO-1)

Recently, it has been shown that increased levels of free Heme produced during malaria infection induces inflammation that damages host vascular endothelium, which contributes to cerebral pathogenesis and acute lung injury (ALI) which are major features of fatal malaria (Epiphanio, Campos et al. ; Hunt and Stocker 2007; Pamplona, Ferreira et al. 2007; Pamplona, Hanscheid et al. 2009). Heme oxygenase (HO) is the rate-limiting step enzyme in the degradation of Heme groups to biliverdin, carbon monoxide (CO), and iron. HO-1 is also known as a heat shock protein 32 (hsp32), which is an integral membrane protein of the smooth endoplasmic reticulum (Lin, Weis et al. 2007), and is the only inducible isoform of HO. The up regulation of HO-1 provides protection against cellular stress including oxidative stress, heavy metal toxicity, UV radiation, and inflammation, thus preventing deleterious effects of Heme and mediating anti-inflammatory and antiapototic functions (Geuken, Buis et al. 2005; Datta, Banerjee et al. 2010). HO-1 may facilitate the repair of injured tissues through inhibition of infiltrating inflammatory cells (Datta, Dormond et al. 2007). Moreover, HO-1 that is induced by reactive oxygen species and nitric oxide (NO) has recently been shown to be involved in the regulation of angiogenesis (Pae, Oh et al. 2005; Bussolati and Mason 2006).

The expression of HO-1 occurs at low levels in most tissues under physiological conditions (Ehrich and Eke 2007). HO-1 can localize to distinct subcellular compartments. Inducible HO activity appeared in the plasma membrane, cytosol, mitochondria (Ryter and Choi 2009), isolated caveolae and the nucleus (Kim, Wang et al. 2004) in cell culture models. Early studies indicate that HO-1 in the mitochondria and caveolae performs important biological and physiological functions (Ryter and Choi 2009), although the function of HO-1 in caveolae and the nucleus is not completely understood. The nuclear form of HO-1 serves potentially as a transcriptional regulator (Ryter and Choi 2009). Upon different stimuli of hypoxia, hemin or

Heme-hemopexin, HO-1 translocates to the nucleus. Nuclear translocation compromises HO activity, but nuclear localization of HO-1 protein functions to up regulate genes that promote cytoprotection against oxidative stress (Lin, Weis et al. 2007).

Heme/HO-1 interactions have moved to center stage in CM research since 2007. At the time, Mota's group reported that HO-1 and carbon monoxide (CO) suppressed the pathogenesis of ECM (Pamplona, Ferreira et al. 2007). HO-1 was then found to be capable of inhibiting vascular occlusion in transgenic sickle mice (another hemolytic disease) (Belcher, Mahaseth et al. 2006; Belcher, Vineyard et al. 2010). From these studies it seems that the ability of individuals to respond strongly in response to an increase in HO-1 may be a crucial endogenous protective factor. However, some studies refute the findings that HO-1 protects the development of ECM (Takeda, Kikuchi et al. 2005). Their data suggests that the frequency of short (GT)n alleles (<28 repeats), which may lead to high levels of HO-1, is markedly higher in CM patients (Takeda, Kikuchi et al. 2005). Moreover, liver stages of malaria infection was remarkably reduced in *Hmox1-/-* mice (Pamplona, Ferreira et al. 2007). These findings suggest that the regulated expression of HO-1 is quite complex in different tissues at different stages of the *Plasmodium* life cycle. Therefore further experimental and epidemiological studies are necessary to unveil the role of Heme/HO-1 in the severity of malaria. Our study (Liu & Stiles, manuscript in review) demonstrated that (1) infection of C57 BL/6 mice with PbA resulted in significant tissue damage. (2) Heme/HO-1 and CXCL10/CXCR3 are involved in the pathogenesis of severe malaria, such that the level of free Heme is linked to PbA infection in mice. (3) Expression of HO-1 in tissues may be protective against PbA induced Heme-associated damage. (4) High levels of CXCL10 are associated with ECM onset in PbA infected mice. (5) Heme up regulates HO-1 and CXCL10 production *in vitro*, and regulates CXCL10 at the transcriptional level *in vitro*. (6) HO-1 transcription was positively regulated by CXCL10. Overall, our results demonstrate that Heme and CXCL10 molecules as well as related signaling pathways play a very important role in inflammation and organ damage in malaria and CM encephalopathy.

5.1.3.2 Arginine/Nitric oxide signaling pathway

The role of Nitric oxide (NO) in malaria pathogenesis has been inconsistent. The relationship between NO activity and inducible NO synthase and pathogenesis is controversial (Anstey, Weinberg et al. 1996; Cramer, Nussler et al. 2005). NO exerts effects in host defense, neurotransmission, and vascular maintenance. NO is an effecter for TNF, and it is thought that inflammatory cytokines increase inducible NO synthase in brain endothelium resulting in increased NO production. NO is permeable to BBB, diffusing into brain tissue, and consequently impairing neurotransmission and may be an explanation for reversible comas (Clark, Rockett et al. 1992). These toxic molecules might contribute to the pathogenesis of severe and cerebral malaria (Clark, Hunt et al. 1986; Clark, Rockett et al. 1991). However, recent clinical and experimental studies in CM have failed to support this belief (Lopansri, Anstey et al. 2003; Gramaglia, Sobolewski et al. 2006; Weinberg, Lopansri et al. 2008). Indeed, they did find good evidence for the protective role of NO in human CM (Lopansri, Anstey et al. 2003; Gramaglia, Sobolewski et al. 2006; Weinberg, Lopansri et al. 2008). Some investigators proposed that severe malaria is associated with reduced NO production and low blood levels of L-arginine, the substrate for NO synthase (Yeo, Rooslamiati et al. 2008). Cell-free hemoglobin produced by hemolysis in *falciparum* malaria quench NO, disrupt endothelial function, increase adhesion receptor expression and impair tissue perfusion (Yeo, Lampah et al. 2009). Adjunctive agents to improve endothelial NO bioavailability including L-arginine are being extensively tested in human patients (Yeo, Lampah et al. 2007; Yeo, Lampah et al. 2008; Yeo, Rooslamiati et al. 2008; Yeo, Lampah et al. 2009) and a safety pharmacokinetics profile has been established (Yeo, Rooslamiati et al. 2008).

5.1.3.3 Coagulation and CM

The role of coagulation cascade in CM is controversial. However, most investigators propose that *P. falciparum* infection is associated with a procoagulant state (Francischetti 2008). Francischetti et al proved that the coagulation cascade played a crucial role in the pathogenetic processes leading to the cerebral complications (Francischetti 2008). Tissue factor expression in the endothelium, and the amplification of the coagulation cascade by pRBCs and platelets at sequestration sites, contribute critically in initiating and maintaining a coagulation–inflammation cycle which leads to cerebral involvement in *falciparum* malaria (Francischetti 2008). In addition to the typical role in the regulation of hemostasis, coagulation factors have an inflammatory role [having cross talk with inflammatory cytokines (Esmon, Taylor et al. 1991) that is important in the pathogenesis of CM (Moxon, Heyderman et al. 2009)]. This finding sheds new insight into potentially novel therapies for CM. The possible pivotal role of platelets was reported recently from Malawian patients with cerebral malaria [(Wassmer, Taylor et al. 2008), see 4.4 Platelets]. Pantethine interrupted the early stages of the coagulation-inflammation cascade and prevented the cerebral syndrome in ECM model (Penet, Abou-Hamdan et al. 2008).

5.2 Gene-expression profiling and CM

cDNA microarray analysis from brain tissue performed in genetically resistant (CM-R) and susceptible (CM-S) mice identified 327 genes discriminated between infection stages, mouse strains and CM-R and CM-S phenotypes (Delahaye, Coltel et al. 2006; Delahaye, Coltel et al. 2007). Analysis of these 327 genes using expression analysis systematic explorer (EASE) software revealed that the clustered genes were biologically relevant to the defense response such as the response to malaria, inflammatory and immune response, and metabolism like oxidative phosphorylation, glycolysis/gluconeogenesis or tryptophan metabolism. The promising areas explored by this analysis shed new light on the key events that control CM pathogenesis and the development of therapeutic strategies. The host transcriptome database changed during pathogenesis of ECM in whole blood (Oakley, Anantharaman et al. 2011). They found over 300 potential biomarkers of ECM detectable in the circulating system by comparing CM-resistant BALB/c mice to those of susceptible C57BL/6 and CBA/Caj mice. Among these, some molecules such as complement component C1q, nonspecific cytotoxic cell receptor protein 1, and prostate stem cell antigen will probably be the main markers related to CM encephalopathy.

5.3 Genetic polymorphisms associated with severe malaria

5.3.1 Common erythrocyte variants and severe malaria

Epidemiological studies in humans and experimental animals have demonstrated that genetic factors are very important in the initiation, progression and development of disease severity as well as the clinical outcome of malaria. Erythrocyte polymorphisms (variants) are biologically relevant to malaria pathogenesis (Min-Oo and Gros 2005). The protective roles of erythrocyte variants are shown in Table 1.

Hb variant	Type of studies	Function	Mechanism	Reference
HbS	*In vivo* case control	Protection: CM, severe anemia, respiratory distress, hyperparasitemia, prostration, acidosis, and hyperlactatemia	N/A	(May, Evans et al. 2007)
	In vivo mouse model C57 BL/6	Protection: ECM	HO-1 activation via Nrf2, and inhibition of CD8+	(Ferreira, Marguti et al. 2011)
HbC	*In vivo* case control	Protection: CM, severe anemia		(Mockenhaupt, Ehrhardt et al. 2004; May, Evans et al. 2007)
HbF	*In vitro* HMVEC cell culture	Protection: malaria	Impairs cytoadherence of pRBCs with EC and monocytes	(Amaratunga, Lopera-Mesa et al. 2011)
G6PD deficiency	*In vivo* case-control	Protection: severe malaria	N/A	(Guindo, Fairhurst et al. 2007)
	In vitro culture of *P falciparum*	Protection: malaria	Inhibits parasite growth under oxidative stress and susceptibility to phagocytosis	(Roth, Raventos-Suarez et al. 1983; Cappadoro, Giribaldi et al. 1998)
α-thalassaemia	*In vivo* case-control	Reduces the risk of severe malaria	Reduces multiplication of parasites	(Mockenhaupt, Ehrhardt et al. 2004)
β-thalassaemia	*In vitro* culture of *P falciparum*	Reduces the risk of severe malaria	Enhances susceptibility of pRBCs to phagocytosis	(Ayi, Turrini et al. 2004)
(PK) deficiency	*In vivo* mouse model, C57BL /6J, A/J, C3H and SJL	Protection: malaria	Enhances susceptibility of pRBCs to phagocytosis	(Min-Oo, Fortin et al. 2003)

Table 1. Common erythrocyte variants and severe malaria

5.3.2 Polymorphisms of the histocompatibility region (HLA)

T-cell recognition of malaria epitopes on infected host cells through class I and II major histocompatibility complex (MHC) antigens is a basic feature of pre-erythrocytic immunity to *P. falciparum* malaria. Therefore high-resolution typing of HLA class I and II loci were performed (Hananantachai, Patarapotikul et al. 2005; Lyke, Fernandez-Vina et al. 2011) to test for associations of human leukocyte antigen (HLA) alleles with malaria severity. HLA-A and HLA-B, DRB1 were identified as potential susceptibility factors for CM, thus providing further evidence that polymorphism of MHC genes results in altered malaria susceptibility.

6. Diagnosis, prognosis and prediction of CM encephalopathy

WHO proposed a definition of CM as a clinical syndrome characterized by coma (inability to localize a painful stimulus) at least 1 h after termination of a seizure or correction of hypoglycaemia, detection of asexual forms of *P falciparum* malaria parasites on peripheral blood smears, and exclusion of other causes of encephalopathy (Idro, Jenkins et al. 2005; WHO, 2000). This definition lacks specificity, and individuals with other underlying causes of coma might be misdiagnosed as CM. The presence of malarial retinopathy is therefore recommended to differentiate patients whose comas are caused by *P. falciparum* or other reasons (See 2.2 Retinal changes associated with CM). MRI may help in the early diagnosis of CM so that early treatment can begin and improve the clinical outcome (Vyas, Gupta et al. 2010; Rasalkar, Paunipagar et al. 2011). Due to unreliable local electricity production, operation of MRI was always interrupted and it might take longer for MRI to become a regular diagnostic technique for malaria in Sub-Saharan Africa where most of CM in children occur. This is the major reason why an NIH-supported project of clinical characterization of pediatric patients with CM using neurological MRI methods in Blantyre, Malaŵi was not successful (Latourette, Siebert et al. 2010). More practically, the histidine-rich protein II (HRP2)-based rapid diagnostic tests has shown high sensitivity compared to conventional microscopy in diagnosis of malaria and therefore may be a suitable screening method for malaria infection (Wilson, Adjei et al. 2008; Batwala, Magnussen et al. 2010).

Clinical scores to predict fatal outcome in severe malaria have been developed previously (Helbok, Kendjo et al. 2009). A recent study in Ghanaian patients demonstrated an association between fatal CM and increased serum and CSF levels of proinflammatory and proapoptotic factors including CXCL10, IL-1ra, sTNFR1, sTNFR2, sFas and decreased serum and CSF levels of neuroprotective angiogenic growth factors (PDGFbb) (Armah, Wilson et al. 2007). Further investigations in Indian patients confirmed findings from Ghana, indicating that CXCL10, sTNFR2 and sFas are positively correlated, VEGF is negatively correlated with mortality associated with CM (Jain, Armah et al. 2008). Most recently, a retrospective case-control study performed by Erdman et al (Erdman, Dhabangi et al. 2011) indicated that host soluble triggering receptor expressed on myeloid cells-1(TREM-1) and soluble FMS-like tyrosine kinase-1 (Flt-1) as the biomarkers of pediatric severe and fatal malaria. In addition, simple biomarker combinations, such as Ang-2+procalcitonin (PCT)+sICAM-1, Ang-2+CXCL10+PCT, and PCT+CXCL10+sTREM could accurately predict death in an African pediatric population. These results suggest the utility of combinatorial biomarker strategies as prognostics methods to assess malaria severity (Erdman, Dhabangi et al. 2011).

7. New therapies for CM

7.1 New treatment or management of cerebral malaria

Because of its effectiveness and cost, chloroquine has been the best and widely used antimalaria drug. Unfortunately *P. falciparum* parasite resistance to chloroquine has been observed in most of malaria-endemic areas (Chinappi, Via et al. 2010). The current recommended new therapies for CM are described in Table 2. These studies on new drugs against CM encephalopathy target not only parasites but the secondary damage induced by parasitemia.

Type of compound	Type of studies		Biological effects reported	Reference
1. Anti-plasmodial drugs				
Artemisinin	ICR or C57BL/6 mice infected by Plasmodium berghei ANKA (PbA).	*In vivo*	Anti-plasmodial activity; disruption of CD4+ and CD8+ T cell inflammatory responses, and VEGF action	(Waknine-Grinberg, Hunt et al. 2010)
Curcumin	ICR or C57BL/6 mice infected by PbA.	*In vivo*	Anti-inflammatory properties and anti-plasmodial activity; inhibition of activity of NF-κB, production of NO and iNOS expression	(Waknine-Grinberg, McQuillan et al. 2010)
2. Immunomodulator therapies				
Fasudil (HA-1077)	Primary human lung endothelial cells (HLECs) infected with *P.falciparum*	*In vitro*	A Rho kinase inhibitor, decreases both NF-kappaB activation and endothelial cell apoptosis	(Taoufiq, Gay et al. 2008)
	Children infected with *P.falciparum*	*In vivo*	Prevents endothelium apoptosis	(Zang-Edou, Bisvigou et al. 2010),
	ICR or C57BL/6 mice infected with PbA (both mouse strains serve as murine models for CM)	*In vivo*	Does not reduce parasitemia, but increases survival, delays or prevents the development of CM	(Waknine-Grinberg, McQuillan et al. 2010)
E6446	Human PBMCs and BALB/c mouse spleen cells	*In vitro*	A synthetic antagonist of nucleic acid-sensing TLRs,Low doses of E6446 specifically inhibits the activation of human and mouse TLR9, high doses inhibits the human TLR8 response to single-stranded RNA	(Franklin, Ishizaka et al. 2011)
	C57 BL/6 mice infected with *P.berghei* iRBCs	*In vivo*	Reduces the activation of TLR9 and modulates cytokine response during acute *Plasmodium* infection, prevents limb paralysis, cerebral vascular leak, and death,	(Franklin, Ishizaka et al. 2011)
rHuEpo	African children	*In vivo*	Prevents brain damage	(Casals-Pascual, Idro et al. 2008)
	C57 BL6 and CBA/J mice infected with PbA	*In vitro*	Epo decreases inflammatory response and neuronal apoptosis in the brain, increases survival, shortens coma recovery times	(Kaiser, Texier et al. 2006; Bienvenu, Ferrandiz et al. 2008; Wiese, Hempel et al. 2008)

Hydroxyurea	HLECs infected by the *P.falciparum* 3D7 clone *in vitro*	*In vitro*	Up regulates ICAM-1 and enhances cytoadherence, but does not induce endothelial cell apoptosis. In contrast, it inhibits parasite growth and prevents mice from developing neurological syndrome	(Pino, Taoufiq et al. 2006)
Statins Simvastatin	C57 BL6 and CBA/J mice infected with PbA	*In vivo*	Failes to extend survival or reduce parasitemia in C57BL/6 mice infected with PbA.	(Helmers, Gowda et al. 2009)
	EAE in C57BL/6 mice	*In vitro*	Simvastatin potentiates production of TNF and IL-6 in vitro murine peritoneal macrophages treated with *Pf*GPI	(Helmers, Gowda et al. 2009)
AVA	*P. falciparum* cultures treated by AVA	*In vitro*	Atrovastatin (AVA) reduces the growth of *P.falciparum in vitro*	(Parquet, Briolant et al. 2009)
Pantethine	C57 BL6 and CBA/J mice infected with PbA	*In vivo*	Reduces the platelet response to activation by thrombin and collagen, microparticle release by TNF-activated endothelial cells and protects against the cerebral syndrome	(Penet, Abou-Hamdan et al. 2008)
LMP-420	HBVEC	*In vitro*	Inhibits endothelial cell activation, i.e., the up regulation of ICAM-1 and VCAM-1 on HBEC, abolishes the cytoadherence of ICAM-1-specific *P. falciparum*-parasitized RBCs on ECs, causes a dramatic reduction of HBEC microparticle release induced by TNF or LT stimulation	(Wassmer, Cianciolo et al. 2005)
N-acetylcysteine amid (AD4)	Case control	*In vivo*	Has no effect on outcomes such as mortality, lactate clearance or coma recovery times	(Agbenyega, Planche et al. 2003; Charunwatthana, Abul Faiz et al. 2009)
Levamisole	Case control	*In vivo*	Decreases sequestration of pRBCs via inhibition of binding of pRBCs to CD36	(Dondorp, Silamut et al. 2007)

Table 2. New treatment or management of cerebral malaria

7.2 Malaria vaccines and CM encephalopathy

Malaria vaccine is urgently needed to sustain the gains of malaria control. A clinical trial (ClinicalTrials.gov number, NCT00380393.) on 894 children conducted in Kenya and Tanzania (Bejon, Cook et al. 2011) demonstrated that RTS,S/AS01E is a very promising malaria vaccine. RTS,S is a circumspozoite protein [CSP repeat region (R)] that targets the pre-erythrocytic cycle of *P. falciparum* in humans (Lusingu, Olotu et al. 2010; Bejon, Cook et al. 2011; Olotu, Lusingu et al. 2011)]. RTS,S-containing vaccines induce pre-erythrocytic immunity, differing from naturally acquired immunity, which largely targets blood-stage parasites (Bejon, Cook et al. 2011; Olotu, Lusingu et al. 2011). RTS,S/AS01E vaccines decrease the concentrations of antibodies to merozoite antigens, which probably reflects reduced exposure to blood-stage infections. Long-term protective efficacy of RTS,S vaccination is more likely to have a direct effect of the pre erythrocytic immunity induced by the vaccine, rather than the result of enhanced acquisition of immunity to blood-stage antigens (Bejon, Cook et al. 2011; Olotu, Lusingu et al. 2011). Although these antibodies were not correlated to clinical immunity, the overall effect of RTS,S vaccines still had a significantly lower incidence of clinical malaria than did unvaccinated individuals. Protection was sustained for at least 15 months (Bejon, Cook et al. 2011). Whole-parasite vaccine strategies (Coban, Igari et al. 2010; Coban, Yagi et al. 2010; Taylor-Robinson 2010) for malaria infection have attracted researchers' attention. They trigger parasite antigen-specific immune responses through TLR9 and NOD-like receptors (NLRs) (Coban, Igari et al. 2010; Coban, Yagi et al. 2010). Heme-detoxification byproduct, hemozoin, is also being considered as a potential vaccine adjuvant against malaria (Coban, Igari et al. 2010; Coban, Yagi et al. 2010).

8. Conclusions

A severe complication of *Plasmodium* infection is cerebral malaria, a condition mainly attributed to sequestration of pRBCs, leukocytes and platelets in cerebral microcirculation and overwhelming inflammatory immune reactions of the host. CM presents as a diffuse encephalopathy caused by *P. falciparum* and remains a major cause of death and disability. Much effort is still needed to understand the pathophysiology of this disease at the cellular and molecular level, to enable the development of more effective therapies aimed at both eliminating parasites as well as the secondary effects they cause.

9. Acknowledgements

This work was supported by the National Institutes of Health grant numbers NIH-FIC (1T90-HG004151-01) for postdoctoral training in Genomics and Hemoglobinopathies, NIH/FIC/NINDS R21 and NIH-RCMI (RR033062).

10. References

(WHO, 2000). "Severe falciparum malaria. World Health Organization, Communicable Diseases Cluster." Trans R Soc Trop Med Hyg 94 Suppl 1(1): S1-90.

Agbenyega, T., T. Planche, et al. (2003). "Population kinetics, efficacy, and safety of dichloroacetate for lactic acidosis due to severe malaria in children." J Clin Pharmacol 43(4): 386-396.

Aloisi, F., G. Borsellino, et al. (1995). "Cytokine regulation of astrocyte function: in-vitro studies using cells from the human brain." Int J Dev Neurosci 13(3-4): 265-274.

Amaratunga, C., T. M. Lopera-Mesa, et al. (2011). "A role for fetal hemoglobin and maternal immune IgG in infant resistance to Plasmodium falciparum malaria." PLoS One 6(4): e14798.

Anstey, N. M., J. B. Weinberg, et al. (1996). "Nitric oxide in Tanzanian children with malaria: inverse relationship between malaria severity and nitric oxide production/nitric oxide synthase type 2 expression." J Exp Med 184(2): 557-567.

Arcasoy, M. O. (2008). "The non-haematopoietic biological effects of erythropoietin." Br J Haematol 141(1): 14-31.

Armah, H. B., N. O. Wilson, et al. (2007). "Cerebrospinal fluid and serum biomarkers of cerebral malaria mortality in Ghanaian children." Malar J 6(147): 147.

Ayi, K., F. Turrini, et al. (2004). "Enhanced phagocytosis of ring-parasitized mutant erythrocytes: a common mechanism that may explain protection against falciparum malaria in sickle trait and beta-thalassemia trait." Blood 104(10): 3364-3371.

Azevedo, L. C., M. A. Pedro, et al. (2007). "Circulating microparticles as therapeutic targets in cardiovascular diseases." Recent Pat Cardiovasc Drug Discov 2(1): 41-51.

Balachandar, S. and A. Katyal (2010). "Peroxisome proliferator activating receptor (PPAR) in cerebral malaria (CM): a novel target for an additional therapy." Eur J Clin Microbiol Infect Dis.

Barry, O. P. and G. A. FitzGerald (1999). "Mechanisms of cellular activation by platelet microparticles." Thromb Haemost 82(2): 794-800.

Batwala, V., P. Magnussen, et al. (2010). "Are rapid diagnostic tests more accurate in diagnosis of plasmodium falciparum malaria compared to microscopy at rural health centres?" Malar J 9(349): 349.

Bauer, P. R., H. C. Van Der Heyde, et al. (2002). "Regulation of endothelial cell adhesion molecule expression in an experimental model of cerebral malaria." Microcirculation 9(6): 463-470.

Beare, N. A., S. Lewallen, et al. (2011). "Redefining cerebral malaria by including malaria retinopathy." Future Microbiol 6(3): 349-355.

Bejon, P., J. Cook, et al. (2011). "Effect of the Pre-erythrocytic Candidate Malaria Vaccine RTS,S/AS01E on Blood Stage Immunity in Young Children." J Infect Dis 204(1): 9-18.

Belcher, J. D., H. Mahaseth, et al. (2006). "Heme oxygenase-1 is a modulator of inflammation and vaso-occlusion in transgenic sickle mice." J Clin Invest 116(3): 808-816.

Belcher, J. D., J. V. Vineyard, et al. (2010). "Heme oxygenase-1 gene delivery by Sleeping Beauty inhibits vascular stasis in a murine model of sickle cell disease." J Mol Med 88(7): 665-675.

Belnoue, E., M. Kayibanda, et al. (2002). "On the pathogenic role of brain-sequestered alphabeta CD8+ T cells in experimental cerebral malaria." J Immunol 169(11): 6369-6375.

Belnoue, E., S. M. Potter, et al. (2008). "Control of pathogenic CD8+ T cell migration to the brain by IFN-gamma during experimental cerebral malaria." Parasite Immunol 30(10): 544-553.

Benveniste, E. N. (1992). "Inflammatory cytokines within the central nervous system: sources, function, and mechanism of action." Am J Physiol 263(1 Pt 1): C1-16.

Bernaudin, M., A. S. Nedelec, et al. (2002). "Normobaric hypoxia induces tolerance to focal permanent cerebral ischemia in association with an increased expression of hypoxia-inducible factor-1 and its target genes, erythropoietin and VEGF, in the adult mouse brain." J Cereb Blood Flow Metab 22(4): 393-403.

Bienvenu, A. L., J. Ferrandiz, et al. (2008). "Artesunate-erythropoietin combination for murine cerebral malaria treatment." Acta Trop 106(2): 104-108.

Birbeck, G. L., M. E. Molyneux, et al. (2010). "Blantyre Malaria Project Epilepsy Study (BMPES) of neurological outcomes in retinopathy-positive paediatric cerebral malaria survivors: a prospective cohort study." Lancet Neurol 9(12): 1173-1181.

Biswas, A. K., A. Hafiz, et al. (2007). "Plasmodium falciparum uses gC1qR/HABP1/p32 as a receptor to bind to vascular endothelium and for platelet-mediated clumping." PLoS Pathog 3(9): 1271-1280.

Boivin, M. J., P. Bangirana, et al. (2007). "Cognitive impairment after cerebral malaria in children: a prospective study." Pediatrics 119(2): e360-366.

Brines, M. and A. Cerami (2005). "Emerging biological roles for erythropoietin in the nervous system." Nat Rev Neurosci 6(6): 484-494.

Brines, M., G. Grasso, et al. (2004). "Erythropoietin mediates tissue protection through an erythropoietin and common beta-subunit heteroreceptor." Proc Natl Acad Sci U S A 101(41): 14907-14912.

Brines, M., N. S. Patel, et al. (2008). "Nonerythropoietic, tissue-protective peptides derived from the tertiary structure of erythropoietin." Proc Natl Acad Sci U S A 105(31): 10925-10930.

Bussolati, B. and J. C. Mason (2006). "Dual role of VEGF-induced heme-oxygenase-1 in angiogenesis." Antioxid Redox Signal 8(7-8): 1153-1163.

Campanella, G. S., A. M. Tager, et al. (2008). "Chemokine receptor CXCR3 and its ligands CXCL9 and CXCL10 are required for the development of murine cerebral malaria." Proc Natl Acad Sci U S A 105(12): 4814-4819.

Campos, F. M., B. S. Franklin, et al. (2010). "Augmented plasma microparticles during acute Plasmodium vivax infection." Malar J 9(327): 327.

Cappadoro, M., G. Giribaldi, et al. (1998). "Early phagocytosis of glucose-6-phosphate dehydrogenase (G6PD)-deficient erythrocytes parasitized by Plasmodium falciparum may explain malaria protection in G6PD deficiency." Blood 92(7): 2527-2534.

Carter, J. A., J. A. Lees, et al. (2006). "Severe falciparum malaria and acquired childhood language disorder." Dev Med Child Neurol 48(1): 51-57.

Carter, J. A., V. Mung'ala-Odera, et al. (2005). "Persistent neurocognitive impairments associated with severe falciparum malaria in Kenyan children." J Neurol Neurosurg Psychiatry 76(4): 476-481.

Casals-Pascual, C., R. Idro, et al. (2008). "High levels of erythropoietin are associated with protection against neurological sequelae in African children with cerebral malaria." Proc Natl Acad Sci U S A 105(7): 2634-2639.

Casals-Pascual, C., R. Idro, et al. (2009). "Can erythropoietin be used to prevent brain damage in cerebral malaria?" Trends Parasitol 25(1): 30-36.

Chaisavaneeyakorn, S., J. M. Moore, et al. (2002). "Immunity to placental malaria. III. Impairment of interleukin(IL)-12, not IL-18, and interferon-inducible protein-10 responses in the placental intervillous blood of human immunodeficiency virus/malaria-coinfected women." J Infect Dis 185(1): 127-131.

Chaiyaroj, S. C., A. S. Rutta, et al. (2004). "Reduced levels of transforming growth factor-beta1, interleukin-12 and increased migration inhibitory factor are associated with severe malaria." Acta Trop 89(3): 319-327.

Charunwatthana, P., M. Abul Faiz, et al. (2009). "N-acetylcysteine as adjunctive treatment in severe malaria: a randomized, double-blinded placebo-controlled clinical trial." Crit Care Med 37(2): 516-522.

Chen, L. and F. Sendo (2001). "Cytokine and chemokine mRNA expression in neutrophils from CBA/NSlc mice infected with Plasmodium berghei ANKA that induces experimental cerebral malaria." Parasitol Int 50(2): 139-143.

Chilongola, J., S. Balthazary, et al. (2009). "CD36 deficiency protects against malarial anaemia in children by reducing Plasmodium falciparum-infected red blood cell adherence to vascular endothelium." Trop Med Int Health 14(7): 810-816.

Chinappi, M., A. Via, et al. (2010). "On the mechanism of chloroquine resistance in Plasmodium falciparum." PLoS One 5(11): e14064.

Clark, I. A., N. H. Hunt, et al. (1986). "Oxygen-derived free radicals in the pathogenesis of parasitic disease." Adv Parasitol 25: 1-44.

Clark, I. A., K. A. Rockett, et al. (1991). "Proposed link between cytokines, nitric oxide and human cerebral malaria." Parasitol Today 7(8): 205-207.

Clark, I. A., K. A. Rockett, et al. (1992). "Possible central role of nitric oxide in conditions clinically similar to cerebral malaria." Lancet 340(8824): 894-896.

Clarke, S. E., M. C. Jukes, et al. (2008). "Effect of intermittent preventive treatment of malaria on health and education in schoolchildren: a cluster-randomised, double-blind, placebo-controlled trial." Lancet 372(9633): 127-138.

Coban, C., Y. Igari, et al. (2010). "Immunogenicity of whole-parasite vaccines against Plasmodium falciparum involves malarial hemozoin and host TLR9." Cell Host Microbe 7(1): 50-61.

Coban, C., K. J. Ishii, et al. (2007). "Pathological role of Toll-like receptor signaling in cerebral malaria." Int Immunol 19(1): 67-79.

Coban, C., M. Yagi, et al. (2010). "The malarial metabolite hemozoin and its potential use as a vaccine adjuvant." Allergol Int 59(2): 115-124.

Collins, T., M. A. Read, et al. (1995). "Transcriptional regulation of endothelial cell adhesion molecules: NF-kappa B and cytokine-inducible enhancers." Faseb J 9(10): 899-909.

Combes, V., N. Coltel, et al. (2005). "ABCA1 gene deletion protects against cerebral malaria: potential pathogenic role of microparticles in neuropathology." Am J Pathol 166(1): 295-302.

Combes, V., F. El-Assaad, et al. "Microvesiculation and cell interactions at the brain-endothelial interface in cerebral malaria pathogenesis." Prog Neurobiol 91(2): 140-151.

Combes, V., F. El-Assaad, et al. (2010). "Microvesiculation and cell interactions at the brain-endothelial interface in cerebral malaria pathogenesis." Prog Neurobiol 91(2): 140-151.

Combes, V., A. C. Simon, et al. (1999). "In vitro generation of endothelial microparticles and possible prothrombotic activity in patients with lupus anticoagulant." J Clin Invest 104(1): 93-102.

Combes, V., T. E. Taylor, et al. (2004). "Circulating endothelial microparticles in malawian children with severe falciparum malaria complicated with coma." Jama 291(21): 2542-2544.

Conroy, A. L., E. I. Lafferty, et al. (2009). "Whole blood angiopoietin-1 and -2 levels discriminate cerebral and severe (non-cerebral) malaria from uncomplicated malaria." Malar J 8(1): 295.

Coppinger, J. A., G. Cagney, et al. (2004). "Characterization of the proteins released from activated platelets leads to localization of novel platelet proteins in human atherosclerotic lesions." Blood 103(6): 2096-2104.

Core, A., C. Hempel, et al. (2011). "Plasmodium berghei ANKA: erythropoietin activates neural stem cells in an experimental cerebral malaria model." Exp Parasitol 127(2): 500-505.

Couper, K. N., T. Barnes, et al. (2010). "Parasite-derived plasma microparticles contribute significantly to malaria infection-induced inflammation through potent macrophage stimulation." PLoS Pathog 6(1): e1000744.

Cox, D. and S. McConkey (2010). "The role of platelets in the pathogenesis of cerebral malaria." Cell Mol Life Sci 67(4): 557-568.

Craig, A. and A. Scherf (2001). "Molecules on the surface of the Plasmodium falciparum infected erythrocyte and their role in malaria pathogenesis and immune evasion." Mol Biochem Parasitol 115(2): 129-143.

Cramer, J. P., A. K. Nussler, et al. (2005). "Age-dependent effect of plasma nitric oxide on parasite density in Ghanaian children with severe malaria." Trop Med Int Health 10(7): 672-680.

Crawley, J., S. Smith, et al. (1996). "Seizures and status epilepticus in childhood cerebral malaria." Qjm 89(8): 591-597.

D'Ombrain, M. C., T. S. Voss, et al. (2007). "Plasmodium falciparum erythrocyte membrane protein-1 specifically suppresses early production of host interferon-gamma." Cell Host Microbe 2(2): 130-138.

Datta, D., P. Banerjee, et al. (2010). "CXCR3-B can mediate growth-inhibitory signals in human renal cancer cells by downregulating the expression of heme oxygenase-1." J Biol Chem.

Datta, D., O. Dormond, et al. (2007). "Heme oxygenase-1 modulates the expression of the anti-angiogenic chemokine CXCL-10 in renal tubular epithelial cells." Am J Physiol Renal Physiol 293(4): F1222-1230.

Deininger, M. H., P. G. Kremsner, et al. (2002). "Macrophages/microglial cells in patients with cerebral malaria." Eur Cytokine Netw 13(2): 173-185.

Delahaye, N. F., N. Coltel, et al. (2007). "Gene expression analysis reveals early changes in several molecular pathways in cerebral malaria-susceptible mice versus cerebral malaria-resistant mice." BMC Genomics 8(452): 452.

Delahaye, N. F., N. Coltel, et al. (2006). "Gene-expression profiling discriminates between cerebral malaria (CM)-susceptible mice and CM-resistant mice." J Infect Dis 193(2): 312-321.

Di Perri, G., I. G. Di Perri, et al. (1995). "Pentoxifylline as a supportive agent in the treatment of cerebral malaria in children." J Infect Dis 171(5): 1317-1322.

Doeuvre, L., L. Plawinski, et al. (2009). "Cell-derived microparticles: a new challenge in neuroscience." J Neurochem 110(2): 457-468.

Dondorp, A. M., K. Silamut, et al. (2007). "Levamisole inhibits sequestration of infected red blood cells in patients with falciparum malaria." J Infect Dis 196(3): 460-466.

Dong, Y. and E. N. Benveniste (2001). "Immune function of astrocytes." Glia 36(2): 180-190.

Dugbartey, A. T., F. J. Spellacy, et al. (1998). "Somatosensory discrimination deficits following pediatric cerebral malaria." Am J Trop Med Hyg 59(3): 393-396.

Eddleston, M. and L. Mucke (1993). "Molecular profile of reactive astrocytes--implications for their role in neurologic disease." Neuroscience 54(1): 15-36.

Ehrich, J. H. and F. U. Eke (2007). "Malaria-induced renal damage: facts and myths." Pediatr Nephrol 22(5): 626-637.

El Kasmi, K. C., J. Holst, et al. (2006). "General nature of the STAT3-activated anti-inflammatory response." J Immunol 177(11): 7880-7888.

Epiphanio, S., M. G. Campos, et al. "VEGF promotes malaria-associated acute lung injury in mice." PLoS Pathog 6(5): e1000916.

Erdman, L. K., G. Cosio, et al. (2009). "CD36 and TLR interactions in inflammation and phagocytosis: implications for malaria." J Immunol 183(10): 6452-6459.

Erdman, L. K., A. Dhabangi, et al. (2011). "Combinations of host biomarkers predict mortality among Ugandan children with severe malaria: a retrospective case-control study." PLoS One 6(2): e17440.

Esmon, C. T., F. B. Taylor, Jr., et al. (1991). "Inflammation and coagulation: linked processes potentially regulated through a common pathway mediated by protein C." Thromb Haemost 66(1): 160-165.

Faille, D., V. Combes, et al. (2009). "Platelet microparticles: a new player in malaria parasite cytoadherence to human brain endothelium." Faseb J 23(10): 3449-3458.

Ferrara, N. (2004). "Vascular endothelial growth factor: basic science and clinical progress." Endocr Rev 25(4): 581-611.

Ferreira, A., I. Marguti, et al. (2011). "Sickle hemoglobin confers tolerance to Plasmodium infection." Cell 145(3): 398-409.

Francischetti, I. M. (2008). "Does activation of the blood coagulation cascade have a role in malaria pathogenesis?" Trends Parasitol 24(6): 258-263.

Franklin, B. S., S. T. Ishizaka, et al. (2011). "Therapeutical targeting of nucleic acid-sensing Toll-like receptors prevents experimental cerebral malaria." Proc Natl Acad Sci U S A 108(9): 3689-3694.

Frei, K., U. V. Malipiero, et al. (1989). "On the cellular source and function of interleukin 6 produced in the central nervous system in viral diseases." Eur J Immunol 19(4): 689-694.

Frei, K., C. Siepl, et al. (1987). "Antigen presentation and tumor cytotoxicity by interferon-gamma-treated microglial cells." Eur J Immunol 17(9): 1271-1278.

Geuken, E., C. I. Buis, et al. (2005). "Expression of heme oxygenase-1 in human livers before transplantation correlates with graft injury and function after transplantation." Am J Transplant 5(8): 1875-1885.

Ghezzi, P. and M. Brines (2004). "Erythropoietin as an antiapoptotic, tissue-protective cytokine." Cell Death Differ 11 Suppl 1(1): S37-44.

Gillrie, M. R., G. Krishnegowda, et al. (2007). "Src-family kinase dependent disruption of endothelial barrier function by Plasmodium falciparum merozoite proteins." Blood 110(9): 3426-3435.

Giulian, D., T. J. Baker, et al. (1986). "Interleukin 1 of the central nervous system is produced by ameboid microglia." J Exp Med 164(2): 594-604.

Giulian, D. and L. B. Lachman (1985). "Interleukin-1 stimulation of astroglial proliferation after brain injury." Science 228(4698): 497-499.

Giulian, D., D. G. Young, et al. (1988). "Interleukin-1 is an astroglial growth factor in the developing brain." J Neurosci 8(2): 709-714.

Gramaglia, I., P. Sobolewski, et al. (2006). "Low nitric oxide bioavailability contributes to the genesis of experimental cerebral malaria." Nat Med 12(12): 1417-1422.

Grau, G. E., L. F. Fajardo, et al. (1987). "Tumor necrosis factor (cachectin) as an essential mediator in murine cerebral malaria." Science 237(4819): 1210-1212.

Guindo, A., R. M. Fairhurst, et al. (2007). "X-linked G6PD deficiency protects hemizygous males but not heterozygous females against severe malaria." PLoS Med 4(3): e66.

Gyan, B., B. Q. Goka, et al. (2009). "Cerebral malaria is associated with low levels of circulating endothelial progenitor cells in African children." Am J Trop Med Hyg 80(4): 541-546.

Hananantachai, H., J. Patarapotikul, et al. (2005). "Polymorphisms of the HLA-B and HLA-DRB1 genes in Thai malaria patients." Jpn J Infect Dis 58(1): 25-28.

Hansen, D. S., N. J. Bernard, et al. (2007). "NK cells stimulate recruitment of CXCR3+ T cells to the brain during Plasmodium berghei-mediated cerebral malaria." J Immunol 178(9): 5779-5788.

Hansen, D. S., M. A. Siomos, et al. (2003). "Regulation of murine cerebral malaria pathogenesis by CD1d-restricted NKT cells and the natural killer complex." Immunity 18(3): 391-402.

Hanum, P. S., M. Hayano, et al. (2003). "Cytokine and chemokine responses in a cerebral malaria-susceptible or -resistant strain of mice to Plasmodium berghei ANKA infection: early chemokine expression in the brain." Int Immunol 15(5): 633-640.

Haque, A., S. E. Best, et al. (2011). "High parasite burdens cause liver damage in mice following Plasmodium berghei ANKA infection independently of CD8(+) T cell-mediated immune pathology." Infect Immun 79(5): 1882-1888.

Haque, A., S. E. Best, et al. (2010). "CD4+ natural regulatory T cells prevent experimental cerebral malaria via CTLA-4 when expanded in vivo." PLoS Pathog 6(12): e1001221.

Haque, A., S. E. Best, et al. (2011). "Granzyme B Expression by CD8+ T Cells Is Required for the Development of Experimental Cerebral Malaria." J Immunol 186(11): 6148-6156.

Hasselblatt, M., H. Ehrenreich, et al. (2006). "The brain erythropoietin system and its potential for therapeutic exploitation in brain disease." J Neurosurg Anesthesiol 18(2): 132-138.

Helbok, R., E. Kendjo, et al. (2009). "The Lambarene Organ Dysfunction Score (LODS) is a simple clinical predictor of fatal malaria in African children." J Infect Dis 200(12): 1834-1841.

Helmers, A. J., D. C. Gowda, et al. (2009). "Statins fail to improve outcome in experimental cerebral malaria and potentiate Toll-like receptor-mediated cytokine production by murine macrophages." Am J Trop Med Hyg 81(4): 631-637.

Hemmer, C. J., H. A. Lehr, et al. (2005). "Plasmodium falciparum Malaria: reduction of endothelial cell apoptosis in vitro." Infect Immun 73(3): 1764-1770.

Hermsen, C., T. van de Wiel, et al. (1997). "Depletion of CD4+ or CD8+ T-cells prevents Plasmodium berghei induced cerebral malaria in end-stage disease." Parasitology 114 (Pt 1)(Pt 1): 7-12.

Ho, M., M. J. Hickey, et al. (2000). "Visualization of Plasmodium falciparum-endothelium interactions in human microvasculature: mimicry of leukocyte recruitment." J Exp Med 192(8): 1205-1211.

Holding, P. A., J. Stevenson, et al. (1999). "Cognitive sequelae of severe malaria with impaired consciousness." Trans R Soc Trop Med Hyg 93(5): 529-534.

Hunt, N. H., J. Golenser, et al. (2006). "Immunopathogenesis of cerebral malaria." Int J Parasitol 36(5): 569-582.

Hunt, N. H. and G. E. Grau (2003). "Cytokines: accelerators and brakes in the pathogenesis of cerebral malaria." Trends Immunol 24(9): 491-499.

Hunt, N. H. and R. Stocker (2007). "Heme moves to center stage in cerebral malaria." Nat Med 13(6): 667-669.

Idro, R., N. E. Jenkins, et al. (2005). "Pathogenesis, clinical features, and neurological outcome of cerebral malaria." Lancet Neurol 4(12): 827-840.

Idro, R., K. Marsh, et al. (2010). "Cerebral malaria: mechanisms of brain injury and strategies for improved neurocognitive outcome." Pediatr Res 68(4): 267-274.

Ikenoue, N., S. Kawazu, et al. (2002). "PCR-amplification, sequencing, and comparison of the var/PfEMP-1 gene from the blood of patients with falciparum malaria in the Philippines." Southeast Asian J Trop Med Public Health 33 Suppl 3: 8-13.

Jain, V., H. B. Armah, et al. (2008). "Plasma IP-10, apoptotic and angiogenic factors associated with fatal cerebral malaria in India." Malar J 7(83): 83.

Jain, V., P. P. Singh, et al. (2009). "A preliminary study on pro- and anti-inflammatory cytokine profiles in Plasmodium vivax malaria patients from central zone of India." Acta Trop 113(3): 263-268.

John, C. C., P. Bangirana, et al. (2008). "Cerebral malaria in children is associated with long-term cognitive impairment." Pediatrics 122(1): e92-99.

John, C. C., R. Opika-Opoka, et al. (2006). "Low levels of RANTES are associated with mortality in children with cerebral malaria." J Infect Dis 194(6): 837-845.

John, C. C., A. Panoskaltsis-Mortari, et al. (2008). "Cerebrospinal fluid cytokine levels and cognitive impairment in cerebral malaria." Am J Trop Med Hyg 78(2): 198-205.

John, C. C., G. S. Park, et al. (2008). "Elevated serum levels of IL-1ra in children with Plasmodium falciparum malaria are associated with increased severity of disease." Cytokine 41(3): 204-208.

Kaiser, K., A. Texier, et al. (2006). "Recombinant human erythropoietin prevents the death of mice during cerebral malaria." J Infect Dis 193(7): 987-995.

Kang, S. S. and D. B. McGavern (2010). "Microbial induction of vascular pathology in the CNS." J Neuroimmune Pharmacol 5(3): 370-386.

Kim, H. P., X. Wang, et al. (2004). "Caveolae compartmentalization of heme oxygenase-1 in endothelial cells." FASEB J 18(10): 1080-1089.

Labbe, K., J. Miu, et al. (2010). "Caspase-12 dampens the immune response to malaria independently of the inflammasome by targeting NF-kappaB signaling." J Immunol 185(9): 5495-5502.

Lackner, P., C. Burger, et al. (2007). "Apoptosis in experimental cerebral malaria: spatial profile of cleaved caspase-3 and ultrastructural alterations in different disease stages." Neuropathol Appl Neurobiol 33(5): 560-571.

Latourette, M. T., J. E. Siebert, et al. (2010). "Magnetic Resonance Imaging Research in Sub-Saharan Africa: Challenges and Satellite-Based Networking Implementation." J Digit Imaging 17: 17.

Lin, Q., S. Weis, et al. (2007). "Heme oxygenase-1 protein localizes to the nucleus and activates transcription factors important in oxidative stress." J Biol Chem 282(28): 20621-20633.

Liu, M., S. Guo, et al. (2011). "CXCL10/IP-10 in infectious diseases pathogenesis and potential therapeutic implications." Cytokine Growth Factor Rev 27: 27.

Lobov, I. B., P. C. Brooks, et al. (2002). "Angiopoietin-2 displays VEGF-dependent modulation of capillary structure and endothelial cell survival in vivo." Proc Natl Acad Sci U S A 99(17): 11205-11210.

Looareesuwan, S., P. Wilairatana, et al. (1998). "Pentoxifylline as an ancillary treatment for severe falciparum malaria in Thailand." Am J Trop Med Hyg 58(3): 348-353.

Lopansri, B. K., N. M. Anstey, et al. (2003). "Low plasma arginine concentrations in children with cerebral malaria and decreased nitric oxide production." Lancet 361(9358): 676-678.

Lucas, R., J. N. Lou, et al. (1997). "Respective role of TNF receptors in the development of experimental cerebral malaria." J Neuroimmunol 72(2): 143-148.

Lusingu, J., A. Olotu, et al. (2010). "Safety of the malaria vaccine candidate, RTS,S/AS01E in 5 to 17 month old Kenyan and Tanzanian Children." PLoS One 5(11): e14090.

Lyke, K. E., M. A. Fernandez-Vina, et al. (2011). "Association of HLA alleles with Plasmodium falciparum severity in Malian children." Tissue Antigens 77(6): 562-571.

Lynch, S. F. and C. A. Ludlam (2007). "Plasma microparticles and vascular disorders." Br J Haematol 137(1): 36-48.

Maiese, K., F. Li, et al. (2005). "New avenues of exploration for erythropoietin." Jama 293(1): 90-95.

Marsh, K., M. English, et al. (1996). "The pathogenesis of severe malaria in African children." Ann Trop Med Parasitol 90(4): 395-402.

Masuda, S., M. Nagao, et al. (1993). "Functional erythropoietin receptor of the cells with neural characteristics. Comparison with receptor properties of erythroid cells." J Biol Chem 268(15): 11208-11216.

Masuda, S., M. Okano, et al. (1994). "A novel site of erythropoietin production. Oxygen-dependent production in cultured rat astrocytes." J Biol Chem 269(30): 19488-19493.

May, J., J. A. Evans, et al. (2007). "Hemoglobin variants and disease manifestations in severe falciparum malaria." Jama 297(20): 2220-2226.

McEver, R. P. (2001). "Adhesive interactions of leukocytes, platelets, and the vessel wall during hemostasis and inflammation." Thromb Haemost 86(3): 746-756.

McQuillan, J. A., A. J. Mitchell, et al. (2011). "Coincident parasite and CD8 T cell sequestration is required for development of experimental cerebral malaria." Int J Parasitol 41(2): 155-163.

Medana, I. M., T. Chan-Ling, et al. (1996). "Redistribution and degeneration of retinal astrocytes in experimental murine cerebral malaria: relationship to disruption of the blood-retinal barrier." Glia 16(1): 51-64.

Medana, I. M., T. Chan-Ling, et al. (2000). "Reactive changes of retinal microglia during fatal murine cerebral malaria: effects of dexamethasone and experimental permeabilization of the blood-brain barrier." Am J Pathol 156(3): 1055-1065.

Medana, I. M., G. Chaudhri, et al. (2001). "Central nervous system in cerebral malaria: 'Innocent bystander' or active participant in the induction of immunopathology?" Immunol Cell Biol 79(2): 101-120.

Medana, I. M., N. P. Day, et al. (2002). "Axonal injury in cerebral malaria." Am J Pathol 160(2): 655-666.

Medana, I. M., N. P. Day, et al. (2003). "Metabolites of the kynurenine pathway of tryptophan metabolism in the cerebrospinal fluid of Malawian children with malaria." J Infect Dis 188(6): 844-849.

Medana, I. M., T. T. Hien, et al. (2002). "The clinical significance of cerebrospinal fluid levels of kynurenine pathway metabolites and lactate in severe malaria." J Infect Dis 185(5): 650-656.

Medana, I. M., N. H. Hunt, et al. (1997). "Early activation of microglia in the pathogenesis of fatal murine cerebral malaria." Glia 19(2): 91-103.

Medana, I. M., N. H. Hunt, et al. (1997). "Tumor necrosis factor-alpha expression in the brain during fatal murine cerebral malaria: evidence for production by microglia and astrocytes." Am J Pathol 150(4): 1473-1486.

Medana, I. M., R. Idro, et al. (2007). "Axonal and astrocyte injury markers in the cerebrospinal fluid of Kenyan children with severe malaria." J Neurol Sci 258(1-2): 93-98.

Medana, I. M. and G. D. Turner (2006). "Human cerebral malaria and the blood-brain barrier." Int J Parasitol 36(5): 555-568.

Metenou, S., B. Dembele, et al. (2009). "Patent filarial infection modulates malaria-specific type 1 cytokine responses in an IL-10-dependent manner in a filaria/malaria-coinfected population." J Immunol 183(2): 916-924.

Min-Oo, G., A. Fortin, et al. (2003). "Pyruvate kinase deficiency in mice protects against malaria." Nat Genet 35(4): 357-362.

Min-Oo, G. and P. Gros (2005). "Erythrocyte variants and the nature of their malaria protective effect." Cell Microbiol 7(6): 753-763.

Mishra, S. K. and L. Wiese (2009). "Advances in the management of cerebral malaria in adults." Curr Opin Neurol 22(3): 302-307.

Miu, J., A. J. Mitchell, et al. (2008). "Chemokine gene expression during fatal murine cerebral malaria and protection due to CXCR3 deficiency." J Immunol 180(2): 1217-1230.

Mockenhaupt, F. P., S. Ehrhardt, et al. (2004). "Hemoglobin C and resistance to severe malaria in Ghanaian children." J Infect Dis 190(5): 1006-1009.

Mockenhaupt, F. P., S. Ehrhardt, et al. (2004). "Alpha(+)-thalassemia protects African children from severe malaria." Blood 104(7): 2003-2006.
Moxon, C. A., R. S. Heyderman, et al. (2009). "Dysregulation of coagulation in cerebral malaria." Mol Biochem Parasitol 166(2): 99-108.
Mucke, L. and M. Eddleston (1993). "Astrocytes in infectious and immune-mediated diseases of the central nervous system." Faseb J 7(13): 1226-1232.
Nagai, A., E. Nakagawa, et al. (2001). "Erythropoietin and erythropoietin receptors in human CNS neurons, astrocytes, microglia, and oligodendrocytes grown in culture." J Neuropathol Exp Neurol 60(4): 386-392.
Nantakomol, D., A. M. Dondorp, et al. (2011). "Circulating red cell-derived microparticles in human malaria." J Infect Dis 203(5): 700-706.
Newton, C. R., J. Crawley, et al. (1997). "Intracranial hypertension in Africans with cerebral malaria." Arch Dis Child 76(3): 219-226.
Newton, C. R., N. Peshu, et al. (1994). "Brain swelling and ischaemia in Kenyans with cerebral malaria." Arch Dis Child 70(4): 281-287.
Ngoungou, E. B. and P. M. Preux (2008). "Cerebral malaria and epilepsy." Epilepsia 49 Suppl 6: 19-24.
Nitcheu, J., O. Bonduelle, et al. (2003). "Perforin-dependent brain-infiltrating cytotoxic CD8+ T lymphocytes mediate experimental cerebral malaria pathogenesis." J Immunol 170(4): 2221-2228.
Nomura, S., A. Shouzu, et al. (2009). "Assessment of an ELISA kit for platelet-derived microparticles by joint research at many institutes in Japan." J Atheroscler Thromb 16(6): 878-887.
Oakley, M. S., V. Anantharaman, et al. (2011). "Molecular correlates of experimental cerebral malaria detectable in whole blood." Infect Immun 79(3): 1244-1253.
Ochola, L. B., B. R. Siddondo, et al. (2011). "Specific receptor usage in Plasmodium falciparum cytoadherence is associated with disease outcome." PLoS One 6(3): e14741.
Olotu, A., J. Lusingu, et al. (2011). "Efficacy of RTS,S/AS01E malaria vaccine and exploratory analysis on anti-circumsporozoite antibody titres and protection in children aged 5-17 months in Kenya and Tanzania: a randomised controlled trial." Lancet Infect Dis 11(2): 102-109.
Omer, F. M. and E. M. Riley (1998). "Transforming growth factor beta production is inversely correlated with severity of murine malaria infection." J Exp Med 188(1): 39-48.
Opoka, R. O., P. Bangirana, et al. (2009). "Seizure activity and neurological sequelae in Ugandan children who have survived an episode of cerebral malaria." Afr Health Sci 9(2): 75-81.
Pae, H. O., G. S. Oh, et al. (2005). "A molecular cascade showing nitric oxide-heme oxygenase-1-vascular endothelial growth factor-interleukin-8 sequence in human endothelial cells." Endocrinology 146(5): 2229-2238.
Pain, A., D. J. Ferguson, et al. (2001). "Platelet-mediated clumping of Plasmodium falciparum-infected erythrocytes is a common adhesive phenotype and is associated with severe malaria." Proc Natl Acad Sci U S A 98(4): 1805-1810.
Pamplona, A., A. Ferreira, et al. (2007). "Heme oxygenase-1 and carbon monoxide suppress the pathogenesis of experimental cerebral malaria." Nat Med 13(6): 703-710.

Pamplona, A., T. Hanscheid, et al. (2009). "Cerebral malaria and the hemolysis/methemoglobin/heme hypothesis: shedding new light on an old disease." Int J Biochem Cell Biol 41(4): 711-716.

Pankoui Mfonkeu, J. B., I. Gouado, et al. (2010). "Elevated cell-specific microparticles are a biological marker for cerebral dysfunctions in human severe malaria." PLoS One 5(10): e13415.

Parquet, V., S. Briolant, et al. (2009). "Atorvastatin is a promising partner for antimalarial drugs in treatment of Plasmodium falciparum malaria." Antimicrob Agents Chemother 53(6): 2248-2252.

Patankar, T. F., D. R. Karnad, et al. (2002). "Adult cerebral malaria: prognostic importance of imaging findings and correlation with postmortem findings." Radiology 224(3): 811-816.

Penet, M. F., M. Abou-Hamdan, et al. (2008). "Protection against cerebral malaria by the low-molecular-weight thiol pantethine." Proc Natl Acad Sci U S A 105(4): 1321-1326.

Penet, M. F., A. Viola, et al. (2005). "Imaging experimental cerebral malaria in vivo: significant role of ischemic brain edema." J Neurosci 25(32): 7352-7358.

Picot, S., A. L. Bienvenu, et al. (2009). "Safety of epoietin beta-quinine drug combination in children with cerebral malaria in Mali." Malar J 8(169): 169.

Pino, P., Z. Taoufiq, et al. (2006). "Effects of hydroxyurea on malaria, parasite growth and adhesion in experimental models." Parasite Immunol 28(12): 675-680.

Pino, P., I. Vouldoukis, et al. (2003). "Plasmodium falciparum--infected erythrocyte adhesion induces caspase activation and apoptosis in human endothelial cells." J Infect Dis 187(8): 1283-1290.

Polack, B., F. Delolme, et al. (1997). "Protective role of platelets in chronic (Balb/C) and acute (CBA/J) Plasmodium berghei murine malaria." Haemostasis 27(6): 278-285.

Potchen, M. J., G. L. Birbeck, et al. (2010). "Neuroimaging findings in children with retinopathy-confirmed cerebral malaria." Eur J Radiol 74(1): 262-268.

Potter, S. M., T. Chan-Ling, et al. (2006). "A role for Fas-Fas ligand interactions during the late-stage neuropathological processes of experimental cerebral malaria." J Neuroimmunol 173(1-2): 96-107.

Rasalkar, D. D., B. K. Paunipagar, et al. (2011). "Magnetic resonance imaging in cerebral malaria: a report of four cases." Br J Radiol 84(1000): 380-385.

Reis, P. A., C. M. Comim, et al. (2010). "Cognitive dysfunction is sustained after rescue therapy in experimental cerebral malaria, and is reduced by additive antioxidant therapy." PLoS Pathog 6(6): e1000963.

Rogerson, S. J., G. E. Grau, et al. (2004). "The microcirculation in severe malaria." Microcirculation 11(7): 559-576.

Romagnani, S. (1997). "The Th1/Th2 paradigm." Immunol Today 18(6): 263-266.

Roos, M. A., L. Gennero, et al. (2010). "Microparticles in physiological and in pathological conditions." Cell Biochem Funct 28(7): 539-548.

Roth, E. F., Jr., C. Raventos-Suarez, et al. (1983). "Glucose-6-phosphate dehydrogenase deficiency inhibits in vitro growth of Plasmodium falciparum." Proc Natl Acad Sci U S A 80(1): 298-299.

Ryter, S. W. and A. M. Choi (2009). "Heme oxygenase-1/carbon monoxide: from metabolism to molecular therapy." Am J Respir Cell Mol Biol 41(3): 251-260.

Sargin, D., A. El-Kordi, et al. (2011). "Expression of constitutively active erythropoietin receptor in pyramidal neurons of cortex and hippocampus boosts higher cognitive functions in mice." BMC Biol 9(27): 27.

Schofield, L. and F. Hackett (1993). "Signal transduction in host cells by a glycosylphosphatidylinositol toxin of malaria parasites." J Exp Med 177(1): 145-153.

Schofield, L., S. Novakovic, et al. (1996). "Glycosylphosphatidylinositol toxin of Plasmodium up-regulates intercellular adhesion molecule-1, vascular cell adhesion molecule-1, and E-selectin expression in vascular endothelial cells and increases leukocyte and parasite cytoadherence via tyrosine kinase-dependent signal transduction." J Immunol 156(5): 1886-1896.

Schroit, A. J., J. W. Madsen, et al. (1985). "In vivo recognition and clearance of red blood cells containing phosphatidylserine in their plasma membranes." J Biol Chem 260(8): 5131-5138.

Seixas, E., J. F. Moura Nunes, et al. (2009). "The interaction between DC and Plasmodium berghei/chabaudi-infected erythrocytes in mice involves direct cell-to-cell contact, internalization and TLR." Eur J Immunol 39(7): 1850-1863.

Serghides, L. and K. C. Kain (2001). "Peroxisome proliferator-activated receptor gamma-retinoid X receptor agonists increase CD36-dependent phagocytosis of Plasmodium falciparum-parasitized erythrocytes and decrease malaria-induced TNF-alpha secretion by monocytes/macrophages." J Immunol 166(11): 6742-6748.

Sharma, Y. D. (1997). "Knob proteins in falciparum malaria." Indian J Med Res 106: 53-62.

Shi, X., L. Qin, et al. (2008). "Dynamic balance of pSTAT1 and pSTAT3 in C57BL/6 mice infected with lethal or nonlethal Plasmodium yoelii." Cell Mol Immunol 5(5): 341-348.

Shirafuji, T., H. Hamaguchi, et al. (2008). "Measurement of platelet-derived microparticle levels in the chronic phase of cerebral infarction using an enzyme-linked immunosorbent assay." Kobe J Med Sci 54(1): E55-61.

Silamut, K., N. H. Phu, et al. (1999). "A quantitative analysis of the microvascular sequestration of malaria parasites in the human brain." Am J Pathol 155(2): 395-410.

Sims, P. J., E. M. Faioni, et al. (1988). "Complement proteins C5b-9 cause release of membrane vesicles from the platelet surface that are enriched in the membrane receptor for coagulation factor Va and express prothrombinase activity." J Biol Chem 263(34): 18205-18212.

Siren, A. L., T. Fasshauer, et al. (2009). "Therapeutic potential of erythropoietin and its structural or functional variants in the nervous system." Neurotherapeutics 6(1): 108-127.

Straus, D. S., G. Pascual, et al. (2000). "15-deoxy-delta 12,14-prostaglandin J2 inhibits multiple steps in the NF-kappa B signaling pathway." Proc Natl Acad Sci U S A 97(9): 4844-4849.

Sun, G., W. L. Chang, et al. (2003). "Inhibition of platelet adherence to brain microvasculature protects against severe Plasmodium berghei malaria." Infect Immun 71(11): 6553-6561.

Szklarczyk, A., M. Stins, et al. (2007). "Glial activation and matrix metalloproteinase release in cerebral malaria." J Neurovirol 13(1): 2-10.

Tada, M., A. C. Diserens, et al. (1994). "Analysis of cytokine receptor messenger RNA expression in human glioblastoma cells and normal astrocytes by reverse-transcription polymerase chain reaction." J Neurosurg 80(6): 1063-1073.

Takeda, M., M. Kikuchi, et al. (2005). "Microsatellite polymorphism in the heme oxygenase-1 gene promoter is associated with susceptibility to cerebral malaria in Myanmar." Jpn J Infect Dis 58(5): 268-271.

Taoufiq, Z., F. Gay, et al. (2008). "Rho kinase inhibition in severe malaria: thwarting parasite-induced collateral damage to endothelia." J Infect Dis 197(7): 1062-1073.

Taylor-Robinson, A. W. (2010). "Regulation of immunity to Plasmodium: implications from mouse models for blood stage malaria vaccine design." Exp Parasitol 126(3): 406-414.

Taylor, T. E., W. J. Fu, et al. (2004). "Differentiating the pathologies of cerebral malaria by postmortem parasite counts." Nat Med 10(2): 143-145.

Togbe, D., P. L. de Sousa, et al. (2008). "Both functional LTbeta receptor and TNF receptor 2 are required for the development of experimental cerebral malaria." PLoS One 3(7): e2608.

Treutiger, C. J., A. Heddini, et al. (1997). "PECAM-1/CD31, an endothelial receptor for binding Plasmodium falciparum-infected erythrocytes." Nat Med 3(12): 1405-1408.

Tripathi, A. K., W. Sha, et al. (2009). "Plasmodium falciparum-infected erythrocytes induce NF-kappaB regulated inflammatory pathways in human cerebral endothelium." Blood 114(19): 4243-4252.

Tripathi, A. K., D. J. Sullivan, et al. (2006). "Plasmodium falciparum-infected erythrocytes increase intercellular adhesion molecule 1 expression on brain endothelium through NF-kappaB." Infect Immun 74(6): 3262-3270.

Ullal, A. J., D. S. Pisetsky, et al. (2010). "Use of SYTO 13, a fluorescent dye binding nucleic acids, for the detection of microparticles in in vitro systems." Cytometry A 77(3): 294-301.

Van den Steen, P. E., K. Deroost, et al. (2008). "CXCR3 determines strain susceptibility to murine cerebral malaria by mediating T lymphocyte migration toward IFN-gamma-induced chemokines." Eur J Immunol 38(4): 1082-1095.

van der Heyde, H. C., I. Gramaglia, et al. (2005). "Platelet depletion by anti-CD41 (alphaIIb) mAb injection early but not late in the course of disease protects against Plasmodium berghei pathogenesis by altering the levels of pathogenic cytokines." Blood 105(5): 1956-1963.

Veerasubramanian, P., P. Gosi, et al. (2006). "Artesunate and a major metabolite, dihydroartemisinin, diminish mitogen-induced lymphocyte proliferation and activation." Southeast Asian J Trop Med Public Health 37(5): 838-847.

Vyas, S., V. Gupta, et al. (2010). "Magnetic Resonance Imaging of Cerebral Malaria." J Emerg Med 11: 11.

Waknine-Grinberg, J. H., N. Hunt, et al. (2010). "Artemisone effective against murine cerebral malaria." Malar J 9(227): 227.

Waknine-Grinberg, J. H., J. A. McQuillan, et al. (2010). "Modulation of cerebral malaria by fasudil and other immune-modifying compounds." Exp Parasitol 125(2): 141-146.

Walker, O., L. A. Salako, et al. (1992). "Prognostic risk factors and post mortem findings in cerebral malaria in children." Trans R Soc Trop Med Hyg 86(5): 491-493.

Wang, J. X., W. Tang, et al. (2007). "Investigation of the immunosuppressive activity of artemether on T-cell activation and proliferation." Br J Pharmacol 150(5): 652-661.

Wang, Z., J. Qiu, et al. (2007). "Anti-inflammatory properties and regulatory mechanism of a novel derivative of artemisinin in experimental autoimmune encephalomyelitis." J Immunol 179(9): 5958-5965.

Wassmer, S. C., G. J. Cianciolo, et al. (2005). "Inhibition of endothelial activation: a new way to treat cerebral malaria?" PLoS Med 2(9): e245.

Wassmer, S. C., V. Combes, et al. (2006). "Platelets potentiate brain endothelial alterations induced by Plasmodium falciparum." Infect Immun 74(1): 645-653.

Wassmer, S. C., V. Combes, et al. (2003). "Pathophysiology of cerebral malaria: role of host cells in the modulation of cytoadhesion." Ann N Y Acad Sci 992: 30-38.

Wassmer, S. C., J. B. de Souza, et al. (2006). "TGF-beta1 released from activated platelets can induce TNF-stimulated human brain endothelium apoptosis: a new mechanism for microvascular lesion during cerebral malaria." J Immunol 176(2): 1180-1184.

Wassmer, S. C., T. Taylor, et al. (2008). "Platelet-induced clumping of Plasmodium falciparum-infected erythrocytes from Malawian patients with cerebral malaria-possible modulation in vivo by thrombocytopenia." J Infect Dis 197(1): 72-78.

Weinberg, J. B., B. K. Lopansri, et al. (2008). "Arginine, nitric oxide, carbon monoxide, and endothelial function in severe malaria." Curr Opin Infect Dis 21(5): 468-475.

Wenisch, C., S. Looareesuwan, et al. (1998). "Effect of pentoxifylline on cytokine patterns in the therapy of complicated Plasmodium falciparum malaria." Am J Trop Med Hyg 58(3): 343-347.

White, V. A. (2011). "Malaria in Malawi: inside a research autopsy study of pediatric cerebral malaria." Arch Pathol Lab Med 135(2): 220-226.

White, V. A., S. Lewallen, et al. (2009). "Retinal pathology of pediatric cerebral malaria in Malawi." PLoS One 4(1): e4317.

Wiese, L., C. Hempel, et al. (2008). "Recombinant human erythropoietin increases survival and reduces neuronal apoptosis in a murine model of cerebral malaria." Malar J 7(3): 3.

Wilson, N. O., A. A. Adjei, et al. (2008). "Detection of Plasmodium falciparum histidine-rich protein II in saliva of malaria patients." Am J Trop Med Hyg 78(5): 733-735.

Wilson, N. O., T. Bythwood, et al. (2010). "Elevated levels of IL-10 and G-CSF associated with asymptomatic malaria in pregnant women." Infect Dis Obstet Gynecol 2010: 12.

Wilson, N. O., M. B. Huang, et al. (2008). "Soluble factors from Plasmodium falciparum-infected erythrocytes induce apoptosis in human brain vascular endothelial and neuroglia cells." Mol Biochem Parasitol 162(2): 172-176.

Wilson, N. O., V. Jain, et al. (2011). "CXCL4 and CXCL10 predict risk of fatal cerebral malaria." Dis Markers 30(1): 39-49.

Xu, H., Y. He, et al. (2007). "Anti-malarial agent artesunate inhibits TNF-alpha-induced production of proinflammatory cytokines via inhibition of NF-kappaB and PI3 kinase/Akt signal pathway in human rheumatoid arthritis fibroblast-like synoviocytes." Rheumatology (Oxford) 46(6): 920-926.

Yanez, D. M., J. Batchelder, et al. (1999). "Gamma delta T-cell function in pathogenesis of cerebral malaria in mice infected with Plasmodium berghei ANKA." Infect Immun 67(1): 446-448.

Yanez, D. M., D. D. Manning, et al. (1996). "Participation of lymphocyte subpopulations in the pathogenesis of experimental murine cerebral malaria." J Immunol 157(4): 1620-1624.

Yeo, T. W., D. A. Lampah, et al. (2007). "Impaired nitric oxide bioavailability and L-arginine reversible endothelial dysfunction in adults with falciparum malaria." J Exp Med 204(11): 2693-2704.

Yeo, T. W., D. A. Lampah, et al. (2008). "Recovery of endothelial function in severe falciparum malaria: relationship with improvement in plasma L-arginine and blood lactate concentrations." J Infect Dis 198(4): 602-608.

Yeo, T. W., D. A. Lampah, et al. (2009). "Relationship of cell-free hemoglobin to impaired endothelial nitric oxide bioavailability and perfusion in severe falciparum malaria." J Infect Dis 200(10): 1522-1529.

Yeo, T. W., I. Rooslamiati, et al. (2008). "Pharmacokinetics of L-arginine in adults with moderately severe malaria." Antimicrob Agents Chemother 52(12): 4381-4387.

Yipp, B. G., M. J. Hickey, et al. (2007). "Differential roles of CD36, ICAM-1, and P-selectin in Plasmodium falciparum cytoadherence in vivo." Microcirculation 14(6): 593-602.

Yipp, B. G., S. M. Robbins, et al. (2003). "Src-family kinase signaling modulates the adhesion of Plasmodium falciparum on human microvascular endothelium under flow." Blood 101(7): 2850-2857.

Yu, H. and R. Jove (2004). "The STATs of cancer--new molecular targets come of age." Nat Rev Cancer 4(2): 97-105.

Zang-Edou, E. S., U. Bisvigou, et al. (2010). "Inhibition of Plasmodium falciparum field isolates-mediated endothelial cell apoptosis by Fasudil: therapeutic implications for severe malaria." PLoS One 5(10): e13221.

Zhu, J., X. Wu, et al. (2009). "MAPK-activated protein kinase 2 differentially regulates plasmodium falciparum glycosylphosphatidylinositol-induced production of tumor necrosis factor-{alpha} and interleukin-12 in macrophages." J Biol Chem 284(23): 15750-15761.

8

Encephalopathy Related to Ivermectin Treatment of Onchocerciasis in *Loa loa* Endemic Areas: Operational Considerations

Takougang Innocent[1] and Muteba Daniel[2]
[1]*Foundation for Health research & Development, Yaoundé,*
[2]*National Programme for Onchocerciasis Control, Kinshasa,*
[1]*Cameroon*
[2]*The Democratic Republic of Congo*

1. Introduction

Human onchocerciasis is a public health problem and an obstacle to socioeconomic development in endemic countries of Africa, Arabian Peninsula and South America (WHO, 1995). The community-directed treatment with ivermectin (CDTI) is the main strategy adopted by the African Programme for Onchocerciasis control (APOC). Severe adverse events with encephalopathy (SAEs) have been associated with mass treatment with ivermectin (Mectizan) in areas where *Loa loa* and onchocerciasis are co-endemic (Duke, 2003; Twum-Danso, 2003). This has caused wide spread concern on the sustainability of CDTI (Amazigo et al., 2002; Addiss et al., 2003). The most important risk encountered in distributing ivermectin for the control of onchocerciasis in areas where *Loa loa* is co-endemic is the development of an encephalopathic syndrome. The pathogenesis of *Loa loa* encephalopathy is not fully understood, but the primary determinant is the level of *Loa loa* microfilaraemia (Gardon et al., 1997; Boussinesq et al., 1998; Gardon et al., 1999; Boussinesq et al., 2001) and the inflammatory response to the dying worms (McGarry et al., 2003).

Post ivermectin treatment encephalopathies with fatal outcome have repeatedly been the subject of clinical and operational investigations. Investigations have targeted aspects of implementing mass drug administration, monitoring and referral of early signs of SAE, improved clinical management in the communities and health facilities.Research for primary prevention have also witnessed the development of operational tools, aimed at identifying high risk communities, using in the communities and health Normalized-Difference Vegetation Index (NDVI) and rapid assessment methods (Diggle et al., 2007). For the later purpose, RAPLOA is used to identify communities at risk of SAEs. The objective of the present chapter is to provide an updated review of gathered evidence on the pathophysiology of *Loa loa* mediated encephalopathy and the existing methods for its prevention and case management at the community level.

2. Epidemiology

Onchocerciasis, also known as river blindness, is caused by a filarial nematode, *Onchocerca volvulus*. The adult worms lives in subcutaneous nodules within surface muscles, mainly around the pericostal and the iliac crest.

There are two mains subtypes of *Onchocerca volvulus*, namely the forest and savanah. In the savanal infections, the nodules are mainly located on the upper part of the body, including the trunk, upper limbs and head. Ocular involvement is frequent. In the forest infections, nodules are found primarily on the lower limbs and iliac crest. Cutaneous alterations are the main manifestations of the disase.

The worm is transmitted through the bite of female blackflies of the genus *Simulium*, which bite during the day. The fly breeds in rapidly flowing rivers and streams.

Onchocerciasis is endemic in most countries in sub-saharan Africa. Isolated endemic foci are also present in the Arabian Peninsula (Yemen) and in the Americas (Brazil, Colombia, Ecuador, Guatemala, southern Mexico, and Venezuela). An estimated 17 million people are infected worldwide.

The distribution of the disease has been substantially narrowed with the successful implementation of the Onchocerciasis Control Programme in West Africa (OPC) and the African Programme for Onchocerciasis Control (APOC). OPC used aerial spray of insecticides for the control of onchocerciasis fly vector from 1974 to 2000 when the programme closed down, after reaching its goal. APOC began its activities in 1995. Its main strategy is the annual or biannual distribution of ivermectin, a safe and effective drug that was licensed for human use in 1987. APOC is a partnership involving international donors, the private sector including pharmaceutical companies, Non-governmental Organizations and communities. The delineation of roles and responsibilities within the partnership has been the subject of extended literature and consultative statutory meetings regularly hold to monitor progress towards the control and elimination of the disease. Unfortunately, progress in the control of onchocerciasis in APOC countries met with difficulties as the programme progressed towards central Africa where the level of endemicity of *Loa loa* is highest. *Loa loa* is a filarial worm that inhabits the subcutaneous tissue of humans. The disease is transmitted from one host to the other through the bite of the *Chrysops* fly. The adult breeds in marshy forested habitats. In areas that are co-endemic for both onchocerciasis and loiasis, the mass administration of ivermectin for treatment of onchocerciasis sometimes leads to the occurrence of Severe Adverse Events (SAE) consisting of a potentially lethal encephalopathy.

Short-term travelers to endemic areas are at low risk for this infection. Travelers who visit endemic areas for extended periods of time (generally >3 months) and live or work near black fly habitats are at risk for *Loa loa* infections.

Infection with *O. volvulus* results in skin lesions, including a highly pruritic, papular dermatitis; subcutaneous nodules; lymphadenitis. Ocular lesions occur in endemic countries and can progress to visual loss and blindness. Historically, the term river blindness was coined from the blindness that occurred along streams that were onchocerciasis transmission sites. Symptoms in travelers are primarily dermatologic and may occur months to years after departure from endemic areas. Immigrants from endemic areas may present with skin or ocular disease.

Onchocerciasis is diagnosed by finding the microfilariae in punch biopsy, adult worms in histologic sections of excised nodules or characteristic eye lesions. Serologic testing is most useful for detecting infection in specific groups, such as expatriates with a brief exposure history, when microfilariae are not identifiable. It is equally expected that serological tests and molecular markers will get into wide use as interventions move towards disease elimination goals.

Ivermectin (150–200 μg/kg orally, once or twice per year) is the drug of choice for onchocerciasis. Repeated annual or semiannual doses may be required. The drug kills the microfilariae but not the adult worms, which can live for 15-17 years. Antibiotic trials with doxycycline (100 mg orally per day) directed against *Wolbachia*, an endosymbiont of *O. volvulus*, have demonstrated a decrease in onchocercal microfiladermia with 6 weeks of therapy. Therefore, some experts recommend treating patients with 1 dose of ivermectin followed by 6 weeks of doxycycline. Several health workers however advocated against the wide use of antibiotics in communities as it could foster specific or cross another constrain is the problematic compliance with the numerous doses treatment regimen.

Subcutaneous nodules can be excised if their anatomic location allows it to be done safely.

No vaccine or drug to prevent *Onchocerca* infection is available. Protective measures include avoiding blackfly habitats and the use of personal protection measures against biting insects.

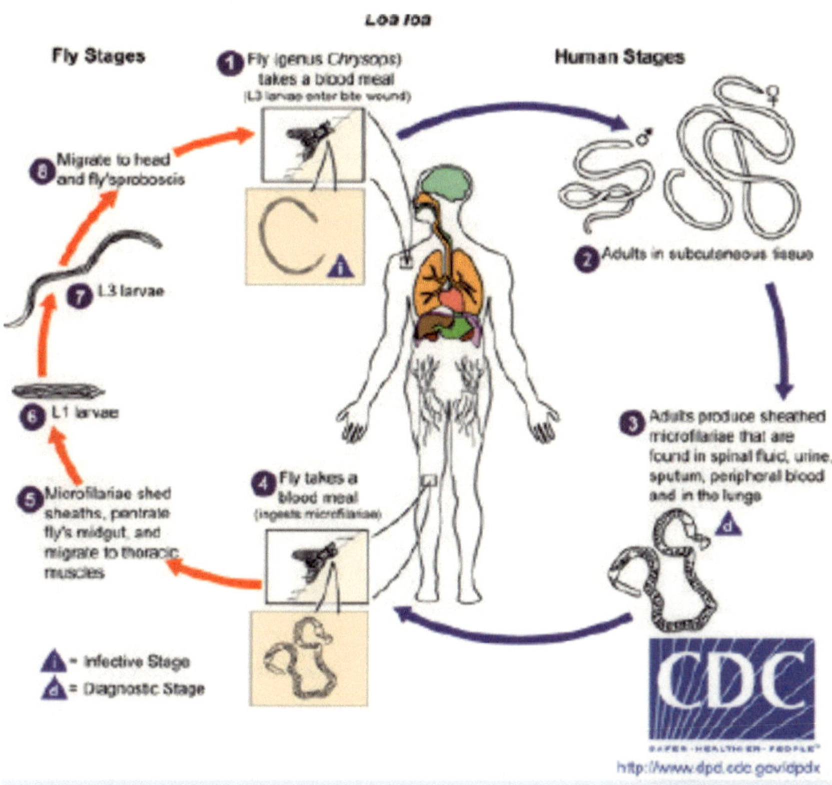

Fig. 1. Life cycle of the Loa loa parasite, involving the human host and the *Chrysops* vector. Reprinted from the CDC webpage.

3. Particularities of the health infrastructure in onchocerciasis and loiasis endemic areas

Populations most affected by onchocerciasis and loiasis live in remote areas of endemic countries where they are poor and underserved by the health system. In fact, despite the Alma Ata Declaration on Primary Health Care (PHC) of 1978 - a system envisaged for improving access to health interventions - equity and access to essential health services remain sub-optimal in sub-Saharan Africa, especially in rural areas. The international community have recognized the potential of PHC (WHO, 2008). There are attempts to its revitalization and PHC has been placed high on the agenda of several international fora (African Review of the Implementation of PHC in Ouagadougou).

Recent efforts by the World Health Organisation (WHO, 2006) emphasized that a significant proportion of the national health budget should focus on interventions linked to the MDGs, targeting those most in need. Unfortunately, African health systems continue to be weak, with fragmented interventions. Health services lack effective mechanisms for making any real impact on the high burden of infectious diseases. Health systems in onchocerciasis endemic countries (mainly in Africa) lack sustainable frameworks to involve partners from other development sectors. However, a functioning health system is the backbone to support sustainable interventions. Community participation enhances the affordability of health interventions compared to conventional, vertical programmes, as recurrent costs become more affordable (Gish, 1992). In order to enhance community participation and engagement in the delivery of health services, many African countries have set up dialogue structures to facilitate communication between the health system and communities. These dialogue structures help bring promotion, prevention and cure together in a safe, effective, socially acceptable and productive way to the population. Its comprehensiveness, integration and continuity, make the dialogue structure a point of entry into the community to build an enduring relationship of trust between people, their health-care providers and the health system. Some of these structures have survived, but others have collapsed. Their poor conception and the exclusion of communities in their inception are some of the reasons of the failure. One of the cornerstones of PHC is working in partnerships. The partnerships that make the greatest impact in the rural population are those that are grounded at the community level. However, the mechanism for bringing together partners to improve their collaboration at this level remains problematic. The Community Directed Treatment with Ivermectin (CDTI), a process in which the community has the responsibility for the organization and delivery of treatment has been adopted by the African Programme for Onchocerciasis Control (APOC) as its strategy to control of onchocerciasis (Brieger et al., 2002). CDTI promotes active community participation in decision making as a means of improving access to the drug, promoting a sense of responsibility and appropriation. It enhances ownership and empowerment of communities (Amazigo et al., 1998). CDTI is a stimulus for developing primary health care in areas with difficult access to formal health services (Hopkins, 1998; Richards *et al.*, 2004). Field trials revealed the efficiency of communities to deliver multiple interventions of various degrees of complexity, thus strengthening the link between communities and the health system (WHO, 2008). Comprehensive revitalization of primary healthcare holds the potential to insure equity in access to health services. Community engagement and involvement in the planning, delivery and monitoring of health interventions, strengthens the interactions between health services and the communities and enhance needs-based and demand-driven provision of services which in turn strengthens PHC delivery schemes (WHO, 2008). The lack of a legal framework and normative orientation also plague optimal community participation and stakeholders' engagement. Community monitoring and referral of SAE cases is crucial in the management of onchocerciasis control programme in areas that are at risk of *Loa loa* mediated encephalopathy.

4. Pathophysiology of *Loa loa* mediated encephalopathy

Loa loa encephalopathy is related to the worm burden, especially the hypermicrofilaremia. Though its mechanism is not sufficiently understood, it is known that Ivermectine (Mectizan)®, in addition to being an effective drug against the microfilariae of *Onchocerca volvulus* (the causative agent of onchocerciasis), is also effective against *L. loa* microfilariae, the rapid killing of which has been associated with this encephalopathy. Encephalopathy may also be linked with higher permeability of brain capillaries as they react to a higher load of worm antigen released after massive destruction of *Loa loa* microfilaria in response to ivermectin administration.

The obstruction of brain capillaries by paralyzed microfilariae lead to local ischemic reactions, increased pressure within the capillaries, rupture of the affected vessels and hemorrhagic suffusion. The hemorrhage equally occurs on the conjunctiva mucosa or on the palpebral area. The last manifestation has been used as a prognostic sign of encephalopathic involvement.

5. Identification of individuals and communities at risk of encephalopathy

5.1 Primary prevention of encephalopathy

The reactions of *Loa loa* to onchocerciasis drugs date back from the use of Diethyl Carbamazine (DEC=Notezine) when severe adverse reactions with encephalopathy were reported. Ivermectin was known as a safe drug for the mass treatment of onchocerciasis until the 1999 when several cases of SAEs occurred as distribution moved to the forest areas of Cameroon and Nigeria, that are breeding environments for Chrysops flies, the vectors of *Loa loa*.

The high number of cases that occurred in Cameroon lead administrative authorities and APOC to stop distribution until clarifications were provided, the causes elucidated and preventive measures laid out. The World Health Organisation special programme for Research and Training in Tropical Diseases (TDR), together with a team of African scientist lead the development of RAPLOA, a rapid assessment method based on the history of migration of the adult *Loa loa* worm through the conjunctiva. Primary prevention equally makes use of community knowledge of *Loa loa*, which is an indicator of the level of endemicity. RAPLOA has been used to map the risk of *Loa loa* encephalopathy, in priority areas for onchocerciasis lymphatic filariasis within the framework of Neglected Tropical Diseases (NTD) control. (Figure 2)

The delivery of RAPLOA entails the administration of a community and individual questionnaires. The RAPLOA community questionnaire helps in getting an onerall view the community experience and endemicity of *Loa loa*. Simple names for eye worm are often associated with high prevalence, while complex and composite names are associated to lower prevalences (Table 1).

Language / ethnic group	*Villages*	Vernacular name	meaning (etymology)
Baya	Bedobo, Mbelibina, Bengue Tiko, Mbile, Belikoungou	*Yolo li* *yolo*=worm *li*=eye	Worm of the eye
Baya	Mbelebina, Camp SODEPA, Bambouti, Garga Sarali, Ndanga Gadima, Dabole,	*Peng li* *peng*=worm *li*=eye	Worm of the eye
Foulbe	Camp SODEPA, Ndanga Gadima, Mbile, Belikoungou	*Guildé guité* *guildé*=worm *guité*=eye	Worm of the eye
Kako	Djal, Djassi	*Ntoro*	Worm of the eye
Kako	Nyamsambo, Kamba Mieri, Ngoura, Ngoulmekong, Letta, Gbabele, Pouyanga, Gaba Letta, Kpangalakonga, Banda, Mbouye, Dem 2	*Kon missi* *kon*=sickness *missi*=eye	Eye sickness
Maka	Bouam, Baktala	*da* *biep* *Naki*	Worm of the eye
Mbimou	Mbiali	*Ntoli*	worm of the eye
Mezime	Kagnol I, Bokendja, Kapang, Djampiel	*Djol*	Worm of the eye
Mvongmvon	Djemba	*Dol*	Worm of the eye
Pol	Grand Pol	*kon mich* *kon*=worm *mich*=eye	Worm of the eye

Table 1. Vernacular names of eye worm in villages of Eastern Cameroon

Several other conditions have been reported to favor encephalopathy in loasis areas and confound with the determinants of SAE. Among these are the consumption of alcoholic beverages, especially the traditional, non standard drinks that contain mixtures of alcohols, some of which may be neurotoxic such as methanol.

Operational guidelines have been provided by the Technical Consultative Committee (TCC) of APOC on the implementation of ivermectin mass distribution in areas that are co-endemic for onchocerciasis and loiasis. Within this scheme, blanked treatment is not recommended and a distribution by axis is advocated based the capabilities of the human resources for health, infrastructure and logistic for the early detection, referral and management of cases.

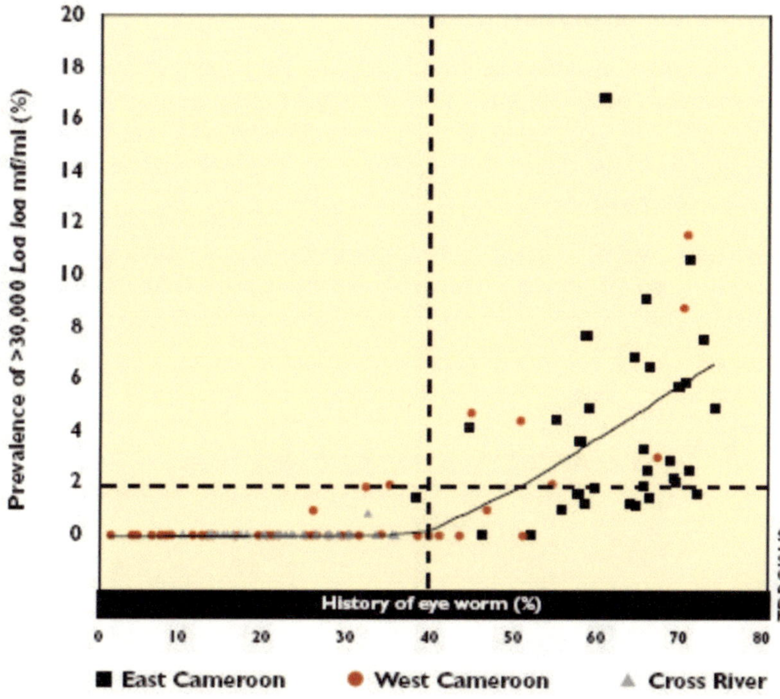

Fig. 2. Relationship between the prevalence of very high microfilarial loads(>30.000 mf/ml) and RAP based on the history of eye worm (From TDR. Guidelines for the Rapid Assessment of Loa loa).

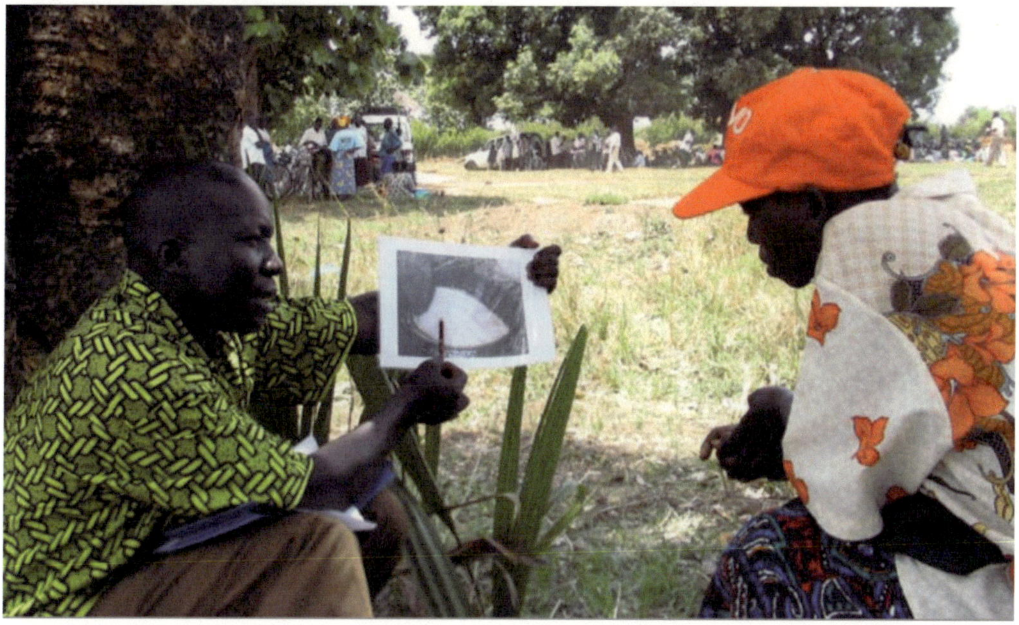

Fig. 3. Delivery of the RAPLOA individual questionnaire to assess the risk of SAE at the community level, using the illustrated eye worm in Southern Sudan (Photo Dr Takougang)

5.2 Secondary prevention of encephalopathy

Not all cases of SAE may be avoided through primary prevention. Thus, early identification and referral of cases of encephalopathy is of paramount importance. Early detection offers improved prognosis. In this regard, ataxia, sub-palpebral hemorrhage have been successfully used, two-three days after treatment, to identify and manage cases of SAEs which would have otherwise developed encephalopathy.

Many lessons have been learned for improved clinical management of cases of encephalopathy in hospital settings. This has lead to improved survival and reduction in mortality among cases.

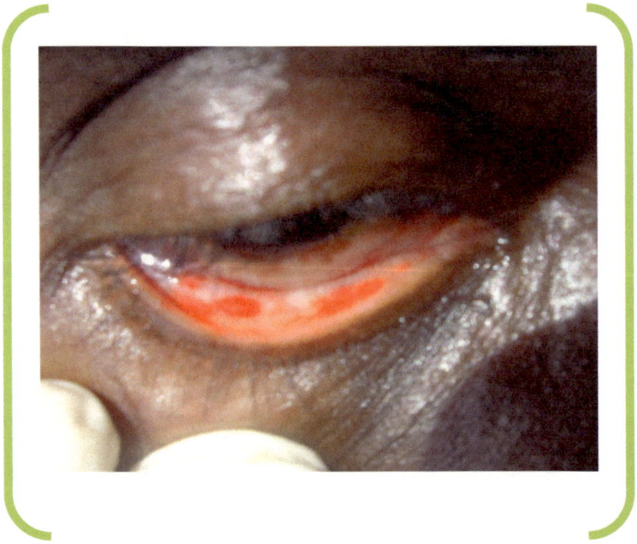

Fig. 4. Sub-palpebral hemorrhage in a case of SAE in Cameroon (Photo Dr J. Kamgno).

5.3 Tertiary prevention of encephalopathy

The literature on the tertiary prevention of encephalopathy is scanty. Apart from clinical data that indicate measures to prevent bed sores, there is very little data on the disabilities that occur following SAE and encephalopathy. The sequelae and their impact on the patient's productivity and quality of life needs to be assessed.

6. Clinical and paraclinical features of *Loa loa* mediated encephalopathy

Post onchocerciasis treatment encephalopathy occurs in people with very high levels of *L. loa* [> 30,000 microfilariae/milliliter blood (mf/ml)] following treatment with Mectizan®. The patient often presents with fever (39-40°C), head ache and ataxia. Signs of central nervous system involvement may follow. Such signs include confusion, omnibulation, lethargy, ataxia, anal and urinary incontinence. Unattented, the patient progresses into into coma.

7. Differential diagnosis

Encephalopathy is a brain disease, damage or malfunction. Encephalopathy presents in a broad spectrum of symptoms that range from mild, such as memory loss or subtle personality changes to dementia, seizures, coma and death. Encaphalopathy on the early is often accompanied by physical manifestations such as poor coordination of limb movements (NINDS, 2011).

A wide range of causes may lead to encephalopathy may be infectious (bacteria, viruses, parasites), anoxia (lack of oxygen to the brain), alcohol consumption, liver failure, kidney failure, metabolic diseases, brain tumors, toxic chemicals, alterations in pressure in the brain, and poor nutrition of nerve cells.

Despite the numerous and varied causes of encephalopathy, an **altered mental state** is usually present. It may be subtle and develop slowly over years or rather rapidly (for example, brain anoxia leading to coma or death in a few minutes). Often, symptoms such as poor judgement or poor coordination of movements are reported. The severity and type of symptoms are related to the underlying cause. Alcohol-induced encephalopathy can result in involuntary hand tremors, while severe anoxia may result in coma with no movement.

The diagnosis of encephalopathy is usually done by clinical tests done during the physical examination (mental status tests, memory tests, coordination tests) that document an altered mental state. Findings on clinical tests either diagnose or presumptively diagnose encephalopathy. Usually, a diagnosis is made when the altered mental state accompanies another primary condition such as chronic liver disease, kidney failure or anoxia.

Many practitioners view encephalopathy as a complication that occurs following a primary underlying health problem. The frame work for the diagnosis and management of cases of encephalopathy includes Complete blood count; search for underlying infections, assessment of blood pressure (high or low blood pressure); blood levels of electrolytes, glucose, lactate, ammonia, oxygen, and liver enzyme levels; drug use or toxin levels (alcohol, cocaine, amphetamines, ..); ceresbrospinal fluid analyses; kidney function (creatinine)

Other diagnostic tools may be useful, but are not often present in *Loa loa* endemic settings. These include Computer Tomography (CT) and Magnetic Resonance Imaging (MRI) scans to assess brain swelling, anatomical abnormalities or infections; Doppler ultrasound to assess blood flow to tissues, encephalogram to assess brain wave patterns.

In the case of *Loa loa* encephalopathies, microfilariae are sought in a standardized finger prick thick blood smear. The presence of such is indicative of the involvement of *Loa loa* in the genesis of encephalopathy. However, under the endemic conditions, infections agents such as *Neisseria meningitidis*, the cause of bacterial meningitis, *Toxoplasma gondii*, and malaria must be ruled out. Cerebral malaria is a likely co-factor in the occurrence of encephalopathy. Clinical orientation, experience, of the treating physician, the specific symptoms and history of the patient are of paramount importance in the early detection and management of cases.

8. Case reports

Several cases of *Loa loa* encephalophathy occur each year in the DRC. During the 2009 Mectizan distribution, the country reported the highest number in the history of participating in activities. Below are a selected number of cases to point out clinical presentation and management.

Case Report #1

Patient WB, aged 33 years old lived in the city of Abuzi in the Abuzi health Zone in the Equateur Province (The Democratic Republic of Congo). He swallowed 3 tablets of ivermectin on the 10/11/2009. He was 149 cm tall and weighed 52 kg. His general state was good before he swallowed ivermectin tablets. He had no history of alcohol consumption 24 hours before or after ivermectin treatment. He presented with fever, altered behavior and coma on 11/11 2009, one day after he swallowed the tablets. He was transferred to the Abuzi reference hospital on the 12/11/2009 and was admitted on same day. At admission, the patient had urinary incontinence. His blood pressure and temperature were within the normal limits. Coma, stage 2 was diagnosed by the attending physician.

Emmergency biomedical investigations revealed a microfilaremia of 2520 *Loa loa* mf/ml from of a thick blood film. The analysis of a concurrent thin blood smear revealed *Plasmodium falciparum* trophozoites.

The diagnosis made by the attending physician was that of cerebral malaria with encephalopathy post ivermectin treatment.

The treatment administered included:

Intravenous drips of quinine in 5% glucose, Ringer lactate serum or physiological saline solutions.

Antibiotics (Ampicilline, Direct intravenous injection) were equally administered was provided for bed sores as appropriate.

Three days after admission, the patient developed bed sores that were unhealed on 14/12/2009, when he was discharged. On discharge, the patient still experienced difficulties walking.

Case report #2:

Patient F., aged 28 years was from the village of Bukarawa , Loko Health Zone in the Equateur Province of the Democratic Republic of Congo. She was admitted in the Loko Health Zone Reference Hospital. At admission, the patient blood pressure was 180/120 mmHg, the Glasgow score was estimated at 5 (coma stage 2) ; Temperature was 39°C.

For her 146 cm height, the patient was reported to have taken 3 tablets of Mectizan 100g on 06 December 2009. The general health status was good prior to the absorption of Mectizan tablets. On 06 December 2009, about 6 hours after absorption, the patient developed intense fever, altered behaviour and fainted. It was in this state that she was transferred to the reference hospital on 08 December 2009. Upon investigations with siblings the patient had not taken any alcoholic drink over the past 24 hours. On admission, the patient had bed sores on the lower part of the lower back, around the sacrum.

The presumptive diagnosis was that of a *Loa loa* encephalopathy related to ivermectin, associated to cerebral malaria or meningitis.

Biomedical evaluation of a thick blood film revealed *Loa loa* microfilariae (620 mf/ml). The glycemia was 186 mg/dl, that decreased to 111 mg/dl on the second day. White blood cell count was 9550/mm3, and the sedimentation coefficient (VS) 91 mm/h.

The following treatment was administered: Intravenous administration of Quinine in 5% Glucose serum for 3 days. Glucose and Ringer Lactate were alternatively use as solutes.

The anti-hypertensive drug Adalate 2X10mg was administered through a nasogastric gavage; Lasilix (Lasix) 40 mg was administered intravenously.

The antipyretic drug Dipyrone was used in an intramuscular injection of 4X1g /day.

For hyperleucocytopenia, an association of Ampicilline and Chloramphénicol was administred through direct intravenous injection 3X 1g /day.

To alleviate bedsores, a nursing protocole for patient mobility was set. Topical antiseptics were used to cleanse the wound of the lower back.

The treatment was followed for 5 days. However, the feverish state persisted, reaching 40,5°C on day 5. Diastolic blood pressure went from 120 down to 100 mm Hg. The systolic Pressure decreased from 190 to 160 mmHg despite the treatment administered.

The patient died on day 5.

9. Management of cases of *Loa loa* mediated encephalopathy

Like all life threatening conditions, *Loa loa* encephalopathy requires prompt medical and nursing care to provide supportive treatment and prevent nosocomial infections. With competent and timely medical care, patients usually recover.

The main features of case management include the monitoring of vital signs, nutrition and nursing care.

Vital signs of importance are blood pressure, pulse, body temperature and respiratory frequency. Nasogastric intubation may be useful in maintaining hydrolytic and nutrients intake for energy support.

Rehydration using Ringer Lactate, physiological solution, hypertonic glucose may be used depending on the patient preexisting health status. Salt and glucose are to be monitored in hypertensive and diabetic patients. Nutrients intake should be shifted from parenteral to per os as soon as the patient is able to sustain feeding. In re-initiating autonomous feeding, preference is given to liquid diets including milk, soups enriched with soja or ground meat.

Nursing care is of utmost importance for the prevention of bed sores that often results from hospital bed pressure. This is reduced through scheduled mobilization of the patient to release circulation and relieve pressure sites. The use of adequate mattresses and bed dressing may be helpful. Care also focuses on the liberation of airways as they are likely to obscure the prognosis. The detection and management of concurrent pathologies may improve the prognosis. This is especially the case for hypertension, diabetes, malaria, meningitis and other health conditions. Malaria may be diagnosed incidentally in standard blood smears that are effected for the confirmatory diagnosis of *Loa loa* infection. It may equally be purposefully sought when there are signs such as fever, omnibulation, diarrhoea or other signs suggestive of simple or cerebral malaria.

Practionners often recommend that corticoid should not be used as they may increase the risk of infection and/or gastrointestinal bleeding after prolonged use.

Because SAE is a medical emergency, all laboratory support tasks should be performed steadily and timely. These include tests for glycemia, blood smears, analyses of cerebro-spinal fluid for *Loa loa* parasites and concurrent infection, such as meningitis.

10. Operational consideration of *Loa loa* interventions in onchocerciasis control

APOC, the leading organization in onchocerciasis control in Africa has led the development of tools for early detection and management of cases of SAE. Todate, mortality associated with the occurrence of encephalopathy is on the decline. As ivermectine is effective against both *Onchocerca* and *Loa loa*, the occurrence of ESG is proportional to the prevalence of high *Loa loa* microfilaremic individuals in affected communities. Thus, the probability of having cases decreases with the duration of effective mass treatment cycles (Figure 5).

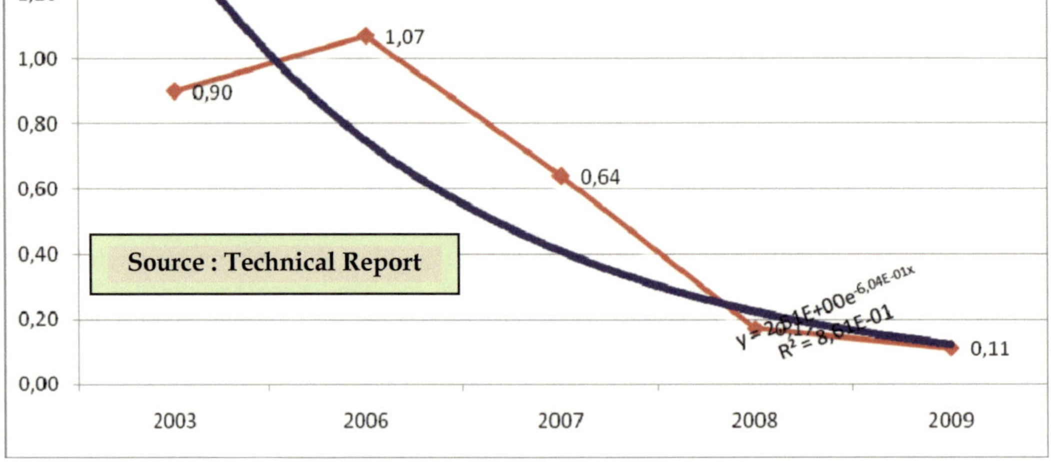

Fig. 5. Evolution of SAE cases following Ivermectine (Mectizan) distribution in onchocerciasis and loiasis co-endemic areas in the Democratic Republic of Congo(2003-2009)

Even though the ESG represent a threat to CDTI operations, especially when encephalopathy triggered deaths are registered, it is still unethical to withhold treatment from thousands of people who live in oncherciasis and loiasis co-endemic areas. In that regard, special guidelines have been developed to inform mass distribution of ivermectine in such areas. Under such circumstances, operational teams are advised to avoid blanket treatment while giving precedence to focal, progressive treatment. The rate of expansion is then proportional to the number of expected cases of SAE, matched to the capacity of the local health infrastructure in available hospital beds, trained personnel and accessibility. Accessibility is a key determinant in countries where the road network is poor. Under some circumstances, mobile teams may be adopted or the capabilities of first line health facilities developed to permit the handling of severe illness resulting from SAE.

11. *Loa loa* mediated encephalopathy and the future of neglected tropical diseases control

Loiasis is a neglected disease that may have great social and economic impact in some endemic areas. Loiasis has for long been regarded as a benign filariasis. Its distribution that is limited to Central Africa has made it a less studied infection. The number of infected individuals was estimated at 2-13 millions (Fain, 1978). Interest in loiasis has been renewed as cases of encephalopathy occurred following treatment of onchocerciasis patients with high coincident *Loa loa* microfilareamia (Chippaux *et al.*, 1996; Gardon *et al.*, 1997; Twum-Danso *and* Meredith, 2003). The occurrence of SAE affects compliance, treatment coverage and the sustainability of CDTI (Amazigo *et al.*, 1998). Data on the distribution of *Loa loa* infection became mandatory to assess the risk of severe adverse events (SAE) as community directed treatment of onchocerciasis with ivermectin (CDTI) was extended to loiasis endemic areas. SAE are a constraint to community participation and compliance with CDTI. Working in Cameroon, the prevalence of *Loa loa* microfilareamia was found to reach rate of 31.5% in adults living in the dense forest area of Yokadouma (Languillon, 1957). Prevalences ranging from 9.6% to 13.5% were reported in the population of Colomines in the savannah area of the Kadei valley (Haumont *et al.*, 1992). A model using satellite mapping of key environmental factors related to the biology of the *Chrysops* vector predicts a high prevalence of *Loa loa* at the regional level (Thomson *et al.*, 2004), but the endemicity of loiasis at the community level may be unexpected (Kamgno and Boussinesq, 2001., Wanji *et al.*, 2001). A study in eastern Cameroon indicated a high morbidity of the disease (Takougang *et al.*, 2002). Loiasis was the second or third cause of medical consultations after malaria and pulmonary diseases in some endemic regions (Boulesteix *and* Carme, 1986; Pinder, 1988). Clinical manifestations of loasis in endemic areas have received little attention (Agbolade *et al.*, 2005). The subconjunctival migration of adult worm, migratory angioedema and pruritus were the most reported signs (Carme et al, 1989; Noireau et al., 1990).

In most areas, the prevalence of eye worm and Calabar swellings were higher than that of microfilareamia. These observations denote that most clinical cases of *Loa loa* filariasis are amicrofilaraemic, and confirm previous observations (Touré *et al.*, 1998; Touré *et al.*, 1999, Pion *et al.*, 2005). The prevalence of *Loa loa* infection that is estimated through the microscopic examination of standard blood film thus leads to an underestimation of the prevalence of loiasis. RAPLOA (Takougang *et al.*, 2002), a tool based on the history of eye worm that is used for the rapid assessment of *Loa loa* infection, may provide a better estimate of the affliction. The term used for the identification of eye worm disease was consistent among the ethnic groups and languages. Most of the local names were composite, derived from the terms for "worm" and "eye". The widespread knowledge of signs and symptoms of *Loa loa* infection are an asset for community involvement in control, health education and promotion activities (Hewlett *et al.*, 1996). The local names for Calabar swellings were less consistent than those of eye worm. Reports of Calabar swellings with intense itching corroborate previous findings (Morrone *et al.*, 2002). The itching that is associated with Calabar swellings can be a cause of distraction from economic activities, and a source of social stigma and low self-esteem (Noireau, 1989). Subconjunctival migration of the worm causes considerable discomfort. It was associated with arthralgia and fatigue (Pinder, 1988; Morrone *et al.*, 2002). These are constrains to productivity and economic development. The morbidity of eye worm disease may be heightened by the reported practices of traditional removal of the worm using a sharp blade, drops from the plants *Allium cepa* or *Tithonia diversifolia*, all of which may further damage the afflicted eye. The risk of physical and chemical damages to the eye consecutive to the local treatment practices, the secondary bacterial infections associated with local treatments may add on to the morbidity of loiasis in endemic populations. *Loa loa* related hypereosinophilia was suspected of playing a role in the aetiology of endocardial fibrosis (Pinder, 1988). In some case histories, glomerulonephritis, cardiomyopathy, retinopathy, lymphadenitis and lymphodoema were reported (Morrone *et al.*, 2002; Agbodale *et al.*, 2005). In a study carried out in Congo, headache and arthralgia were associated with *Loa loa* infection (Carme *et al.*, 1989). The risk of SAE that has motivated most recent studies on *Loa loa* may therefore be a limited view of its health risks spectrum. There is an urgent need of interventions to prevent its health consequences. In that regard, albendazole may be a useful tool (Tabi *et al.*, 2004). The mass distribution of ivermectin and albendazole within CDTI projects within the Global Programme to Eliminate Lymphatic Filariasis (GPELF) will have an incidental impact on *Loa loa* infection (Chippaux et al., 1998; Tsague-Dongmo, 2002).

Field observations have pointed out the effect of alcohol as a co-factor in the determination of ivermectin mediated SAE, but the information available is conflictive. Food and alcohol are known to alter ivermectin bio-availability (Baraka et al., 1996). The contra-indication of alcohol consumption around Ivermectine (Mectizan) intake as indicated by Merck & Co., Inc. have safety concerns, but may unnecessarily deter some people from taking ivermectin (The Mectizan Expert Committee, 2000). Shu *et al.* (2000) failed to establish any enhanced occurrence of side effects in patients who consumed alcohol. .In a study carried out in Cameroon where some local beverages are produced from uncontrolled fermentation, with obviously higher alcohol content and diversity, Takougang *et al.* (2006) reported that the risk of SAE was higher when Ivermectine (Mectizan) was taken for the first time. Males were more likely than females to develop SAE. The occurrence of SAE was not associated with the timing of the last alcohol consumption, indicating that alcohol intake is not a major determinant of SAE. Because of the limited number of cases, the authors did not separate the different types of alcohols consumed. High content distilled alcohols may contribute to SAE, as these beverages contain a variety of alcohols which may be neurotoxic. Still the local palm and raphia wines, are blended with plant adjuvants, some of which may be potent neurotoxics. The plant *Paullina pinnata (Salpindaceae)* – locally called 'Mbami', 'Mbarbi' or 'lianes' – is known to cause head ache. The influence of these adjuvants as determinants of SAE deserves further investigations.

It is possible that some participants (cases) could have denied alcohol consumption for fear of loosing the coverage of hospital costs as practiced by the National Onchocerciasis Control Programme.

One of the determinants of alcohol use and abuse contribution to ill health is the type of alcoholic beverage. Ethanol that is found in beverages may not be a key factor in SAE (Shu *et al.*, 2000), but other alcohols such as methanol or buthanol of the locally produced "Arki", "Odontol" or "Hah" could contribute. The plant adjuvants of beverages may be at least co-factors. In one instance, a community distributor reported that a patient who developed SAE had ingested palm wine after ivermectin treatment. A similar case was quoted by Boussinesq et al. (2003). While there is an increased bioavailability of ivermectin following its co-administration with ethanol (Edwards et al., 1988; Cerkvenik and Grabnar, 2002), it is unlikely that the level of Ivermectin reached is high enough to cause SAE. The adjuvants of palm wine reported by Takougang et al., 2006 contain tannins, alkaloids and saponins which are all potent on the nervous system. Tannins increase capillary resistance, reduce capillary permeability of the red blood cells and are vasoconstrictors. Vasoconstriction of the extracranial arteries causes headache, restlessness and dizziness. Saponins are characterised by their tensio-active properties. Many saponins speed up haemoglobin degradation through their interaction with sterols of the membrane of the red blood cells. Alkaloids are complex nitrogenous substances with a bitter taste, that which is most preferred by consumers of palm wine. Alkaloids can be stimulants or depressors of the central nervous system (Bruneton, 1999). It is therefore required that the role of plant used as adjuvants in alcoholic drinks, as co-factors in SAE should be further assessed.

12. Conclusion

Early detection, operational adjustment and research based decision-making has contributed to improved management of SAE and encephalopathy in the control of onchocerciasis. However, further investigations are warranted on the sequelae and impact of encephalopathies on patient's productivity and quality of life. As the implementation of integrated control of Neglected Tropical Diseases progresses outside the onchocerciasis endemic areas, more challenges will be faced in lymphatic filariasis elimination areas. Implementation research will be needed to address operational issues, compliance, detection of novel side effects resulting from the co-administration of ivermectin, Albendazole and Praziquantel in previously naïve areas. Scaling up these interventions will equally face the genetic variability of human hosts and their cultural and behavioral correlates. Multidisciplinary collaborative research including epidemiology, social science, clinical and biological sciences will be warranted to address these issues.

13. References

Agbodale O.M., Akinboye D.O., Ogunkolo O.F. (2005). *Loa loa* and *Mansonella perstans*: Neglected human infections that need control in Nigeria. *African Journal of Biotechnology*, 4(13):1554-1558.

Amazigo U. 2008. APOC. Annals of Tropical Medicine and Parasitology 102(Suppl. 1): 19-22.

Amazigo UV., Noma M., Boatin BA., Etya'ale DE., Seketeli A & Dadzie KY. (1998). Delivery systems and cost recovery in Mectizan treatment for onchocerciasis. *Annals of Tropical Medicine and Parasitology*, 92(Suppl.1) :S23-S31.

Amazigo UV, Obono OM, Dadzie KY, Remme J (2002). Monitoring community - directed treatment programmes for sustainability: lessons from the African programme for onchocerciasis control (APOC). Annals of Trop Med. Parasitol. 96 (1):575 - 592.

Baraka OZ, Mahmoud BM, Marschke CK, Geary TG, Homeida MM A, Williams JF (1996). Ivermectin distribution in the plasma and tissues of patients infected with *Onchocerca volvulus. Eur.* J. Clin. Pharmacol. 50:407-410.

Boulesteix G. & Carme B. (1986). Encéphalite au cours du traitement de la filariose à *Loa loa* par la diéthylcarbamazin. A propos de 6 observations. *Bulletin de la Société de Pathologie Exotique*, 79 : 649-654.

Boussinesq M, Gardon J, Gardon-Wendel, N, Chippaux JP (2003). Clinical picture, epidemiology and outcome of Loa-associated serious adverse events related to mass ivermectin treatment of onchocerciasis in Cameroon. Filaria Journal 2:1-4.

Boussinesq M, Gardon J, Gardon J, Gardon-Wendel N, Kamgno J, Ngoumou P, Chippaux JP (1998). Three probable cases of *Loa loa* encephalopathy following ivermectin treatment for onchocerciasis. Am. J. Trop. Hyg. 58(4):461-469.

Boussinesq M., Gardon J., Kamgno J., Pion S.D., Gardon-Wendel N., Chippaux JP. (2001). Relationship between the prevalence and intensity of *Loa loa* in the Central Province of Cameroon. *Annals of Tropical Medicine and Parasitology*, 95(5):495-507.

Brieger W R. 2000. Implementation and sustainability of community-directed treatment of Onchocerciasis with ivermectin. Geneva, UNDP/World Bank/WHO Special Programme for Research and Training in Tropical Diseases.

Bruneton J (1999). Pharmacognosie. Phytochimie- Plantes Médicinales. Ed. Lavoisier., London.

Cerkvenik Flajs V, Grabnar I (2002). Ivermectin pharmacokinetics. Slov. Vet. Res. 39(3/4):167-178.

Carme B., Nambouéni J.P., Copin N., Noireau F. (1989). Clinical and biological study of Loa loa filariasis in Congolese. *American Journal of Tropical Medicine and Hygiene*, 41(3):331-337.

Chippaux JP., Boussinesq M., Gardon J., Gardon-Wendel N. & Ernould J-C. (1996). Severe adverse reaction risks during mass treatment with ivermectin in loiasis endemic areas. *Parasitology Today*, 12(11): 448-50.

Diggle P. J., Thomson M. C., Christensen O. F., Rowlingson B., Obsomer V., Gardon J., Wanji S., Takougang I., Enyong P., Kamgno J., Remme J. H, Boussinesq M.And Molyneux D. H. 2007. Spatial modelling and the prediction of Loa loa risk: decision making under uncertainty. Annals of Tropical Medicine & Parasitology, Vol. 101, No. 6, 499–509

Duke BOL (2003). Overview: Report of a scientific working group on serious adverse events following Mectizan treatment of onchocerciasis in *Loa loa* endemic areas. Filaria Journal 2:1-4.

Edwards G, Dingsdale A, Helsby N, Orme ML, Breckenridge AM (1988). The relative systemic availability of ivermectin after administration as capsule, tablet, and oral solution. Eur. J. Clin. Pharmacol. 35:681-684.

Fain, A. (1978). Les problèmes actuels de la loase. *Bulletin of the World Health Organization*, 56:155-167.

Gardon J, Gardon-Wendel N, Demanga-Ngangue, Kamgno J, Chippaux JP, Boussinesq M (1997). Serious reactions after mass treatment of onchocerciasis with ivermectin in an area endemic for *Loa loa* infection. The Lancet 3(50):18-22.

Gardon J., Gardon-Wendel N., Demanga-Ngangue, Kamgno J., Chippaux J.P., Boussinesq M. (1997). Serious reactions after mass treatment of onchocerciasis with ivermectin in an area endemic for *Loa loa* infection. *Lancet;* 350:18- 22.

Gish. O. 1992. Malaria Eradication and the Selective Approach to Health Care: Some Lessons from Ethiopia. *International Journal of Health Services*, 22(1): 179-192.

Hopkins A D. 2005. Ivermectin and Onchocerciasis : Is it all solved? Eye 19: 1057–1066.

Haumont G., Tribouley-Duret J., Villard H., Guy M., Lucchese F., Same Ekobo A. & Ripert C. (1992). Etude épidémiologique des filarioses (onchocercose, loase, mansonellose) dans la vallée de la Kadéïi (Cameroun). *Bulletin de Liaison et de Documentation de l'OCEAC*, 99 :34-39.

Hewlett B.S., Kollo B. & Cline B.L. 1996. Ivermectin distribution and the cultural context of forest onchocerciasis in South Province, Cameroon. *American Journal of Tropical Medicine and Hygiene*, 54(5):517-522.

Kamgno J, Boussinesq M (2001). Hyperendémicité de la loase dans la plaine Tikar, région de savane arbustive du Cameroun. Bull. Soc. de Patho. Exot. 94(4):342-346.

Languillon J. (1957). Carte des filaires du Cameroun. *Bulletin de la société de Pathologie Exotique,* 50:417-427.

Morrone A., Franco G., Tchangmena O.B., Marangi M. (2002). A case of loiasis in Rome. *Journal Européen de l'Académie de Dermatologie et de Vénérologie,* 16(3):280-283.

National Institute of Neurological disorders and Stroke. NINDS Encephalopathy Information Page. Ninds.nih.gov/disorders/encephalopathy/encephalopathy.htm. Downloaded on 10 October 2011.

Noireau, F., Carme, B., Apembet, D. J. & Gouteux, J. (1989). Loa and Mansonella filariasis in Chaillu mountains, Congo: parasitological prevalence. Transactions of the Royal Society of Tropical Medicine and Hygiene, 83, 529–534.

Pinder M. (1988). *Loa loa* - A Neglected Filaria. *Parasitology Today*, 4(10):279-284.

Pion S.D.S., Demanou M., Oud*in B.,* Bouss*inesq M. (2005).* Lo*iasis* : the i*ndividual factors associated with the p*resence of microfilareamia. Ann*als of Tropical Medicine and Parasitology, 99(5):*491-500.

Richards F O., Boatin B., Sauerbrey M., Seketeli A. 2004. Control of Onchocerciasis_Today: Status and challenges. Trends in Parasitology 17: 558–563.

Shu EN, Onwujekwe EO, Okonkwo PO (2000). Do alcoholic beverages enhance availability of ivermectin ? Eur. J. Clin. Pharmacol. 56:437-438.

Tabi E.T., Befidi-Mengue R., Nutman T.B., Horton J., Folefalk A., Pensia E., Fualem R., Fogako J., Gwanmesia P., Quakyi I., Leke R. (2004). Human loiasis in a Cameroonian village: A double-blind, placebo controlled, crossover clinical trial of a three-day albendazole regimen. *American Journal of Tropical Medicine and Hygiene,* 71(2):211-215.

Takougang I., Meremikwu M., Wanji S., Yenshu E.V., Aripko B., Lamlenn S.B., Eka I.B., Enyong P., Meli J., Kale O., Remme J.H. (2002). A rapid assessment method for *Loa loa* endemicity. *Bulletin of the World Health Organization*, 80(11):852-858.

Takougang I, Meli J, Lamlenn S, Tatah Pn & Ntep M. 2007. Loiasis, a Neglected and Underestimated Affliction: Endemicity, Morbidity and Perceptions in Eastern Cameroon. Annals of Tropical Medicine and Parasitology. 101(2):151-160.

The Mectizan Expert Committee. 2000. Recommendations for the treatment of onchocerciasis with Mectizan in areas co-endemic for onchocerciasis and loiasis.

Thomson M.C., Obsomer V., Kamgno J., Gardon J, Wanji S., Takougang I., Enyong P., Remme J.H., Molyneux D.H. & Boussinesq M. (2004). Mapping the distribution of Loa loa in Cameroon in support of the African Programme for Onchocerciasis Control.Filaria Journal, 3:7

Touré F.S., Deloron P., Egwang T. G., Wahl G. (1999). Relation entre intensité de la transmission de la filaire *Loa loa* et prévalence des infections. *Médecine Tropicale,* 59(3): 249 - 252.

Touré F.S., Mavoungou E., Kassambara L., Williams T., Wahl G.M., Egwang T.G. (1998).Human occult loiasis: field evaluation of a nested polymerase chain reaction assay for the detection of occult infection. *Tropical Medicine and International Health,* 3(6): 505 - 511.

Tsague-Dongmo L., Kamgno J., Pion SD., Moyou-Somo R., Boussinesq M. (2002). Effects of a 3-day regimen of albendazole (800 mg daily) on *Loa loa* microfilareamia. *Annals of Tropical Medicine and Parasitolology,* 96(7) :707-715.

Twum-Danso NAY, Meredith SEO (2003). Variation in incidence of serious adverse events after onchocerciasis treatment with ivermectin in areas of Cameroon co-endemic for loiasis. Trop. Med. and Internat. Health. 8(9):820-831.

WHO (1992). The Alcohol Use Disorders Identification Test : Guidelines for use in Primary Healthcare. Programme on Substance Abuse. World health Organization. WHO/PSA/92.4.

WHO (1995). Onchocerciasis and its control. Report of a WHO Expert Committee on Onchocerciasis Control. WHO Tech. Rep. Ser. N°852. Geneva.

WHO 2006. Report -working together for health. Geneva.

WHO. 2008. Primary Health Care - Now More than Ever. Geneva.

9

Past and Future of Diagnosis and Therapy of Transmissible Spongiform Encephalopathy

Chih-Yuan Tseng and Jack Tuszynski
*Department of Oncology, University of Alberta
Edmonton, AB,
Canada*

1. Introduction

Transmissible spongiform encephalopathies (TSEs), also known as prion diseases, including Creutzfeldt-Jakob disease (CJD) in human, Bovine Spongiform Encephalopathy (BSE) in cow, and scrapie in sheep, represent diseases with complex and still poorly understood molecular mechanisms (Prusiner, 1998). The protein-only hypothesis postulates a possible pathogenic mechanism involving the prion protein. The α–helix rich normal prion protein (PrPC) is found to be infected by its β-sheet rich abnormal proteinase K (PK)-resistant form, PrPSc, and is converted into PrPSc (Prusiner, 1998). This infection will lead to the aggregation of PrPSc-based amyloid fibrils that accumulate in the peripheral and invade to the central nervous system and damage neurons.

In this chapter, we discuss current understanding of pathogenic mechanisms in this prion-only hypothesis based disease in Section 2. This understanding then leads to the discussions of the past and present developments in both diagnosis and therapy for these diseases in Section 3. Based on the understanding of pathogenic mechanisms and current diagnosis and therapeutic strategies, we propose an alternative strategy. The proposal considers an aptamer-based theranostic approach to detect and prevent the aggregation of amyloid plaques in Section 4. Note that aptamer is defined as short nucleic acid sequences, and designed through Systematic Evolution of Ligands by EXponential enrichment (SELEX) (James, 2000). It is hoped that this proposal will open a novel research direction and eventually lead to a better diagnosis and treatment of prion diseases in the future.

2. The infectivity of prion diseases

Numerous models have been developed to provide better understanding of the pathogenesis of the prion diseases. One of models advanced is the template-assistance model (Prusiner, 1998; Horiuchi & Caughy, 1999; Tompa et al., 2002). This model assumed that PrPC, which is normally more stable than PrPSc in isolation, would in the presence of PrPSc convert to the latter via a transient catalytic interaction with it. The implication is that a dimer of PrPSc's is energetically more stable than a system of non-interacting PrPC and PrPSc. This was supported by Morrissey and Shakhnovich's computational analyses (Morrissey & Shakhnovich, 1999). When there are other PrPSc's present, the initial autocatalytic process would then lead to a propagation of PrPC to PrPSc conversion. Therefore, many studies have been focused on investigating possible mechanisms of this triggering event. For example, Zou and Cashman report in their studies that acidic environment increases the chance of triggering conversion (Zou & Cashman, 2002). Several groups have searched for the potential sites responsible for the conversion, referred to as hot spots, in PrPC (Guilbert, et al, 2000; Kuwata et al., 2007; Tseng et al., 2009).

Furthermore, experimental evidences suggest that the infectivity of BSE cross-strains may associate with a host-independent molecule (Somerville, 2002). Gale showed that a phospholipid is most likely to be this molecule through the strain thermostability studies (Gale, 2006). Recent studies of prion diseases in membrane environments suggest that Phosphatidylserine (PS) is a molecule capable of altering amyloid aggregation pathways and increasing aggregation rates (Robinson & Pinheiro, 2010). This finding is further supported by the identification of the endosome recycling compartment as the potential conversion site (Marijanovic et al., 2009; Thellung et al., 2011).

In addition to exploring pathogenic mechanisms, another fundamental issue is how PrPSc based amyloid aggregation leads to the development of clinical symptoms and neuropathology. Chiesa et al. have designed a series of experiments based on Tg(PG14) mice models to resolve this issue (Chiesa et al., 2000). They demonstrated that one of the most obvious symptoms in neuropathology is massive loss of cerebellar granule cells due to apoptosis. Apoptosis is a vital, highly regulated, natural process that contributes to the development and maintenance of human and animal cells and tissues (Kerr et al., 1972; Weinberg, 2007). Apoptosis plays multiple roles in the normal development of organisms extending from embryonic development to the maintenance of normal cell homeostasis (Reed & Tomaselli, 2000; Elmore, 2007; Rastogi et al., 2009). Chiesa et al.'s discovery is supported by a recent study by Thellung et al. (Thellung et al., 2011), in which SH-SY5Y human neuroblastoma cells were used. They observed that accumulation of human PrPSc90-231 in membrane triggers lysosome dependent apoptosis and leads to neuronal cells death.

These insights seem open a route that differs from modern approaches as will be discussed below and which could lead to novel detection and "treatment" methods of prion diseases. However, before we propose this alternative solution, we first need to understand how modern approaches work including their advantages and shortcomings.

3. Past and current developments of diagnosis and treatment of prion diseases

3.1 Diagnosis

According to the WHO manual for surveillance of human TSEs (WHO, 2003), current diagnosis methods can be categorized into two groups based on pathological characteristics of TSEs at microscopic and macroscopic levels. First, because of the diverse etiology of prion diseases in humans and animals, many studies have focused on the search for common mechanisms of these diseases at the molecular (microscopic) level in order to detect their onsets. The key question in this search is to ask if one can distinguish PrPSc from PrPC based on pathological changes and how this can be accomplished. The crux of the matter hinges on the conventional belief that specific prion protein types correlate with phenotypes of the disease. Second, several pathological characteristics of TSEs at the brain (macroscopic) level are generally recognized, can one distinguish signals or patterns generated by diseased brains from those present in normal brains. The key to correct diagnosis of TSEs then depends on the specificity and sensitivity of sensors

Regarding to the first group of diagnoses, three characteristics of PrPSc including prion protein gene (PRNP) codon 129 polymorphisms (Quadrio et al., 2011), Tyr-Tyr-Arg exposure (Paramithiotis et al., 2003) and over-expression of brain protein 14-3-3 (P14-3-3) (Hsich et al., 1996) were found to be distinctive from PrPC. Regarding to first characteristic, codon 129 was shown to be responsible for determining the variants of PK-resistant PrPSc in CJD (Parchi et al., 1996, 1999). Note that codon 129 encodes for two amino acids, methionine (M) and valine (V). A phenotypic influence in inherited prion diseases associated with codon 129 has been investigated and summarized in (Kovacs et al., 2002; Capellari et al., 2011). Regarding to second characteristic, Paramithiotis et al. showed that the Tyr-Tyr-Arg motif in PrP, which is a hydrophilic-like fragment, will be exposed to solvent when PrPC is converted into PrPSc. Regarding the third characteristic, P14-3-3 has been studied because of its potential as a bio-marker (Hsich et al., 1996). Basically, they found the presence of proteins 130 and 131, which are P14-3-3 type proteins, in cerebrospinal fluid from patients with CJD and little amount in normal patients. This result has led to the development of P14-3-3 immunoassays to aid in the diagnosis of prion diseases.

Regarding the second group, several noninvasive tools such as electroencephalography (EEG) and magnetic resonance imaging (MRI) have been investigated to detect abnormal onsets of prion diseases in brain besides biopsy. Tschampa et al. have shown that periodic sharp wave complexes appear in neuronal electric signals measured by non-invasive EEG in patients with CJD. These complexes are most likely the consequence of parvalbumin-positive neurons being reduced in the majority of thalamic nuclei (Tschampa et al., 2002). Namely, the damage to these neurons determines the generation of this typical clinical feature of CJD. World Health Organization (WHO) has standardized a protocol using EEG in diagnosis in 1998 (WHO, 2003). For MRI-related methods such as fluid attenuation inversion recovery (FLAIR) and diffusion-weighted MRI imaging (DWMRI), these are still relatively new techniques that have been introduced (Appel et al., 2011). These methods are based on the detection of abnormal signals from the basal ganglia, thalamus and cortex of patients. However, since most studies have investigated using only small samples it is still impossible to firmly confirm the usefulness of MRI in this context. Nevertheless, it was shown that MRI may be able to better locate abnormal patterns in deep gray matter while EEG may be more sensitive in the cortex. Both methods may have a complementary role in diagnosing prion diseases.

In summary, there are three tools commonly considered to aid in the diagnosis of prion diseases at present. Regarding codon 129 (genetic analysis), there are more and more studies that support the findings of a reproducible phenotypic spectrum of CJD variants and that the codon 129 genotype acts as the main determinant of the disease phenotype. Namely, DNA sequencing of the coding region of the PRNP may detect the onset of the disease. Regarding P14-3-3 (immunoassay), although it is not specific to prion diseases, it is a marker of neuronal damage and has been available *in vivo*. Regarding the periodic sharp wave complexes (EEG analysis), it indicates a footprint of neuronal electric signals from neurons damaged by PrPSc aggregation. It has been found that incorporation of non-invasive EEG analysis and P14-3-3 detection increases the sensitivity of detection and improves diagnostic criteria (Zerr et al., 2000). Furthermore, Quadrio et al. suggest that conducting genetic analysis focusing on PRNP in addition to the combination of P14-3-3 detection and EEG analysis provides an extensive strategy to better diagnose prion diseases because these methods are sensitive to specific variants of PrP (Quadrio et al., 2011). Because the current molecular-based diagnoses hinge on the specificity and sensitivity of distinguishing between PrPC and PrPSc, the variants of PrP lower the success rate of these methods. Searching for more universal footprints of these variants will be one way to better detect the onset of prion diseases. Note that there are many other methods not mentioned here including in vivo biomarkers in blood and urine and tissue-based analysis which are currently under investigation (refer to (WHO, 2003; Quadrio et al., 2011) for more details).

3.2 Treatments

3.2.1 Rationale

Although there are no effective therapies for prion diseases yet, one can still summarize the current strategies as being divided into three categories based on various concepts of choosing therapeutic targets. Note that the discussions below are based on the assumption that the blood-brain barrier penetration issue is overcome. Moreover, an additional issue in treating prion diseases, administration methods was shown by Doh-ura et al. (Doh-ura et al., 2004) to be equally crucial as designing better inhibitors. These authors have demonstrated intra-ventricular administration of pentosan polysulfate (PPS, an FDA approved drug originally designed for anti-malaria treatments) through an infusion device can inhibit PrPSc aggregation. However, based on our expertise in drug discovery, we will limit our discussion to addressing the issue of effective inhibitor design in this section.

Based on the prion hypothesis, researchers in this field have focused on three targets, which include PrPC, PrPSc and PrPSc-producing cells. First, regarding the selection of PrPC as a target, Mallucci et al's study provides strong evidence in support of this choice (Mallucci et al., 2007). They showed that when PrPc is depleted at an early stage of the disease in mouse, damaged neuronal functions are recovered. Furthermore, the recovery is independent of PrPSc aggregation, which implies novel mechanisms of neurotoxicity and therapeutic possibilities. Second, for choosing PrPSc as a target, the idea is simply to stop PrPSc aggregation. Many studies pointed out that PrPSc is replicated and accumulated in the lympho-reticular system during the initial stage of extra-cerebral prion infection (Mabbott & MacPherson, 2006). Furthermore, because Korth et al. discovered a unique epitope in PrPSc (Korth et al, 1997), this finding makes PrPSc a promising target to prevent prion infection at an early stage through immunotherapy. Third, for choosing PrPSc-producing cells as a target, the goal is to stop the infection in the peripheral nervous system and to prevent the plaque from being transmitted to the central nervous system. Several studies suggest dendritic cells as a potential target to inhibit neuronal invasion because of the role of dendritic cells in up-regulating follicular dendritic cells (FDCs), in which PrPSc are replicated and accumulated in diseased mice (Huang et al., 2002; Brown et al., 2009).

Various bio-materials including antibodies, chemical compounds and aptamers have been investigated as inhibitors for these three targets. For example, targeting PrPC includes anti-PrP antibody development (Fe´raudet-Tarisse et al., 2010) and PPS (Doh-ura et al., 2004) etc.

Targeting PrPSc includes anti-PrP monoclonal antibody development (Mab) IgM (Paramithiotis, 2003) and 6D11 (Sadowski, 2009) and RNA aptamer design (Weiss et al., 1997; Proske et al., 2002; Rhie et al., 2003). For PrPSc-producing cells, cytotoxic T cells, antibody raised based on dendritic cells are used (Rosset et al. 2009). Although the results obtained from the immunotherapy focused on either PrPC, PrPSc or PrPSc-producing cells remain controversial, the immunotherapy is still a widely investigated strategy and has been shown to have an anti-prion effect in cellular and animal models (Paramithiotis et al., 2003; Sadowski et al., 2009; Fe´raudet-Tarisse et al., 2010). Because of the controversial issues in immunotherapy, many other groups continue searching for novel small molecule inhibitors including those either mimicking negative inhibition of prion replication by Perrier et al. (Perrier et al., 2000) or those targeting protease-resistant PrP by Charvériat et al. (Charvériat et al., 2008).

Since currently immunotherapy is the most developed and promising treatment, we will only focus on this modality in order to learn more about the key issues involved and to gain better understanding of the features of prion diseases revealed through these studies as discussed in the following sections.

3.2.2 Immunotherapy

Basically, immunotherapy hinges on inducing anti-PrP antibodies in appropriate hosts and utilizes these anti-PrP antibodies to activate the host's immune system's response against PrPSc aggregation. Several approaches of generating antibodies are employed including either bacterially-expressed full length PrP, PrP-PrP polyproteins, synthetic PrP peptides etc. However, studies have shown these approaches result in a low anti-PrP titer and immune-effects are moderate (Heppner & Aguzzi, 2004).

Nevertheless, immunotherapy still attracts the attention of many investigators. While much effort has been made to determine more factors responsible for prion conversion as potential drug targets, as mentioned previously, even more work is focused on targeting either PrPC, PrPSc or PrPSc-producing cells. A strategy that applies anti-PrP antibodies directly against PrPC has been shown to delay PrPSc peripheral accumulation (Fe´raudet-Tarisse et al., 2010). Fe´raudet-Tarisse et al. (2010) further studied pharmacokinetics and pharmacodynamics of several anti-PrP antibodies to examine their immunotherapeutic effects in mice. Another strategy in immunotherapy is to target PrPSc peripheral replication in the lympho-reticular system before the central nervous system (Bessen et al. 2009). The follicular dendritic cells are the major target of prion infection. Sadowski et al. showed that Mab 6D11 raised against PrPSc fibrils from brains of terminally ill CD-1 mice infected with 139A strain (Kascsak et al, 1987) prevents infection of FDC-P1 cells and removes PrPSc from the infected FDC-P1/22L cell line (Sadowski et al., 2009). However, Sadowski et al. also showed that time-limited treatment, which is more practical from the clinical point of view, using Mab 6D11 is not capable of preventing prion diseases. This result is also supported by the findings of Fe´raudet-Tarisse et al. (Fe´raudet-Tarisse et al., 2010). Therefore, one can conclude that the currently available anti-PrP antibodies are likely to only temporarily control PrPSc aggregation.

In summary, several issues hinder the practical implementation of immunotherapy in prion diseases. It includes a low anti-PrP antibody titer and moderate immuno-effects.

Furthermore, additional issues such as the expressed full length PrP approach are discussed below. First, the products failed to recognize the cell-surface PrPC, which is believed to directly associate with prion conversion, in wild type mice (Heppner & Aguzzi, 2004) and second, the full length antibodies when encountering the blood-brain barrier, are unable to cross it and enter into brain (Campana et al., 2009). The molecular mechanisms in the issue of low titer and moderate immuno-effects require more studies for better understanding. The latter issue may be resolved based on the work of Campana et al., in which they proposed a protocol to develop antibody fragments for prion diseases (Campana et al., 2009).

To develop a more promising immunotherapy for prion diseases in the future, it will require further investigations into various key areas. As shown in the works (Heppner & Aguzzi, 2004; Sadowski et al., 2009; Fe´raudet-Tarisse et al., 2010), these key areas include understanding the mechanisms of antibody resistance, identification of better antibodies against either PrPC or PrPSc (or other immune effectors such as dendritic cells (Rosset et al. 2009)) and designing proper administration methods (not addressed here) etc.

4. Aptamer-based theranostic approach to targeting phosphatidylserine

4.1 Logic

In the diagnosis and treatment of prion diseases, as mentioned previously, two questions need to be answered, i.e.: (a) what are "good" factors that would allow detectors to distinguish between PrPC and PrPSc and (b) what are appropriate therapeutic targets. In diagnosis, Protein P14-3-3 was shown to be a marker for neuronal damage and its use in detecting the onset of prion diseases has been demonstrated *in vivo* (Hsich et al., 1996). The question emerges if there are any other markers one can utilize to detect neuronal damage due to PrPSc aggregation? In terms of therapy, we have previously stated that three targets, PrPC (Mallucci et al., 2007), PrPSc (Huang et al., 2002; Brown et al., 2009) and PrPSc-producing cells (Bessen et al. 2009) are commonly considered as proper targets that could be used to prevent the disease. However, there are no effective prophylactic or therapeutic treatments available at present (Fe´raudet-Tarisse et al., 2010). Even for immunotherapy, its effects remain controversial (Heppner & Aguzzi, 2004). Since this controversial issue is yet to be resolved, we argue that targeting conversion factors rather than either PrPC, PrPSc, or PrPSc-producing cells may emerge as a viable strategy to avoid this problem and treat prion diseases.

As discussed in Sec. 2, Gale has shown that PS is the host-independent molecule associated with enhancing PrPSc aggregation (Gale, 2006). Robinson and Pinheiro have recently reported that PSs alter amyloid aggregation pathways by increasing aggregation (Robinson & Pinheiro, 2010), which suggests an alternative approach for therapeutic treatment of prion diseases. Namely, we may be able to delay or even stop PrPSc aggregation by directly inhibiting the interactions between PSs and PrPSc amyloid.

Furthermore, Chiesa et al and Thellung et al. have shown intracellular PrPSc aggregation in membranes triggers apoptosis (Chiesa et al, 2000; Thellung et al., 2011). Since we know that an early marker of apoptosis is the redistribution of PS between inner and outer plasma membranes (PS externalization) (Reutelingsperger et al., 1995; Blankenberg, 2009), PS externalization is specific to apoptotic cells with the exception of activated platelets and erythrocytes. Therefore, it is an attractive target for apoptosis detection (Blankenberg, 2008, 2009; Smrz et al., 2008) and as means of providing an early indication of the success or failure of therapy for prion diseases.

4.2 Aptamer design

Recently, aptamers have attracted great attention and may provide a viable alternative in the diagnosis and treatment of prion diseases (Weiss et al., 1997; Proske et al., 2002; Rhie et al., 2003). Aptamers are in many aspects, such as binding specificity and strong affinity, equivalent to antibodies. There are several advantages of using aptamers over antibodies. First, the selection of aptamers using SELEX can target any system while identification of antibodies depends on animal systems. Second, once an aptamer is selected, it can be easily synthesized and manipulated.

Based on their characteristics, aptamers appear to be a viable material, other than antibodies, to be implemented as either inhibitors or detectors of cellular events such as apoptosis. Aptamers are selected through SELEX to bind to specific bio-molecular targets including small molecules, proteins, nucleic acids, phospholipids as well as complex structures such as cells, tissues, bacteria and other organisms. Because aptamers have strong and specific binding affinity through molecular recognition and low toxicity, they are generally recognized as having potential therapeutic and diagnostic clinical applications (Nimjee et al., 2005; James, 2000). SELEX consists of a number of rounds of *in vitro* selection in which the RNA/DNA pool is incubated with the binding target. In practice, multiple rounds of selection and expansion are required in SELEX before unique tightly binding sequences can be identified. Additionally, isolated aptamers will often need to be re-engineered to reduce their sequence length and impart additional favorable biological properties. These issues pose a challenge for the efficient identification of correct aptamers.

Despite the issues involved in the use of SELEX, several groups have successfully identified RNA aptamers to bind specifically to either PrPC (Weiss et al., 1997; Proske et al., 2002) or PrPSc (Rhie et al., 2003). Proske et al. have utilized PrPC protein comprising amino acid residues 90-129, which belong to a short epitope (90-141) as the target. The resulting RNA aptamer has been shown to recognize the full-length PrPC and to reduce PrPSc formation in prion-infected neuroblastoma cells. On the other hand, Rhie et al. have selected RNA aptamers targeting scrapie-associated fibrils. They have shown an at least 10-fold higher binding affinity for PrPC. Although this aptamer has not been tested for its ability to inhibit the prion conversion in either cell lines or animal models, the studies in a cell-free model system do show the inhibition of the conversion due to the presence of this aptamer.

Even though we cannot dismiss the applicability of the above two examples in prion diseases, the issues involving SELEX still impede practical implementations of aptamer structures in various directions in both diagnosis and therapeutics. We have developed an information-driven theoretical approach, called Entropic Fragment Based Aptamer design (EFBA), in order to resolve these issues and design aptamers based solely on the structural information regarding molecular targets. Basically, our approach is based on a seed-and-grow strategy to determine the aptamer that has the highest probability to interact with the target of interest. Details of the approach and its validation are discussed in (Tseng et al., 2011).

Because of the molecular characteristics of aptamers and our validated aptamer design algorithm, we can apply the algorithm to computationally design aptamer-based theranostic agents that can specifically bind to any targets that are associated with either prion conversion or PrPSc aggregation. Thereafter, we can computationally and experimentally investigate its binding properties and apply the results to improve the designed sequence.

4.3 Aptamer-based theranostic approach targeting PS

4.3.1 Strategy

As we know, PS is shown to increase PrPSc aggregation, which is independent of the host, and PrPSc aggregation triggers apoptosis. Furthermore, when apoptosis is initiated, an early indication of this process is PS externalization. Therefore, we propose to design an aptamer simply targeting PS to inhibit interactions between PrPSc and PS. The inhibition may also delay accumulation. Besides, we can monitor the changes of PS externalization to not only detect the onset of the disease but also to estimate therapeutic effects.

The advance of aptamer design of our algorithm allows us to computationally design an aptamer-based theranostic agent aimed at prion diseases. The application of aptamers will likely be free from difficulties of using other materials such as a well-studied apoptotic probe, annexin V, a small peptide (Blankenberg, 2009). For example, annexin V has a high uptake in normal tissues, especially liver and kidney, a long biological half-life in non-target tissues, a high radiation burden for ^{111}In and ^{124}I analogs and laborious radiochemistry for the labeling (Boersma et al., 2005). Therefore, an aptamer attached with a fluorescence tag that specifically binds to PS can both inhibit the interactions between PrPSc aggregation and PS and detect the changes of PS externalization at the same time using fluorescence imaging.

In the following, we will only demonstrate the application of our aptamer design algorithm in designing a DNA aptamer to bind specifically to PS. Furthermore, wet lab investigations in both imaging properties and therapeutic effects will not be presented here because of resource limitations at present.

4.3.2 The PS DNA-aptamer

In our earlier work (Tseng et al., 2011), the design of a PS aptamer has been briefly addressed. Basically, we start with the molecular model of PS, which was manually constructed using the MOLDEN program (Schaftenaar & Noordik, 2000). The resulting structure was then minimized with the GAMESS-US (Schmidt et al., 1993) program using the AM1 semi-empirical method (Dewar & Dieter, 1986; Dewar et al., 1985). The PS structure was further equilibrated using molecular dynamics simulation for 1 ns for DNA aptamer design. Two top sequences, namely 5′-AAAAGA-3′ (PS-aptamer I) and AAAGAC (PS-aptamer II), were selected from our design for experimental binding assays and *in silico* experiments (*in silico* results are not shown here). The structure of the PS-aptamer I in new ribbons format and the potential location of its binding site are shown in the left panel of Fig. 1. Note that the aptamer structure has not been energy equilibrated yet.

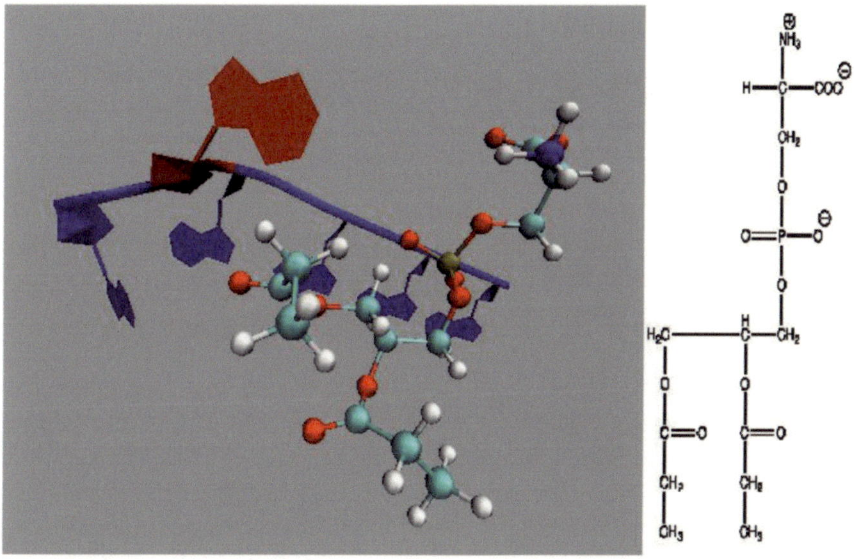

Fig. 1. The tertiary structure (on the left) of the designed PS-aptamer I generated using VMD (Humphrey et al., 1996) and the two-dimensional structure (on the right) of PS are shown. Note adenine is colored by blue and guanine is red.

Two liposomes were prepared in order to study both the designed PS aptamer binding affinity and specificity. The first one uses DPPC and DPPS at a 10:1 DPPC/DPPS molar ratio and the second one uses DPPC alone. In both cases cholesterol exists at the DPPC/cholesterol molar ratio of 2:1. The latter served as a control without PS available for binding. The results are shown in Fig. 2. The low fluorescent level shown in the right-hand panel indicates that the PS-aptamer II binds either poorly or not at all to DPPC. Conversely, the left-hand panel shows a relatively high fluorescence level while DPPS is present. It suggests that both DNA aptamers bind specifically to DPPS. Second, although both DNA aptamers bind to DPPS, the results show that the PS-aptamer II has a higher fluorescence level than the PS-aptamer I when the concentrations of DNA aptamers are increased beyond 0.165 nmol. This suggests that the PS-aptamer II has a relatively better or stronger binding affinity than PS-aptamer I.

Since the fluorescence studies did not show any saturation point for both aptamers, it is definitely required to further re-engineer this PS aptamer template to enhance its binding affinity before one can consider implementing it to become a theranostic agent. Furthermore, more studies in model systems and cell lines, are required to further investigate the theranostic effects of this aptamer. Nevertheless, given an appropriate drug delivery technique such as the exosome-based drug delivery technique (Alvarez-Erviti et al., 2011), which has the ability to carry therapeutic agents including nucleic acid across the blood-brain-barrier, to deliver PS aptamer into cells, it is likely that this PS aptamer-based theranostic agent will open new possibilities in the development of a successful therapy for prion diseases.

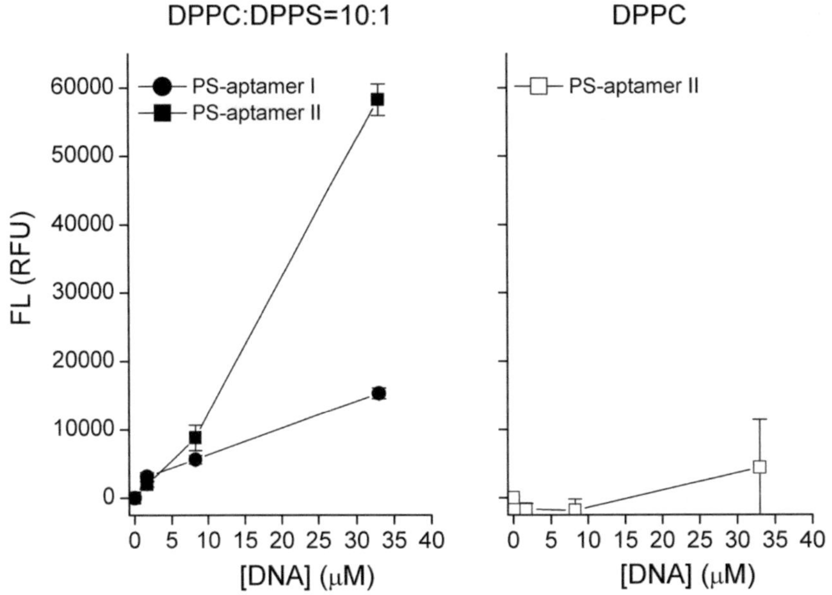

Fig. 2. Fluorescence (FL) measured in relative fluorescence units (RFU) versus DNA aptamer concentration. Left panel: selective binding of two designed DNA aptamers with liposomes containing PS. Right panel: low non-specific binding of designed DNA aptamer with liposome containing only PC.

5. Conclusions

We have reviewed current understanding of infectivity of prion diseases and recent developments in the area of diagnosis and therapeutic strategies involving various types of biochemical and chemical agents. In particular, we discussed the advantages and challenges involved in three tools, genetic (codon 129), P14-3-3 in the cerebrospinal fluid and EEG analysis, in diagnosis and a widely investigated treatment, immunotherapy. Based on these insights into the search for a detector to diagnose the onset of prion diseases and treatments aimed at either stopping prion conversion or PrPSc aggregation, a prion conversion factor, PS, has recently attracted our attention. In those studies, PS has been shown to increase PrPSc aggregation. This aggregation then activates neuronal cell apoptosis, which in turn triggers PS externalization as an early marker. We argue that these two discoveries may suggest a potential theranostic target.

An aptamer-based theranostic approach targeting PS is proposed here. Based on our recently proposed aptamer design algorithm, a promising result in designing a specific PS binding aptamer is demonstrated. A series of wet lab studies will be designed to validate and implement this proposal including both imaging of apoptosis events and inhibition of PrPSc aggregation. Finally, given this PS DNA aptamer template, we hope this proposal will trigger a ripple effect in the research community and lead to a solution which will assist us in diagnosing and preventing prion diseases.

6. Acknowledgment

This research was funded by the Alberta Cancer Foundation, the Allard Foundation, NSERC, the Canadian Breast Cancer Foundation and Alberta Advanced Education and Technology.

7. References

Alvarez-Erviti, L.; Seow, Y.; Yin, H; Betts, C.; Lakhal, S. & Wood, M. J. A. (2011). Delivery of siRNA to the mouse brain by systemic injection of targeted exosomes. *Nature Biotecnology*, Vol. 29, No. 4, (March 2011), pp. 341-345, ISSN 1087-0156

Appel, S. A; Chapman, J.; Prohovnik, I.; Hoffman, Chen.; Cohen, O. S.; Blatt, I. (2011). The EEG in E200K familial CJD: relation to MRI patterns. *Journal of Neurology*, DOI: 10.1007/s00415-011-6208-5, (August 2011), ISSN 1432-1459

Bessen, R. A.; Martinka, S.; Kelly, J. & Gonzalez, D. (2009). Role of the Lymphoreticular System in Prion Neuroinvasion from the Oral and Nasal Mucosa. *Journal of Virolology*, Vol. 83, No. 13, (July 2009), pp. 6435–6445, ISSN 0022-538X

Blankenberg, F. G. (2008). In vivo imaging of apoptosis. *Cancer Biology & Therapy*, Vol. 7, No. 10, (October 2008), pp. 1525-1532, ISSN 1538-4047

Blankenberg, F. G. (2009). Imaging the molecular signatures of apoptosis and injury with radiolabeled annexin V. *Proceedings of the American Thoraic Society*, Vol. 6 No. 5, (August 2009), pp. 469-476, ISSN 1546-3222

Boersma, H. H.; Kietselaer, B. L.; Stolk, L.M.; Bennaghmouch, A.; Hofstra, L.; Narula, J.; Heidendal, G. A. & Reutelingsperger, C. P. (2005). Past, present, and future of annexin A5: from protein discovery to clinical applications. Journal Nuclear Medicine, Vol. 46, No.12, (September 2005), pp. 2035-2050, ISSN 2159-662x

Brown, K. L.; Stewart, K.; Ritchie, D. L.; Mabott, N. A.; (1999). Scrapie replication in lymphoid tissues depends on protein prion-expressing follicular dendritic cells. Nature Medicine, Vol. 5, No. 11, (November 1999), pp. 1308–1312, ISSN 1078-8956

Campana, V; Zentilin, L; Mirabile, I; Kranjc, A; Casanova, P; Giacca, M; Prusiner, S. B.; Legname, G & Zurzolo, C. (2009). Development of antibody fragments for immunotherapy of prion diseases. *Biochemical Journal*, Vol. 418, No. 3, (March 2009), pp. 507-515, ISSN 0264-6021

Capellari, S.; Strammiello, R.; Saverioni, D.; Kretzschmar, H. & Parchi, P. (2011). Genetic Creutzfeldt-Jakob disease and fatal familial insomnia: insights into phenotypic variability and disease pathogenesis. *Acta Neuropathologica*, Vol. 121 No. 1 (January 2011), pp. 21-37, ISSN 0001-6322

Charvériat, M.; Reboul, M.; Wang, Q.; Picoli, C.; Lenuzza, N.; Montagnac, A.; Nhiri, N.; Jacquet, E.; Guéritte, F.; Lallemand, J.-Y.; Deslys J.-P. & Mouthon, F. (2009). New inhibitors of prion replication that target the amyloid precursor. *Journal of General Virology*, Vol. 90 No. 5 (May 2009), pp.1294–1301, ISSN 0022-1317

Chiesa, R.; Drisaldi, B.; Quaglio, E.; Migheli, A.; Piccardo, P.; Ghetti, B. & Harris, D. A. (2000). Accumulation of protease-resistant prion protein (PrP) and apoptosis of cerebellar granule cells in transgenic mice expressing a PrP insertional mutation. *Proceedings of the National Academy of Sciences*, Vol. 97, No. 10, (May 2000), pp. 5574-5579, ISSN 1091-6490

Dewar, M. & Dieter, K. (1986). Evaluation of AM1 calculated proton affinities and deprotonation enthalpies. *Journal* of the *American Chemical Society*, Vol. 108, No. 25, (December 1986), pp. 8075-086, ISSN 0002-7863

Dewar, M., Zoebisch, E., Healy, E. & Stewart, J. (1985). Development and use of quantum mechanical molecular models. 76. AM1: A new general purpose quantum mechanical molecular model. *Journal* of the *American Chemical Society*, Vol. 107, No. 13, (June 1985), pp. 3902-3909, ISSN 002-7863

Doh-ura, K.; Ishikawa, K.; Murakami-Kubo, I.; Sasaki, K.; Mohri, S.; Race, R. & Iwaki, T. (2004) Treatment of Transmissible Spongiform Encephalopathy by Intraventricular Drug Infusion in Animal Models. *Journal of Virology*, Vol. 78, No. (2004), pp. 4999–5006, ISSN 0022-538X

Elmore, S. (2007). Apoptosis: a review of programmed cell death. *Toxicologic Pathology*, Vol. 35, No. 4, (2007), pp. 495–516, ISSN 0192-6233

Fe´raudet-Tarisse, C.; Andre´oletti, O.; Morel, N.; Simon, S.; Lacroux, C.; Mathey, J.; Lamourette, P.; Relaño, A.; Torres, J. M.; Créminon, C. & Grassi, J. (2010). Immunotherapeutic effect of anti-PrP monoclonal antibodies in transmissible spongiform encephalopathy mouse models: pharmacokinetic and pharmacodynamic analysis. *Journal of General Virology*, Vol. 91, No. 6 (June 2010), pp.1635–1645, ISSN 0022-1317

Gale, P. (2006). The infectivity of transmissible spongiform encephalopathy agent at low doses: the importance of phospholipid. Journal of Applied Microbiology, Vol. 101, No. 2, (August 2006), pp. 261-274, ISSN 1364-5072

Guilbert, C.; Ricard, F. & Smith, J. C. (2000). Dynamic simulation of the mouse prion protein. *Biopolymers*, Vol. 54, No. 6, (November 2000), pp. 406–415, ISSN 1097-0282

Heppner, F. L. & Aguzzi, A. (2004). Recent developments in prion immunotherapy. *Current Opinion in Immunology*, Vol. 16, No. 5, (October 2004), pp. 594–598, ISSN 0952-7915

Horiuchi, M. & Caughey, B. (1999). Prion protein interconversions and the transmissible spongiform encephalopathies. *Structure*, Vol. 7, No. 10, (October 1999), R231-R240, ISSN 0969-2126

Hsich, G.; Kenney, K.; Gibbs, C. J.; Lee, K. H. & Harrington, M. G. (1996). The 14-3-3 brain protein in cerebrospinal fluid as a marker for transmissible spongiform encephalopathies. *The New England Journal of Medicine*, Vol. 335, No. 13, (September 1996), pp. 924-30, ISSN 1533-4406

Huang, F. P.; Farquhar, C. F.; Mabott, N. A; Bruce, M. E. & MacPherson, G. G. (2002). Migrating intestinal dendritic cells transport PrPSc from the gut. *Journal of General Virology*, Vol. 83, No. 1, (January 2002), pp. 267–271, ISSN 0022-1317

Humphrey, W.; Dalke, A. & Schulten, K. (1996). VMD - Visual molecular dynamics. *Journal of Molecular Graphics*, Vol. 14, No. 1, (February 1996), pp. 33-38, ISSN 1093-3263

James, W. (2000). Aptamer, In: *Encyclopedia of Analytical Chemistry*, pp. 4848-4871, Wiley& Sons Inc., ISBN 9780470027318, Hoboken, NJ, USA.

Kascsak, R. J.; Rubenstein, R.; Merz, P. A.; Tonna-DeMasi, M.; Fersko, R.; Carp, R. I.; Wisniewski, H. M. & Diringer, H. (1987). Mouse polyclonal and monoclonal antibody to scrapie-associated fi bril proteins. *Journal of Virology*, Vol. 61, No. 12, (December 1987), pp. 3688–3693, ISSN 0022-538X

Kerr, J. F.; Wyllie, A. H. & Currie, A. R. (1972). Apoptosis: a basic biological phenomenon with wide-ranging implications in tissue kinetics. *British Journal of Cancer*, Vol. 26, No. 24, (August 1972), pp. 239–257, ISSN 0007-0920

Kovacs, G. G.; Trabattoni, G.; Hainfellner, J. A.; Ironside, J. W.; Knight, R. S. & Budka, H. (2002). Mutations of the prion protein gene phenotypic spectrum. *Journal of Neurology*, Vol. 249, No. 11, (November 2002), pp. 1567-1582, ISSN 0340-5354

Korth, C.; Stierli, B.; Streit, P.; Moser, M.; Schaller, O.; Fischer, R.; Schulz-Schaeffer, W.; Kretzschmar, H.; Raeberk, A.; Braun, U.; Ehrenspergerl, F.; Hornemann, S.; Glockshuber, R.; Riek, R.; Billeter, M.; WuÈthrich, K. & Oesch, B. (1997). Prion (PrP Sc)-specific epitope defined by a monoclonal antibody. *Nature*, Vol. 390, No. 6, (November 1997), pp. 74-77, ISSN 1078-8956

Kuwata, K.; Nishida, N. & Matsumoto, T.; Kamatari, Y. O.; Hosokawa-Muto, J.; Kodama, K.; Nakamura, H. K.; Kimura, K.; Kawasaki, M.; Takakura, Y.; Shirabe, S.; Takata, J.; Kataoka Y. & Katamine, S. (2007). Hot spots in prion protein for pathogenic conversion. *Proceedings of the National Academy of Sciences*, Vol. 104, No. 29, (July 2007), pp. 11921-11926 ISSN 1091-6490

Mabbott, N.A. & MacPherson, G.G. (2006). Prions and their lethal journey to the brain. *Nature Reviews Microbiology*, Vol. 4, (March 2006), pp. 201–211 ISSN 1740-1526

Marijanovic, Z.; Caputo, A.; Campana, V. & Zurzolo, C. (2009). Identification of an Intracellular Site of Prion Conversion. *PLoS Pathogens*, Vol. 5, No. 5, (May 2009), pp. e1000426, ISSN 1553-7374

Mallucci, G. R.; White, M. D.; Farmer, M.; Dickinson, A.; Khatum, H.; Dickinson, A.; Khatun H.; Powell, A. D.; Brandner, S.; Jefferys, J. G. & Collinge, J. (2007). Targeting cellular prion protein reverses early cognitive deficits and neurophysiological dysfunction in prion-infected mice. *Neuron*, Vol. 53, No. 3, (February 2007), pp. 325–335, ISSN 1740-925X

Morrissey, M. P. & Shakhnovich, E. I. (1999). Evidence for the role of PrPC helix 1 in the hydrophilic seeding of prion aggregates. *Proceedings of the National Academy of Sciences*, Vol. 96, No. 20, (September 1999), pp. 11293-11298, ISSN 1091-6490

Nimjee S. M.; Rusconi C. P. & Sullenger B. A. (2005). Aptamers: An emerging class of therapeutics. *Annual Review of Medicine*, Vol. 56, (2005), pp. 555-583, ISSN 0066-4219

Paramithiotis, E.; Pinard, M.; Lawton, T.; LaBoissiere, S.; Leathers, V. L.; Zou, W. Q.; Estey, L. A.; Lamontagne, J.; Lehto, M. T.; Kondejewski, L. H.; Francoeur, G. P.; Papadopoulos, M.; Haghighat, A.; Spatz, S. J.; Head, M.; Will, R.; Ironside, J.; O'Rourke, K.; Tonelli, Q.; Ledebur, H. C.; Chakrabartty, A. & Cashman, N. R. (2003) A prion epitope selective for the pathologically misfolded conformation. *Nature Medicine*, Vol. 9, No. 7, (July 2003), pp. 893-899, ISSN 1078-8956

Parchi, P.; Castellani, R.; Capellari, S.; Ghetti, B; Young, K.; Chen, S. G.; Farlow, M.; Dickson, D. W.; Sima, A. A.; Trojanowski, J. Q.; Petersen, R. B. & Gambetti, P. (1996). Molecular basis of phenotypic variability in sporadic Creutzfeldt-Jakob disease. *Annals of Neurolology*, Vol. 139, No. 6, (June 1996), pp. 767-78, ISSN 0364-5134

Parchi, P.; Giese, A.; Capellari, S.; Brown, P.; Schulz-Schaeffer, W.; Windl, O.; Zerr, I.; Budka, H.; Kopp, N.; Piccardo, P.; Poser, S.; Rojiani, A.; Streichemberger, N.; Julien, J.; Vital, C.; Ghetti, B.; Gambetti, P. & Kretzschmar, H. (1999). Classification of sporadic Creutzfeldt-Jakob disease based on molecular and phenotypic analysis of 300 subjects. *Annals of Neurolology*, Vol. 46, No. 2, (August 1999), pp. 224-33, ISSN 0364-5134

Perrier, V.; Wallace, A. C.; Kaneko, K.; Safar, I.; Prusiner, S. B. & Cohen, F. E. (2000). Mimicking dominant negative inhibition of prion replication through structure-based drug design. *Proceedings of the National Academy of Sciences*, Vol. 97, No. 11, (March 2000), pp. 6073-6078, ISSN 1091-6490

Proske, D.; Gilch, S.; Wopfner, F.; Schätzl, H. M.; E. Winnacker, L. & Famulok, M. (2002). Prion-protein-specific aptamer reduces PrPSc formation. ChemBioChem Vol. 3, No. 8, (August 2002), pp. 717-725, ISSN 1439-7633

Prusiner, S. B. (1998). Prions. *Proceedings of the National Academy of Sciences*, Vol. 95, No. 23, (November 1998), pp. 13363-13383, ISSN 1091-6490

Quadrio, I.; Perret-Liaudet, A. & Kovacs, G. G. (2011). Molecular diagnosis of human prion disease. *Expert Opinion on Medical Diagnostics*, Vol. 5, No. 4, (July 2011), pp. 291-306, ISSN 1753-0059

Rastogi, R. P.; Richa & Sinha, R. P. (2009). Apoptosis: molecular mechanisms and pathogenicity. *EXCLI Journal*. Vol. 8, (August 2009), pp. 155-181, ISSN 1611-2156

Matrin, S. J.; Reutelingsperger, C. P. M.; McGahon, A. J.; Rader, J. A.; van Schie, R. C. A. A.; LaFace, D. M. & Green, D. R. (1995). Early Redistribution of Plasma Membrane Phosphatidylserine Is a General Feature of Apoptosis Regardless of the Initiating Stimulus: Inhibition by Overexpression of Bcl-2 and Abl. *Journal of Experimental Medicine*, Vol. 182, No. 5, (November 1995), pp, 1545-1556, ISSN 0022-1007

Reed, J. C. & Tomaselli, K. J. (2000). Drug discovery opportunities from apoptosis research. *Current Opinion in Biotechnology*, Vol. 11, No. 6, (December 2000), pp. 586-592, ISSN 0958-1669

Rhie, A.; Kirby, L.; Sayer, N.; Wellesley, R.; Disterer, P.; Sylvester, I.; Gill, A.; Hope, J.; James, W. & Tahiri-Alaoui, A. (2003). Characterization of 2-Fluoro-RNA Aptamers That Bind Preferentially to Disease-associated Conformations of Prion Protein and Inhibit Conversion. *Journal of Biological Chemistry*, Vol. 278, No. 41, (October 2003), pp. 39697–39705, ISSN 0021-9258

Robinson, P. J. & Pinheiro, T. J. (2010). Phospholipid Composition of Membranes Directs Prions Down Alternative Aggregation Pathways. *Biophysical Journal*, Vol. 98, No. 8, (April 2010), pp. 1520-1528, ISSN 0006-3495

Rosset M. B.; Sacquin A.; Lecollinet, S.; Chaigneau, T.; Adam, M.; Crespeau, F. & Eloit, M. (2009). Dendritic Cell-Mediated-Immunization with Xenogenic PrP and Adenoviral Vectors Breaks Tolerance and Prolongs Mice Survival against Experimental Scrapie. *PLoS One*, Vol. 4, No. 3, (March 2009), pp. e4917, ISSN 1932-6203

Sadowski, M. J.; Pankiewicz, J.; Prelli, F.; Scholtzova, H.; Spinner, D. S.; Kascsak, R. B.; Kascsak, R. J. & Wisniewski, T. (2009). Anti-PrP Mab 6D11 suppresses PrP Sc replication in prion infected myeloid precursor line FDC-P1/22L and in the lymphoreticular system in vivo. *Neurobiology of Disease*, Vol. 34, No. 2, (March 2009), pp. 267–278, ISSN 0969-9961

Schaftenaar, G. & Noordik, J. (2000). Molden: A pre- and post-processing program for molecular and electronic structures. *Journal of Computer-Aided Molecular Design*, Vol. 14, No. 2, (February 2000), pp. 123-134, ISSN 0920-654X

Schmidt, M. W.; Baldridge, K. K.; Boatz, J. A.; Elbert, S. T.; Gordon, M. S.; Jensen, J. H.; Koseki, S.; Matsunaga, N.; Nguyen, K. A.; Su, S.; Windus, T. L.; Dupuis, M. & Montgomery, J. A. (1993). General atomic and molecular electronic structure system. *Journal of Computational Chemistry, Vol.* 14, No. 11, (November 1993), pp. 1347-363, ISSN 0192-8651

Smrz, D.; Lebduska, P.; Dráberová, L.; Korb, J. & Dráber, P. (2008). Engagement of phospholipid scramblase 1 in activated cells: implication for phosphatidylserine externalization and exocytosis. *Journal of Biological Chemistry,* Vol. 283, No. 16, (April 2008), pp. 10904-10918, ISSN 0021-9258

Somerville, R. A. (2002). TSE agent strains and PrP: reconciling structure and function. *Trends in Biochemical Sciences,* Vol. 27, No. 12, (December 2002), pp. 606-612, ISSN 0968-0004

Thellung, S.; Corsaro, A.; Villa, V.; Simi, A.; Vella, S.; Pagano, A. & Florio, T. (2011). Human PrP90-231-induced cell death is associated with intracellular accumulation of insoluble and protease-resistant macroaggregates and lysosomal dysfunction. *Cell Death and Disease,* Vol. 2, (March 2011), pp. e138, ISSN 2041-4889

Tompa, P.; Tusnady, G. E.; Friedrich, P. & Simon, I. (2002). The role of dimerization in prion replication. *Biophysical Journal,* Vol. 82, No. 4, (April 2002), pp. 1711-1718, ISSN 0006-3495

Tschampa, H. J.; Herms, J. W.; Schulz-Schaeffer, W. J.; Maruschak, B.; Windl, O.; Jastrow, U.; Zerr, I.; Steinhoff, B. J.; Poser, S. & Kretzschmar, H. A. (2002). Clinical fndings in sporadic Creutzfeldt Jakob disease correlate with thalamic pathology. *Brain,* Vol. 125, No. 11, (November 2002), pp. 2558-2566, ISSN 0006-8950

Tseng, C.-Y.; Yu, C.-P. & Lee, HC. (2009). Integrity of H1 helix in prion protein revealed by molecular dynamic simulations to be especially vulnerable to changes in the relative orientation of H1 and its S1 flank. *European Biophysics Journal,* Vol. 38, No. 5, (February 2009), pp. 601-611, ISSN 0175-7571

Tseng, C.-Y.; Ashrafuzzaman, Md; Mane, J. Y.; Kapty, J.; Mercer, J. R. & Tuszynski, J. A. (2011). Entropic fragment based approach for aptamer design. *Chemical Biolology & Drug Design,* Vol. 78, No. 1, (May 2011), pp. 1-13, ISSN 1747-0285

Weiss, S.; Proske, D.; Neumann, M.; Groschup, M. H.; Kretzschmar, H. A.; Famulok, M. & Winnacker, E. L. (1997). RNA aptamers specifically interact with prion protein PrP. *Journal of Virolology,* Vol. 71, No. 11, (November 1997), pp. 8790-8797, ISSN 0022-538X

Weinberg, R. A. (2007). *The biology of Cancer* (1st), Garlan Science, ISBN 9780815340782, NY USA

WHO. (2003). WHO manual for surveillance of human transmissible spongiform encephalopathies including variant Creutzfeldt-Jakob disease, WHO, ISBN 9241545887, Geneva, Switzerland

Zerr, I.; Pocchiari, M.; Collins, S.; Brandel, J. P.; de Pedro Cuesta, J.; Knight, R. S.; Bernheimer, H.; Cardone, F.; Delasnerie-Lauprêtre, N.; Cuadrado Corrales, N.; Ladogana, A.; Bodemer, M.; Fletcher, A.; Awan, T.; Ruiz Bremón, A.; Budka, H.; Laplanche, J. L.; Will, R. G. & Poser, S. (2000). Analysis of EEG and CSF 14-3-3 proteins as aids to the diagnosis of Creutzfeldt–Jakob disease. *Neurology,* Vol. 55, No. 6, (September 2000), pp. 811-815, ISSN 0028-3878

Zou, W. Q. & Cashman, N. R. (2002). Acidic pH and detergents enhance in vitro conversion of human brain PrPC to PrPSc-like form. *Journal Biological Chemistry,* Vol. 277, No. 46, (November 2002), pp. 43492–43947, ISSN 0021-9258